CONTEMPORARY FEMINIST RESEARCH FROM THEORY TO PRACTICE

Also Available

Handbook of Arts-Based Research
Edited by Patricia Leavy

Handbook of Emergent Methods
Edited by Sharlene Nagy Hesse-Biber
and Patricia Leavy

Method Meets Art, Second Edition:
Arts-Based Research Practice
Patricia Leavy

Research Design: Quantitative, Qualitative,
Mixed Methods, Arts-Based,
and Community-Based Participatory
Research Approaches
Patricia Leavy

Contemporary Feminist Research from Theory to Practice

Patricia Leavy
Anne Harris

𝄞

THE GUILFORD PRESS
New York   London

To all those around the globe
who are standing up for gender equality through speaking out,
marching, activism, art, and scholarship;
and to those committed to microactivism in their homes,
workplaces, and everyday lives—we salute you

Copyright © 2019 The Guilford Press
A Division of Guilford Publications, Inc.
370 Seventh Avenue, Suite 1200, New York, NY 10001
www.guilford.com

Printed in the United States of America

This book is printed on acid-free paper.

Last digit is print number: 9 8 7 6 5 4 3 2 1

Library of Congress Cataloging-in-Publication Data

Names: Leavy, Patricia, 1975- author. | Harris, Anne M., author.
Title: Contemporary feminist research from theory to practice / Patricia
  Leavy, Anne Harris.
Description: New York : Guilford Press, [2019] | Includes bibliographical
  references and index.
Identifiers: LCCN 2018025852| ISBN 9781462520251 (pbk. : alk. paper) | ISBN
  9781462536283 (hardcover : alk. paper)
Subjects: LCSH: Women's studies. | Women's studies—Methodology. |
  Feminism—Research—Methodology.
Classification: LCC HQ1180 .L43 2019 | DDC 305.4—dc23
LC record available at *https://lccn.loc.gov/2018025852*

Preface

Feminist research is not like many other forms of research, because it holds explicit social commitments at the forefront. Beginning with the status of girls and women, but not ending there, feminism is an engaged human rights position that seeks to expose and remedy gender inequities. Feminist research suggests ways forward to a better world in which critical scholarship plays an active role in inspiring and enacting social change. We use the term "feminism" as opposed to a general "human rights" label to acknowledge, as Chimamanda Ngozi Adichie does, "the specific and particular problem of gender" and how female humans are targeted by these inequities (2015, p. 42). However, working from an intersectional approach coupled with a nonbinary understanding of gender, we provide a layered view of the problem of "gender" as it is lived by diverse individuals and groups.

Contemporary Feminist Research from Theory to Practice offers a comprehensive inter- and transdisciplinary introduction to contemporary feminisms. This book provides a historical context for understanding feminist research, presents the major theories feminist researchers develop and use globally, describes methods for conducting research and practical strategies for "doing" feminist research, and provides information on writing and publishing feminist research in various forms, and on incorporating social activism and advocacy into feminist practice. The literature on feminist research practice often focuses narrowly on traditional approaches to research and Western perspectives. We sought to offer a different kind of text, one that highlights the multiperspectival and socially constructed nature of contemporary feminist research, including global feminisms, transnational collaboration, digital media and virtual embodiment, and feminist "publics."

Our perspective is grounded in critical scholarship, intersectionality, and a nonbinary understanding of gender. This book understands contemporary feminist research as that which addresses inequality with an agenda for social change. We believe that critical scholarship—that which problematizes social conditions as they are—can only be addressed intersectionally, or, in other words, in the interwoven ways that it gets played out in real life. Not only are we in bodies that are gendered, but, rather, we simultaneously occupy race, ethnicity, social class, sexuality, and other positionalities. In order to be wide awake as feminist researchers, we must not only ask about gender, but we must also ask: What about race? What about sexuality? What about ableism? What about class (socioeconomic) inequity? How do these conditions and positions work together or against one another? This book asks you to think about doing research that is embedded in and accountable to "real life," and making real life better—not just for women, but for all—and to realize that these are not separate projects but interconnected ones.

Further, contemporary feminist research is concerned not only with the conditions of girls and women, but with all gender-based inequities, and today particularly with the highly visible but contested terrain of transgender and noncisgender human rights and the ways in which changing definitions of gender impact all genders and all who fall outside the "gender spectrum" or somewhere fluid within it. In this vein, we are troubling the common he/she binary and instead using he/she/they in this text.

Why This Book Is Needed

We wrote this book because we are both committed to the promise and practice of contemporary, inclusive feminist research. We also believe that it's difficult to find a comprehensive overview and guide to feminist research. Many books focus either on theory or methods, or on particular genres of feminist research. In writing this book, we hope to offer a robust introduction to feminist research that inspires you to delve further into topics of interest. We also wrote this book because as the world has changed rapidly, so too have the academic and social/cultural landscapes. In turn, feminisms have changed. From increasingly nonbinary understandings of gender to the digital landscape that increasingly impacts our personal and research lives, great changes have occurred. We felt a feminist text that pays homage to the past, but is firmly grounded in contemporary concerns and practices, was needed.

Special Features of This Book

Key Terms Highlighted with Call-Out Bubbles

Throughout this book, we have identified a number of key terms as central to contemporary feminist research. Throughout this text when there are examples of a specific term, we provide call-out bubbles highlighting the term. We review the significance some of these highlighted terms in Chapter 1, but the box below previews the list.

Ally	Girls and women
Cisgender	Intersectionality
Critical theory/approaches	Methodologies
Ethics	Ontology
Feminist digital media	Power sharing
Feminist epistemologies	Reflexivity
Gender	Representation
Genderqueer, gender-creative, gender-fluid	Socially constructed (gender) categories

Profiles of Prominent Feminist Researchers and Online Video Interviews

In Part I, we offer profiles of prominent feminist researchers, addressing both their overall body of work and individual approaches, and their more recent work. Links to short online video interviews with the researchers themselves accompany the written text.

Discussion Questions and Activities

Discussion questions and more engaged activities are provided at the end of every chapter to help you review the chapter material and take it further.

Suggested Resources

While we have attempted to draw on a wide range of feminist voices in this text, we fully recognize that not all voices can be included. Our own voices, those of two White, Western feminists, have shaped every aspect of this text. Therefore, we've included a list of suggested resources at the end of each chapter so that you can invite more authors into your study of feminist research.

Audience for the Book

This book is appropriate for undergraduate and graduate courses in feminism(s), feminist research, research methods, qualitative inquiry, theory, and women's or gender studies. It may also be of value to individual students and researchers working on a thesis, a dissertation, a research study, or public writing, or those who wish to engage in activism.

Organization

This book is divided into three parts. Part I focuses on the historical context of feminist research and the major theoretical frameworks, analyzed from a global perspective. Part II focuses on research praxis, offering chapters on ethics, research with participants (quantitative, qualitative, and community-based), and research with nonliving data in the case of content or media analysis and evaluating programs or other interventions. Part III addresses what happens after research has occurred. We detail the process of writing and publishing feminist research, offering writing instruction for formal academic writing as well as artistic and popular forms. We conclude with a chapter on public scholarship and what it means to be a feminist researcher in the world. Chapters can be read out of order, and chapters not of interest can be omitted.

Acknowledgments

First and foremost, we are grateful to our brilliant publisher and editor, C. Deborah Laughton. Thank you for your unwavering support of this project.

We extend a spirited thank you to the entire team at The Guilford Press. In particular, thank you to Seymour Weingarten, Bob Matloff, Katherine Sommer, Jeannie Tang, Judith Grauman, Katherine Lieber, Marian Robinson, Lucy Baker, Martin Coleman, Rosalie Wieder, Paul Gordon, Carly DaSilva, Andrea Sargent, Oliver Sharpe, and Robert Sebastiano.

Thank you to the leading feminist scholars who graciously shared their time and wisdom with us. To be able to sit down with you, face to face, and understand, person to person, once again why this work is so very important, we thank Professor Cynthia Dillard, Associate Professor Eve Tuck, and Professor Aimee Carrillo Rowe, as well as Professor Jack Halberstam, Professor Jessica Ringrose, Dr. Amy Shields Dobson, and others whose expertise and passion informed this text but were not captured on video.

Thank you to the formerly anonymous reviewers: Stacie Craft DeFreitas, Department of Social Sciences, University of Houston–Downtown; Venus E. Evans-Winters, Department of Educational Administration and Foundations, Illinois State University; and Angela J. Hattery, Women and Gender Studies Program, George Mason University.

We also thank Patricia's awesome assistant, Shalen Lowell, for their assistance with locating literature, formatting, and more. And we deeply thank the incomparable Alta Truden, whose brilliance in film editing is matched only by her commitment and passion for social inclusion and creative projects—thank you, Alta!

Patricia's Personal Acknowledgments

Anne Harris, thank you. This book was a do-over for me and I'm truly grateful for the opportunity. Thank you for your understanding when the world made it hard for me to put pen to paper. I'm proud of what we wrote. Sincere thanks to my friends and colleagues for lending their support during the process. Special thanks to Melissa Anyiwo, Celine Boyle, Pam DeSantis, Sandra Faulkner, Ally Field, Jessica Smartt Gullion, Libby Hatlan, Monique Robitaille, and Adrienne Trier-Bieniek. I'm also grateful to my family for their support during the long process of putting this book together. Thank you, Mark, for all of the advice along the way. Having a thoughtful and wise springboard for ideas is a rare and priceless gift. Last, but never least, thank you, Madeline, for reminding me why our generation has to do better for your generation. You fueled this writing.

Anne's Personal Acknowledgments

Thank you, Patricia, for being that writer friend of whom I always dreamed, the one that I could go stay with and actually write with through the day, and cook with at night—I love and respect you, especially when we get to do do-overs, on the page and in life. This book is for Stacy, because you inspire me to be a better scholar, activist, and researcher, and because you remind me every day that research without heart is not research that matters. I also dedicate this book to Haddie, because you don't yet know how much you need these feminist histories, and how much they have made it possible for you to be who you are right now, and perhaps who you will be able to become tomorrow. But I also rejoice in thanking the feminist artists, activists, herstorians, and scholars who have touched my life personally, and made me realize why I needed feminism, even after my well-meaning mother made me promise to never become one when I came out to her as a dyke in 1983: first and foremost, the steadfast Sarah Schulman, who is a modern-day Cassandra—even when it makes the blind hate her, she always speaks the well-informed truth, #Respect; Lesbian Herstory Archives cofounder and femme fatale Joan Nestle, who taught me about the first out lesbian on Broadway, Eva Le Gallienne; the women of WOW

Café and Dixon Place, even when you broke my heart; the feminist gay-boys on Broadway (Craig Lucas, Tony Kushner, Christopher Durang, and others); my beloved and brilliant theater guru and intersectional activist fairy godperson Morgan Jenness; Young Playwrights comrades Sheri M. Goldhirsch (rest in power) and Brett Reynolds—a couple of badass feminist theater bitches; Lola Pashalinski, who inspired our first LOLA Awards; the 5 Lesbian Brothers; all the trans* and nonbinary others who put their lives on the line for gender equalities every single day; and all the people who got off their asses in my formative years in 1980s and '90s New York City and showed me that marching and resistance mean something. Because they do. I salute you all.

Contents

PART II. Feminist Approaches to "Doing Research"

Purchasers of this book can access online videos
at *www.guilford.com/leavy-harris* for personal use
or use with students.

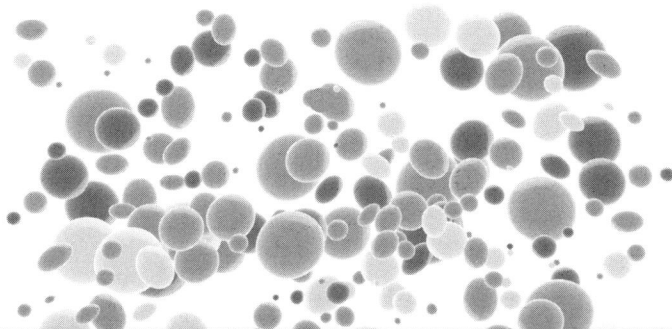

PART I

Feminist Theoretical Frameworks

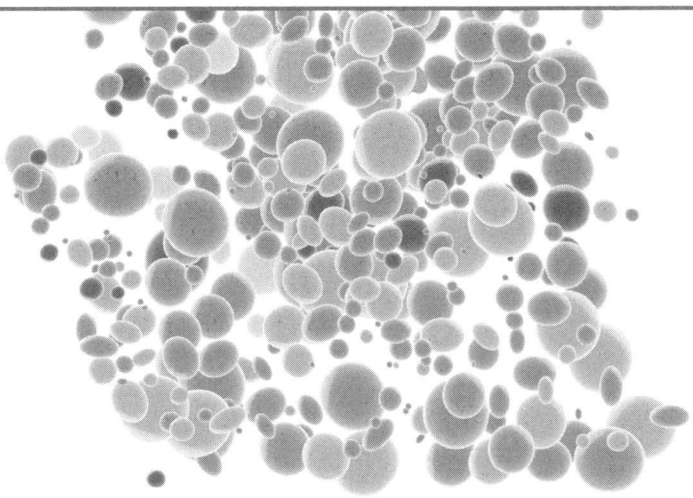

CHAPTER 1

Introduction

I think of feminism as poetry; we hear histories in words;
we reassemble histories by putting them in words.
—SARAH AHMED (2017, p. 12)

LEARNING OBJECTIVES

- To introduce you to the idea of feminist research from a critical, intersectional perspective
- To foreshadow what is coming in this text

What Is Feminist Research?

The gun massacre at the Pulse nightclub in Orlando, Florida, on June 12, 2016, which killed 49 people and wounded 52, was the deadliest attack on lesbian, gay, bisexual, transgender, questioning (LGBTQ) people in U.S. history. On July 22, presidential hopeful Hillary Clinton visited the site of the attack and rightly acknowledged that "it's still dangerous to be LGBTQ in America," calling the massacre a "targeted attack on the Latino LGBTQ community" (Ogles, 2016).

Clinton also acknowledged that members of the LGBTQ community "are more likely than any other group in our country to be the targets of hate crimes" (Ogles, 2016). People of color still constitute a majority of those victims—a fact that should build ally solidarity between feminist, queer, and people-of-color activist movements, but single-issue media coverage seems incapable of bringing intersectional attention to the racist and anti-trans*/queer violence that Orlando represents. Since the shooting, most of the coverage has been about Omar Mateen and his motivations, his history, his orientations, his thoughts and feelings. He was quickly proven to have no formal links with ISIL or other terrorist organizations, yet the coverage continues to focus on him and the specter of terrorism, rather than the victims as minoritarian subjects, on homophobic and transphobic violence, or on gun violence in the U.S. more generally. (Harris & Holman Jones, 2016)

Gender, according to Judith Butler (1990a), is a repetition of stylized acts, which challenges earlier research claiming that there is some "essential" pre-existing gendered self that is then communicated or "revealed" socially; rather, Butler theorized that gender is a co-constructed and ephemeral performance of emergent selves. Gender is importantly significantly different from sex and sexuality.

Beginning with the status of girls and women, but not ending there, feminism is an engaged human rights position that seeks to expose and remedy gender inequities. The study of gender, as a starting point for approaching feminist research, cannot be understood without consideration of other aspects of human existence that influence the ways in which human beings interact socially, including race, physical ability, class, geolocations, and sexuality. We are not bodies that are only gendered, but rather, we simultaneously occupy race, ethnicity, social class, sexuality, and other positionalities. Feminist research recognizes the inescapable need to approach the study of gender in a way that recognizes the simultaneous nature of our complex selves, and the ways in which multiple aspects of privilege or oppression are being exercised at once.

Such multithreaded oppressions require collaboration between the minorities who suffer and allies to the cause. (Adopting the position of "ally" reminds us that we are not the authority on other people's experiences.) The response to the Orlando tragedy exemplifies just such intersectionality and "allyship," and a commitment to intersectionality is what is different about this text: while contemporary feminist research texts abound, this one invites readers to engage with the rapid and diverse evolutions of feminism today, as well as to participate in the kind of intersectional critical scholarship that feminism was established to address.

As you might imagine, **gender** is central to defining what feminist research does and believes, yet gender is not the only focus of feminist research. These intersectional commitments of feminist research as a field constitute a **feminist research ethics**—the political, methodological, and in some cases spiritual beliefs that underpin this area of scholarly research.

But this feminist research ethics is not just an abstract idea—it points to additional feminist concerns, including **ontology** (the nature of knowledge itself), **epistemology** (what counts as knowledge and how that knowledge is represented), and **methodology** (the theories and tools of doing research). As a **critical research approach** it also suggests a range of ways in which feminist researchers believe in changing the world. "Critical" in this sense does not imply "to criticize," but rather to *challenge* the status quo. Feminist research is by its nature a critical research approach, because it challenges the gender-based inequities that are still pervasive around the globe. For example, the gender pay gap (unequal pay for equal work, based on gender) is a social justice issue concerning both gender *and* economics. But gender pay inequity is an issue that also intersects with geography, race, religion, and other conditions. For example, it is easy to find gender pay gap statistics for the United States or Europe, such as those shown in Figure 1.1, but not as easy to find such statistics for other global regions, yet we are told that the gender pay gap is an important indicator to monitor injustices and unfair working conditions.

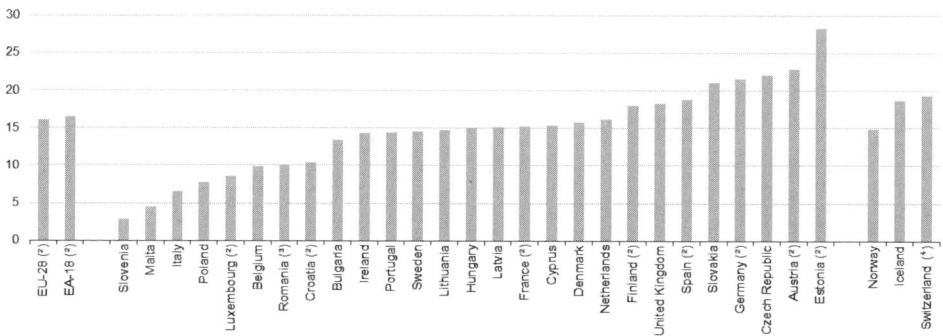

(¹) Enterprises employing 10 or more employees, NACE Rev. 2 B to S (-O).
(²) Provisional data; Ireland: 2012 data
(³) Estimated data
(⁴) 2013 data
No data for Greece

FIGURE 1.1 The unadjusted gender pay gap. The unadjusted gender pay gap 2014, published online March 2016 by Eurostat. The gender pay gap is the average difference between a man's and a woman's pay. There are two distinct numbers regarding the pay gap—the unadjusted versus the adjusted pay gap. The latter takes into account differences in hours worked, occupations, education and job experience. Accessed at *http:// ec.europa.eu/eurostat/statistics-explained/index.php/File:The_unadjusted_gender_pay_ gap,_2014_(¹)_(difference_between_average_gross_hourly_earnings_of_male_and_ female_employees_as_%25_of_male_gross_earnings_new.png#filelinks.*

This book will look closely at these key terms and areas of inquiry from a range of perspectives.

In examining the Orlando tragedy, for example, it is impossible to understand the crime without seeing how race, gender, sexuality, and even religion conflate in ways that inform one another. This intersectionality is the kind of complex understanding that we are encouraging readers of this book to use as a lens through which to approach the theories and methodological innovations of feminism that follow. Contemporary feminist research has the ability through intersectionality and other postmodern and poststructuralist frameworks to foreground the complexity of these areas of inquiry in ways that the mainstream media is routinely unable to convey. As a result, feminist research work offers an important alternative to the often one-dimensional accounts we experience through popular culture. Wouldn't it be wonderful if all fields of scholarship could allow us to understand ourselves and our work better and make an intellectual contribution, while at the same time improving the material conditions of our shared communities and lives? We think so.

This book approaches feminist research from just that point of view. But before we can ask, *What is feminist research?* we must ask ourselves, *What is critical scholarship?*

This book understands contemporary feminist research as that which addresses inequality with an agenda for social change. Again, we believe that **critical scholarship**—that which problematizes social conditions as they are—can only be addressed intersectionally, or in other words, in the interwoven ways that it gets played out in real life. For example, oppressions almost never appear alone—they are usually expressed in multiples. Where there's racism, there is often also sexism, classism, ableism. So in order to be wide awake as feminist researchers we must also ask ourselves the questions *What is race? What is ableism? What is class (socioeconomic) inequity? How do these conditions and positions work together or against one another?* This book asks readers to think about doing research that is embedded in and accountable to "real life," and that aspires to make real life better—not just for women, but for all—and to realize that these are not separate projects but interconnected ones.

This book also asks readers to consider the question *What does it mean to do feminist research?* Feminist research is not like many other forms of research, because it holds social commitments in the front of our work. Feminist research is not just abstract scholarship that analyzes how things are, but rather it suggests ways forward to a better world in which this kind of critical scholarship plays an active role in inspiring and enacting social change. Perhaps most importantly, feminist research is not just concerned with the conditions of girls and women, but with all gender-based inequities, and today in particular, with the highly visible but contested terrain of transgender and cisgender human rights and the ways in which changing definitions of gender impact all genders and all who fall outside the "gender spectrum" or somewhere fluid within it.

What Is an Ally?

As feminist researchers we must also ask, as we suggested was needed in response to the Orlando massacre, *What is an ally?* Feminist research committed to fighting against intersectional and multiple oppressions requires that we recognize that while we might inhabit some of those minority positions, we cannot inhabit them all, and that we still have a scholarly, political, and interpersonal commitment to fight equally for them all. Being an ally also requires **reflexivity** and **power sharing** in our research practice. We must critically interrogate our own positions within the research process and let go of the false idea that we are the all-knowing authority. In praxis—the "doing" of research—being an ally can take many shapes, including setting research agendas in collaboration with community partners, engaging in reciprocal relationships with research participants, using collaborative and participatory designs, disseminating research findings in popular forms, and putting research findings to use (to influence public policy, create programming, etc.). In other words, we are there to support the agendas of those directly oppressed, or oppressed differently from ourselves.

What Is Gender?

We must ask ourselves in a serious way, *What is gender?* It may seem obvious, but as 21st-century feminist research is showing, it's not. Many longtime feminist researchers are learning new terms or new concepts for familiar terms, such as **cisgender,** a term that denotes identification with the gender one is biologically assigned at birth. Males who have come out as transgender females have often been mistreated, even within feminist circles, and these communities and assemblages represent one way in which feminist research is reexamining much of what it does and stands for politically and interpersonally. Many mainstream feminist texts continue, surprisingly, to focus only or primarily on "girls and women," without problematizing these as socially constructed (not "innate") categories, or pay insufficient attention to **genderqueer, gender-creative, gender-fluid,** or **trans*** girls, women, and feminists. This book is different: We go back to basics and ask once again—in utterly new and contemporary ways—that most primary of feminist questions: *What is gender, and therefore what is required to gain gender equity?*

What about the Digital?

This moment is perhaps the most exciting time in history to be doing feminist research. Why? Because definitions and practices of feminism are—like so much else—changing so rapidly and in so many diverse directions. Today more than ever we have culturally diverse feminisms that have different understandings and enactments of feminist ideals while holding common commitments with other feminists around the globe. Today, feminist digital media makes it possible to have feminist memes, concepts, and incidents "go viral" and drum up support almost instantaneously—this has never before been possible in the long history of the fight for gender equality. For example, the #MeToo movement and Time's Up initiative have gained incredible momentum, prompting immediate change, thanks to the Internet. And today, definitions and practices of gender itself are more fluid than ever—and moving rapidly toward even more fluidity. What could be a more engaging and exciting area of research in the current era?

While some would trace the exploration of diverse gender performance to Eve Sedgwick's first articulation of a **queer theory** that went beyond sexuality, others would point out that in the non-Western world, gender fluidity and diversity have been long recognized and long integrated into cultures more generally, as in, for example, the Samoan identity known as *Fa'afafine,* the Tongan *fakaleiti,* Native American "two-spirit identities," Tahitian *Mahu,* and indigenous Australians known as Sistergirls. We begin our engagement with feminist research in the 21st century with girls and women as a starting point but move beyond traditional cisgender definitions and identifications of gender presentation and their alignment with feminist research and politics. In this book we are looking at gender in more complicated and always evolving ways, including feminism for nonbinary gender orientations and identifications. This up-to-date understanding and approach to feminisms for the 21st century is what sets this book apart.

What about Representation?

Also central to our contemporary approach to feminist research is the notion of representation. This is no accident, as both feminist digital media and contemporary gender studies highlight the performative nature of gender. Feminist research is no different. As gender is a socially constructed category, research on feminism across the gender spectrum, including research on girls and women, continues to highlight the ways in which representation reinforces gender inequity and the social justice needs of feminist research.

While a generation ago feminist research focused on the "means of production" of representation, today feminist researchers and our allies and collaborators can create our own images through digital media, video, and social media. We can engage with traditional forms of scholarly representation, subverting the standard forms, and we can also engage with new forms intended to reach popular audiences, and at times inspire social activism. Does that mean that there is equity of representation, either online or off-line? Not at all. What it does mean is that there is a new round of concerns for the curation, production, consumption, and circulation of gendered images that are impacting gender equity concerns in online/off-line worlds, and the need for critical feminist research is only growing. Therefore, we invite you to explore the methodological, theoretical, and popular cultural resources this book has to offer through the range of questions, activities, and additional digital resources available in each chapter. What you can be sure of is that this book and its studies/examples are just as up to date, just as evolving, and just as diverse as feminist research today.

CONCLUSION

As we hope you are beginning to see, feminism is an engaged position from which to conduct research. While feminism begins with the status and circumstances of girls and women, it does not end there. Throughout this book we review the historical context for feminist research, theoretical frameworks, methods for conducting research, writing for different audiences, and activism. We hope to provide you with the basic tools to engage in your own feminist practice, as current events provide the need and inspiration.

DISCUSSION QUESTIONS

1. What does it mean to say that gender is central to feminist research but that gender is not the only focus of feminist research?

2. Select a recent event and reflect on how an intersectional approach is important for analyzing and responding to the event.

ACTIVITIES

1. Find two newspaper articles about the Pulse nightclub massacre. What are the main points of each article? How are the victims and perpetrator characterized? Is an intersectional analysis offered? Please explain your response with examples from the articles.

2. Conduct online research to learn about the #MeToo movement or Time's Up initiative. How did digital media fuel the movement? (Up to 1 page).

SUGGESTED RESOURCES

📚 Books

Ngozi Adichie, C. (2015). *We should all be feminists*. New York: Anchor Books.

　　This is a widely regarded and inspirational statement on the importance of feminism.

Collins, P. H., & Blige, S. (2016). *Intersectionality*. Cambridge, UK: Polity.

　　A comprehensive review of intersectionality including what it is, how to enact it as a part of critical inquiry, and the historical development of the concept.

🖥 Digital Resources

Feminism in Nigeria
www.cddc.vt.edu/feminism/nig.html

An amazing resource page/bibliography on the history, economics, and politics of feminism in Nigeria.

Tales of Passion
www.ted.com/talks/isabel_allende_tells_tales_of_passion

The Chilean American author Isabelle Allende's TED Talk on women, creativity, and the definition of feminism has had nearly 3.6 million views at the time of this writing. Allende is a world-renowned author, one of the most widely read writers in Latin America, and also a self-described feminist and gender warrior. Her

TED Talk is a powerful and articulate commentary on doing this work as a Latina woman, and in Latin America.

Flickering Feminism

www.feminisminchina.com/#daughtersofchina

Flickering Feminism is an archiving project on the history of feminism in China, including a series of excellent videos.

Why I'm a Feminist

www.youtube.com/watch?v=UwJRFClybmk

This video by Laci Green has had over 3.8 million views at the time of this writing. Laci Green is an American internet sensation and YouTube personality, and a trailblazer in the internet video form called vlogs ("video blogs"). She was one of the first vloggers to "go viral," to get commercial backing, and for her internet series to translate into "offline" star status as well. Green has been vocal about the gender constraints that online broadcast upholds, and about the challenges to doing "serious" vlogging as a female presenter. Her YouTube broadcasts (now her own channel) have evolved from a teenage hobby to her later feminist sex education work, and she remains followed by millions.

CHAPTER 2

The Feminist Research Landscape

> There are no safe spaces . . . Bridging is the work of opening
> the gate to the stranger, within and without.
> —GLORIA ANZALDÚA (2002, p. 3)

LEARNING OBJECTIVES

- To establish in broad terms the field of feminist research
- To offer guidance regarding the different geographies, political orientations, and theoretical developments of each major strand of feminist research
- To provide an overview of the relationship between feminist politics and feminist scholarship
- To offer insight into the diverse approaches within the field of feminist research

Feminist research is no longer a singular field, if ever it was. From the vast and sweeping range of its diverse core concepts, concerns, leading figures, and guiding principles, feminist research praxis is—more than ever—a multiplicity, a bridge across difference and a thread between perspectives. It questions in new ways for this era the very notions of truth and truth claims, multiple perspectives, and the knowledge creation that sits at the heart of research practice. Feminist scholarship is no longer defined only as research that concerns itself with gender, but a component of all scholarship concerned with social change and its real-world applications. Indeed, feminist scholar Elizabeth Grosz argues that any contemporary social justice research agenda or project must address how understandings of freedom are now fundamentally linked to "our habitual relations to the material world, [and] may serve feminist and other radical political thought" (2011, p. 5). These kinds of approaches to feminist research highlight the ways in which its disciplinarity and theoretical multiplicity make feminism a most generative and exciting area of contemporary social research today.

Feminist Research Similarities and Differences

There are vast differences across the current feminist research landscape between more established and emergent feminist scholars from every field and methodological approach. One established leader in feminist research, Alison Jaggar, and her pivotal contribution *Just Methods: An Interdisciplinary Feminist Reader* (2014), are significant for the ways in which they advance feminist research, interweaving methods, disciplines, approaches, and their interrelationship with issues of power and research ethics. Jaggar's text (and Halsanger, 2005, among others), like this one, focuses on research methodologies, epistemologies, and dissemination through (and beyond) public and popular cultural channels, yet ours also offers readers a critical discussion of the transformative potential of digital and social media.

Others have moved non-Western feminisms forward over the past 15 years in exciting and expansive ways.[1] Still others continue to expand more traditional approaches to feminist research subdisciplines, including Sprague's (2016) comprehensive attention to positivist and sociological theories and methods. One thing is for sure: feminist research has never been more alive and diverse, in part due to the proliferation of forms of research output and dissemination, but also due to the political and socioeconomic moment in which we find ourselves. In this text, we hope readers will find our robust and accessible theoretical, methodological, ethical, and practical approaches useful, as the "doing" of feminist scholarship and reflexive praxis continues to expand.

Setting the Scene

This chapter will set out an overview of the feminist research landscape until now, and as such it sets the scene for the more focused theoretical and

---

[1] See, for example, Lee-Koo and D'Costa (2008), who use feminist frameworks and research to address feminisms and activisms in international contexts, in an edited volume focused solely on the Asian Pacific, a most welcome contribution.

methodological chapters to follow. As part of that landscape survey, it is important to note the activist history of feminism as a social and political movement, which laid the foundations of feminist research as it became institutionalized in universities, colleges, and even schools. Feminism has certainly changed since its beginning in the 19th century, and continues to change, as well as continuing an interdependent relationship with its activist manifestations. While some disagree with the value of tracing this history in "waves" (first-wave feminism, second-wave feminism, etc.), it is still useful to have a clear and simple picture of these main sections of feminist history that underlie the 21st-century feminist research practices addressed in this book, and so we draw on this metaphor but also map beyond it.

One of the most rewarding (and also challenging) aspects of being a feminist researcher today is the vast array of texts and other sources that feminist research engages with—not only the long ongoing history of previous feminist works, but also other contemporary volumes addressing the wide range of concerns covered by the broad umbrella of "21st-century feminist scholarship" that inform and co-construct the landscape for this one. This text seeks to draw on, celebrate, and complement other volumes on feminist theory and research practice. Such rapidly evolving areas of study within the large rubric of feminist research include more recent attention to the broad spectrum of transgender and nonbinary gender identifications, and how they are influencing ideas about "feminisms." Adding to this, books on feminism and global development, online/off-line feminist activist movements and scholarship, and volumes focusing on new forms of feminist research methods, all make feminist scholarship an exciting place to work. In this chapter we trace a feminist research landscape that we hope will offer both new and experienced researchers a way into the many approaches to contemporary feminist research.

Feminist Research Methods and Disciplines

Feminist research is a thoroughly interdisciplinary area of study, spanning a range of theoretical frameworks such as film and performance theory, psychology, poststructuralism, linguistics, sociology, and art theory. A short survey of some of the most prominent areas in which feminist research is altering discipline-based landscapes includes those listed in the box on page 15.

Feminist Research across the Disciplines
· ·

- **Education:** Dillard, 2000, Hickey-Moody, 2007; Lather, 2007, 2008; Fine, 1994, 1992; Steinberg and Cannella, 2012

- **Philosophy:** Harding, 2012, 2004; Haraway, 1991, 2014; Boler, 1997, 1999; Grosz, 2011

- **New materialism:** Barad, 2007; van der Tuin, 2015; Thiele, 2014; Hinton et al., 2015

- **Youth studies:** Harris, 2004; Holland, Renold, Ross, and Hillman, 2010

- **Geography education:** Bhog et al., 2012; Bondi, 2002

- **Organizational feminism:** D'Enbeau and Buzzanell, 2013; Gouin, Cocq, and McGavin, 2011; Mackay, Kenny, and Chappell, 2010

- **Higher education and adult learning:** Carpenter, 2012

- **Religion and theology:** Fiorenza, 2013; Gebara, 2008; Hopkins, 2009; Scholz, 2010

- **Power, capitalism, and social work:** Karnieli-Miller, Strier, and Pessach, 2009; Holland et al., 2010; Deepak, 2011; Gulbrandsen and Walsh, 2012; Majic, 2014

- **Art:** Meagher, 2011; Toye, 2010; Tyner and Ogle, 2009

- **Social research:** Franks, 2002; MacGregor, 2009

- **War, criminology, violence, and military studies:** Henry, 2014; DeKeseredy, 2011; Basile, Hall, and Walters, 2013; Stachowitsch, 2012; Wattanaporn and Holtfreter, 2014; Weber, 2012

- **Activism studies:** Gulbrandsen, 2012; Hemmings, 2012

- **Globalization, transnationalism, race, and whiteness:** Deepak, 2011; Puar, 2007; Mitra, 2011; White, 2006

- **Sociology:** Bhavnani, 2001; Collins, 2011; Skeggs, 2005; Ward and Schneider, 2009; Ringrose, 2013

- **Mixed methods including triangulation:** Hesse-Biber, 2012; Carroll, 2013; Keary, 2013; Smart, 2009; Spierings, 2012

- **Feminist rhetorical studies:** Royster and Kirsch, 2012

- **Gender and queer studies:** Puar, 2007; Pillow and Mayo, 2007; Ahmed, 2017; Halberstam, 2012; Hesford, 2005; Landström, 2007; Vernet, Vala, and Butera, 2011; Lombardo, Meier, and Verloo, 2010

- **Technology:** Schuster, 2013

- **Psychology:** Sheriff and Weatherall, 2009; Yoder, Snell, and Tobias, 2012

- **Intersectionality:** Crenshaw, 1989; Alexander-Floyd, 2012; Carbin and Edenheim, 2013

- **Health:** Hankivsky et al., 2010

- **Social work and family studies:** Archer, 2009; Basile et al., 2013

- **Postcolonial studies:** Harding, 2012; Anzaldúa and Keating, 2002; Falcon, 2008; Rio, 2012

A Brief History of the Field

The feminist philosopher Megan Boler (1991) noted that

> Radical feminism's challenge to the gendered spheres of "public vs. private" has forever changed Western thought, culture and legislative, judicial and political paradigms. . . . The radical feminist slogan "the personal is political" symbolized the revolutionary reconceptualization of what counts as personal (women's lives, feelings, experience, and labor) and what counts as political (e.g., men's experience and rationality as the governing structure of political and public spaces). The emphasis on women's experiences, including her feelings, as *political* and not merely personal, was a key feature of the radical feminist agenda. (p. 81)

Some feminist scholars still question whether we have progressed beyond arguing for the political importance of women's experiences, observations, scholarship, and other feminist human capital, which continues to be sidelined or invisibilized in the academy. Today, feminist scholarship still systematically argues the possibilities and problematics of women's feelings (and emotions and feelings more generally) as "valid" research and posits their place in rigorous scholarship.

Contemporary feminist research includes now well-worn questions about the defining of feminist theory, as well as the "doing" of feminist research. Is there a feminist method? it asks. Indeed, feminism in qualitative, quantitative, arts-based, participatory, and other emergent paradigms continues to demand attention to how feminist approaches and lenses might help us think differently about a range of age-old questions. What is the role of feminism in the great range of so-called scientific research? How might feminist and decolonial geographies be changing and promise to accelerate in this change over the next ecologically unstable 20 or 30 years?

Margaret Somerville and other scholars of space, place, and belonging continue to look to nonhuman others for multisensory answers to (or further questions for) these investigations. Feminist new materialisms, posthumanism, and new hybrid forms of feminist research are appearing in works like Anna Hickey-Moody's "femifesta" feminist manifesto for arts education in *Posthuman Research Practices in Education* (Taylor & Hughes, 2016) and beyond. But even a cursory glance through scholarship limited to the human world (and not concerned with the posthuman or more-than-human) reveals an ever greater diversity of platforms, approaches, and subjectivities: as just one example, transgender and cisgender feminisms are in dynamic conversation as never before.

The Early Years

When feminism as a scholarly field began around the beginning of the 1970s, the emphasis was firmly fixed on "sex differences and the extent to which such differences might be based on the biological properties of individuals" (Sprague, 2016, p. vii). Fifteen years later, however, by feminist research's second stage, "the focus [had] shifted to the individual sex roles and socialization, exposing gender as the product of specific social arrangements, although still conceptualizing it as an individual trait" (Sprague, 2016, p. vii). The so-called third stage of feminist research is typified by a

> recognition of the centrality of gender as an organizing principle in all social systems, including work, politics, everyday interaction, families, economic development, law, education, and a host of other social domains. As our understanding of gender has become more social, so has our awareness that gender is experienced and organized in race- and class-specific ways. (Sprague, 2016, p. vii)

If **epistemology** is the study of theories of knowledge, *feminist* epistemology is the study of knowledge from a feminist perspective; that is, the production of knowledge through a feminist lens. In this

> **Epistemology** is the systematic study of the theory of knowledge.

volume, we address both epistemology and **ontology,** interrelated aspects of research knowledge creation that are both pivotal in understanding exactly why feminism in research has been so fundamentally challenging to the academic establishment.

This chapter (and this book) offers researchers an accessible approach to understanding feminist epistemologies and ontologies, or what some feminist researchers refer to as "onto-epistemologies"[2] and their implications. In what ways is gender "experienced and organized"?—in *all ways*. To that end, the remainder of this chapter is devoted to a brief overview of the ways in which feminism has moved beyond a field of research

> **Ontology** is the study of existence, and how we describe what we have come to know.

---

[2]The term was coined (or at least conjoined) by new materialist scholar Karen Barad, who has theorized a concept of agential realism. She argues that the theoretic is at once an epistemology (theory of knowing), an ontology (theory of being), and an ethics. They are mutually informing and co-constructive, so she uses "onto-epistemology" to represent their interdependence.

and proliferated as an epistemological lens through which researchers can both *see* and *do* any and all kinds of research. Throughout this chapter's overview of pivotal moments and key figures are scattered highlights of field-defining epistemologies and conceptual leaps that have moved the field forward and expanded it outward like the circles that emanate from a stone tossed into a pond.

Feminist Research Leaps Forward

One pivotal example of this widening out of feminist lenses into all realms of research is the work of educational, race, feminist, and social justice scholar Cynthia Dillard (discussed in detail in Chapter 3, and with a video to view Dillard's contribution in her own words). Dillard's concept of an endarkened feminist epistemology addresses identity, difference, and the politics of representation through the field of education by offering a critical theoretical lens through which readers see how these areas of study are impossible to disentangle.

Patti Lather (2008), a noted feminist scholar in her own right, has paid homage to Cynthia Dillard's work in noting the ways it has crossed educational, racialized, and gendered boundaries, enriching multidisciplinary research as it goes. For example, even though Dillard's primary discipline is education and literacy, her particular way of approaching the study of literacies and education has influenced critical race theory (the study of the impact of race on all walks of life), feminism, and qualitative research[3] more generally. Through Lather's own notion of "getting lost as a methodology" (Lather, 2007), she seeks to clarify from Dillard's work what a "feminist epistemology" actually might look and move like. To do so, she draws on the foundational queer and gender theorist Eve Kosofsky Sedgwick's (1997) notion of "reparative critique." In this example, we purposefully link three pivotal feminist scholars whose works are in conversation with one another in order to begin highlighting the genealogy of a field that some still claim has no discernible scholarly history or trajectory of its own.

---

[3] Most research today falls into two main "paradigms" or structural ways of doing things: qualitative and quantitative (although scholars including the coauthors have noted that arts-based research offers a new paradigm that goes beyond this simple binarism, while other scholars are developing the notion of postqualitative research as well). Qualitative research primarily attends to small, in-depth studies at the individual level and gathers information that is not in numerical form, for example, diary accounts, open-ended questionnaires, unstructured interviews, and unstructured observations. Quantitative data is usually numerical (statistical) and more focused on large-scale studies, large data sets, and generalizable claims. As shorthand, many say qualitative research "goes deep," while quantitative research "goes wide."

Feminist research has rapidly evolved and promises new directions in a 21st-century research landscape that is increasingly concerned with feminist geographies, posthuman others, and gender-expansive borders. In addition to Judith Butler, Donna Haraway (and others, discussed in detail in Chapters 3 and 4), Sedgwick can be counted among the foundational scholars of a 21st-century feminist scholarship, and one whose works have been applied in diverse ways by those like Dillard working cross-disciplinarily.

Lather (2008) values, as we do, the ways in which Dillard's work "examines the 'life notes' of three African American female academics in order to develop a cultural standpoint epistemology out of the intersectionalities of identities 'and the historical and contemporary contexts of oppression and resistance' for such women (Dillard, 2000: 661)" (p. 219). Evolving from her own cultural, racial, and gendered experience and scholarship, Dillard positions her "endarkened feminist epistemology" as a tool for moving toward more ethical, decolonizing methodologies (Tuhiwai Smith, 1999) and away from traditional Western ways of knowing. Decolonizing methodologies refer to the intersections of imperialism and research and make transparent the ways in which imperialism is embedded in scholarly work, and what is considered scholarly knowledge. Dillard's work is just one example of the layered and multidisciplinary nature of contemporary feminist research.

Like feminist scholars writing from queer, (dis)ability, and religiously minoritarian subjectivities, Dillard (and Lather in discussing her) advocate a more transparent and critically self-reflexive acknowledgment of the intersectionalities of our research selves and projects, which shape our (and all) research agendas; one tool offered by Dillard in practical terms is her "six assumptions to guide culturally relevant inquiry" (in Lather, 2008, p. 219). We highlight this part of Dillard's work to make particular note of the need for both theoretically robust and practically efficient tools in feminist research and scholarship, a goal toward which this book contributes.

Tracking Innovations

Other important feminist scholarship innovations in the late 20th and early 21st centuries include feminist science, physics and its evolution into/with **new materialist theory** (which looks at the independent agency of nonhuman objects and subjects), **posthumanism** (scholarship focused on the more-than-human), **postfeminism** (evolutions in feminist social codes), **affect theory** (study of emotions and feelings), and **digital feminisms** (online and off-line), all of which will be explored in detail throughout the subsequent chapters.

Much feminist scholarship over the past 20 years can be characterized by either a social science approach or a postmodern one (see Chapters 3 and 4 for more on this). This volume, like any comprehensive feminist research text today, includes discussions of feminist standpoints, feminist ethnography, postmodern, poststructural, and critical epistemologies, social movement research, activism, globalization and globalizing feminist research, health and social work, feminist pedagogies and praxis, authority and representation in feminist research, science and feminism, and gender diversity. We note the value of, and need to be in, dialogue with a wide range of research and teaching perspectives, student perspectives, policy makers and activists—as all contemporary research and research texts must be, whether they are methodological or conceptual (Sprague, 2016; Hesse-Biber, 2012).

We also want to highlight that the nature of feminist knowledge production is inherently global, and decentred from traditional White, Western, global North, and often still male producers of "legitimate" academic knowledge.

It's a great time to be a feminist researcher. Just at the time when a notion of " 'postfeminism" seems to suggest that we have attained our goals and feminism is no longer needed, along comes a proliferation of antifeminist and antiwomen backlash, bringing a rich tide of new feminist research and passion.

To Wave or Not to Wave

> Activism is the courage to act consciously on our ideas, to exert power in resistance to ideological pressure—to risk leaving home. Empowerment comes from ideas—our revolution is fought with concepts, not with guns, and it is fueled by vision. By focusing on what we want to happen, we change the present. The healing images and narratives we imagine will eventually materialize. (Anzaldúa & Keating, 2002, p. 5)

While the history of feminist thought, activism, and economics is still largely framed in terms of its three-plus "waves" to date, here we ask whether it is useful to talk about waves of feminist research anymore. Why not?

For one reason, scholarship by its nature draws not only *upon* what has come before it, but also draws those predecessors *in* and remains in dialogue with that previous scholarship. In addition, epistemological dialogues and movements are seldom linear, and seldom completely (or sometimes even discernibly) different from one another. But because this is a book for feminist researchers who may be new to this area of inquiry, as well as those who have been engaging with it for some time, we offer an historical overview of the most commonly known three waves of feminism, as well as a snapshot of what post-third-wave feminism (or what some are calling *postfeminism*) may be about (see Figure 2.1).

From postfeminism to digital feminist activism, feminism is definitely "back." High-profile feminist activist groups like Pussy Riot, the Gorilla Girls, and Femen have reminded a new generation of women and men why feminism is still needed. With the advent of digital (and particularly social) media platforms, new social movements—including 21st-century feminism—are getting more coverage than ever before. Whether we are considering the earliest days of "first-wave feminism" around the turn of the 20th century, or today's new feminism for the 21st century, activists for the rights of women have always seen and addressed the intersection of sexual, gender, education, and economic politics. This has lent feminism its historically layered character, especially in increasingly diverse geographical and cultural contexts. Black Feminisms, uneven global "development," and gender/sexuality research in lower-income regions have introduced new groups of coexistent oppressions, known as intersectionalities, in feminist

First Wave	Second Wave	Third Wave	Postfeminism
Late 19th–early 20th century	1960s–1970s	1990s–present	2000–present
Known as the "**suffrage**" period, and its activists as "suffragettes," as it focused on securing voting and basic equal rights for women.	Focused on the right to education, work, equal pay. Challenged traditional representations and roles of women.	Challenged and to some degree broadened the pervasively White, middle-class orientation and agendas of second-wave feminism, including not only working-class women and women of color, but also non-"feminine" women's concerns, such as **queer feminisms**, "girl power," and "ladette" culture in the United Kingdom.	Addresses the perception that feminism is either "over" or no longer relevant to the younger generation. Postfeminism celebrates sexuality, "femininity," and the impossibility of essentializing "women" under a feminist banner.

FIGURE 2.1 Timeline of the feminist movement.

research and activism. A strength of feminist research is its ability to cross disciplinary lines but also epistemological ones, including, most recently, **posthumanism,** affect and emotion, embodiment in the age of technology, aesthetics, organizational change, global cultures, feminist materialisms, and personal relationships. As you can see, no one researcher or single book can address this wide and rich range of applications and disciplines of feminist research in every field it touches and informs, so our goal in this book is to introduce readers to the macrofeminist landscape in which the ever-evolving microfeminisms emerge, thrive, and inform all others. In the next sections, we offer a broad historical overview of feminism across the 20th century and into the 21st.

First-Wave Feminist Research/Feminism (1900–1950)

It's hard to remember today that women have only had the right to vote and participate fully in the governments of their countries for just over 100 years (rights that were won very slowly, incrementally, and unevenly). In 1893, New Zealand became the first nation to legislate voting rights for all women, what was then called "women's suffrage," yet there were several other regions, states, and territories that had partial rights extended (sometimes temporarily).

The right to vote was never won without extended activism and sustained petition to government. It was achieved through the intellectual and public work of many men and women, including, famously, Susan B. Anthony in the United States and Mary Wollstonecraft and Emmeline Pankhurst in the United Kingdom. Women who fought for the vote during this time were called "suffragettes," and it was one of the biggest fights of the day. Huge marches were held, public talks given and attended, and (mostly male) scholars wrote about the pros and cons of conferring this dangerous power upon women, whose power was previously only exerted in the private home. Thus, suffrage became a crucial step in giving women a public voice, power, and role that was then advanced even further during the two world wars, when women were needed for work in the factories because all able-bodied men were sent away to war. Readers should note the not-incidental link between economics, politics, gendered power relations, and the public sphere, as embodied by the seminal figure of Rosie the Riveter.

There were some activists like Constance de Markievicz (an Irish activist of English origin) who were privileged and well educated enough to help document the role of feminist labor in social movements like the Easter Rising in Dublin in 1916. However, the labor of feminists then, as today, remains invisible. And when World War II came to an end in 1945, many men *and* women were happy to go back to the way things before the war, and the working woman and the politics and economics that affected her and her family became somewhat dormant until the more widespread social unrest of the 1960s. The worldwide political upheaval of that decade revealed changing social codes along racial, economic, gender, and sexual lines.

Second-Wave Feminist Research (Early 1960s–1980s)

By the 1970s, feminism's second, most defining, wave was breaking. This was the "burn your bra" era of women who fought back with the battle cry "Equality now!" This second-wave feminist era was typified by marches and a range of forms of civil (and domestic) disobedience, but it was also a time of enormous economic change. For feminist research, it is the birth of the era of women's studies departments in universities, where those who wished to study the "consciousness raising" of the feminist and civil rights movements could explicitly draw out the interconnectedness of these movements, in both political strategies and training of activists.

These strategies came quickly to inform feminist scholarship, which moved from an analysis of social movements to a poststructuralist questioning of how the self (the subject) is formed, and how socially constructed, ubiquitous, and gender defined that interrelationality is. Feminism had finally reached the academy, and it brought the study of sexuality along with its focus on gender, highlighting the inextricability of the two.

But the intersection of gender and sexuality in the second-wave feminist movement also seemed to highlight issues of class and race, for the feminist movement was largely a White and middle-class endeavor. Non-White feminists quickly knew they must point out that they had been marginalized in the civil rights movement by their female gender, and were now being sidelined in the women's movement due to their race. Scholar-activists like Angela Davis and Minnie Bruce Pratt have worked to show the ways in which the feminist movement failed to be as inclusive as it had promised, yet how necessary it was to begin moving in that direction.

Who Were They?

What is generally known as "second-wave feminism" refers mainly to a social movement led by primarily White feminists of the 1970s and '80s (a point that gave it some economic force but also brought it great criticism both from within and without). Throughout the 1970s and '80s, Gloria

Steinem, Betty Friedan, Jill Johnston, Audre Lorde, Gloria Anzaldúa, Alice Walker, and others were instrumental in their searing scholarship, which made visible institutionalized racism and sexism that had plagued them for so long, but also in providing the (again) invisible labor of setting up the first institutional higher education "homes" for the study of the women's movement—women's studies departments—sometimes against great odds and at high personal cost.

Megan Boler has written widely about the "invisible labor" of women and feminist activists, which, in many ways, remains invisible even in hybrid online/offline digital media and social movement scholarship. Boler has documented not only the emotional and affective labor of women in the academy, but also the contribution of feminist scholarship (such as that of Haraway and others) to the field of philosophy of education. Boler provides valuable historicity to the trajectory of the women's movement that both preceded and extended beyond women's studies departments in the academy.

> In the late 1960s and early 1970s in the United States, women who had been involved with the civil rights and New Left movements began a grassroots movement of their own. Frequently, women were denied leadership positions . . . while men planned strategies and headed the public debates. Many women were frustrated with the lack of gender analysis . . . the left movements generally reinscribed traditional patriarchal distinctions of public and private, and perpetuated a definition of the "political" as the economic, public, and legislative realms occupied by men. (Boler 1999, p. 64)

Rather than recognize women's labor (both invisible and visible) as human capital and labor that contributed to the surplus profit required by capitalism, Boler has traced the ways in which women's labor remains sidelined or unseen altogether.

Boler (1999) has argued that

> feminist theories and practices "step up" to this difficult question of how material and economic oppression reveal themselves in our daily lives and consciousness. What I call the "feminist politics of emotion" is a theory and practice that invites women to articulate and publicly name their emotions, and to critically and collectively analyze these emotions not as "'natural," "private" occurrences but rather as reflecting learned hierarchies and gendered roles. The feminist practices of consciousness-raising and feminist pedagogy powerfully reclaim emotions out of the (patriarchally enforced) private sphere and put emotions on the political and public map. Feminist politics of emotions recognize emotions not only as a site of social control, but of political resistance. (p. 47)

The kinds of feminist research that predominated during this period bear out Boler's claims. While poststructuralist scholars like Judith Butler and Gilles Deleuze have come to typify the era of third-wave or post-third-wave feminism (discussed in detail in Chapter 4), back in the late days of second-wave feminism the seeds were already being planted for challenging the "business as usual" of White-male-dominated academic research by those like Donna Haraway working in feminist philosophy, emotions, and the nature of human consciousness.

Third-Wave Feminist Research (1985–Present)

While third-wave feminism has its roots firmly in the activism and consciousness raising of second-wave feminism, it shifted toward the experiences of women of color and race-informed feminist inequalities, and was typified by small presses such as Kitchen Table Press, theater projects and programs by feminists of color, and scholarship on "third-world feminisms." During this time, women's studies departments were thriving but increasingly amalgamated with "gender studies departments," which many feel dealt the first major blow to having a "department of one's own" in academic contexts. Once so-called women's issues were conflated with other scholarly attention to gender and sexuality in gender studies and eventually **queer theory** units/departments, increasing diffusion plagued not only the momentum of feminist activism but also its scholarship at times as well.

Feminist Theory or Gender Theory?

By the mid-1980s, feminism was expanding beyond hegemonic issues of White Western (and largely hetero- or homosexual) women, as women of color (and others) saw it increasingly not meeting their particular needs. Queer, "sex-positive," SlutWalk, sex-worker, and trans* activists, and those of other sexual and gender diversities fought to loosen what they felt was the policing of feminist sexuality and gender expressions. Joan Nestle, Minnie Bruce Pratt, Holly Hughes, and others opened scholarship on queer femme sexuality, while Leslie Feinberg and others spoke out about trans* and female masculinities, all within feminist communities and discourses.

Many of these scholars felt (and still do feel) unwelcome in feminist scholarly, activist, and social circles. Perhaps the most famous flashpoint for some of these inclusion/exclusion debates has been in regard to the Michigan Womyn's Music Festival, and the kind of queer theater and performative representation typified by the scholarship of Sue Ellen Case. In addition, Latina, African American, and subaltern feminist voices were growing and demanding room at the feminist (scholarly, activist, and artistic) table. Of these, one of the greatest was Gloria Anzaldúa.

Writing a few months before her death, in the updated edition of her pivotal feminist text, and reflecting back on its original publication in 1983, Anzaldúa acknowledged that the time had come to look beyond victimhood to what we are doing to one another within feminist communities—not only locally, but in "distant countries, and to the earth's environment" (Anzaldúa & Keating, 2002). She invites us to share her recognition of the need to act collaboratively. In the box below, she paints a beautiful, compelling, and, not incidentally, thoroughly second-wave activist picture of what might be possible if we can try again to come together.

Fighting against a diminishment of humanness is still the project of feminism, and postfeminisms. Each era needs its own call to the barricades, and intergenerational respect is now offered to Anzaldúa and her contribution, which was "carved out for us with [her] fingernails," by a brand-new generation of feminists. Feminism and feminist scholarship, like all social justice projects, are an evolving and infinite commitment, just as working against and into racisms, ageisms, and other oppressions.

Feminist Solidarity

As swells break against the Santa Cruz mudstone promontories I feel that we who struggle for social change are the waves cutting holes in the rock and erecting new bridges. We're loosening the grip of outmoded methods and ideas in order to allow new ways of being and acting to emerge, but we're not totally abandoning the old—we're building on it. We're reinforcing the foundations and support beams of the old *puentes*, not just giving them new paint jobs. While trying to hold fast to the rights feminists, progressives, and activists have carved out for us with their fingernails, we also battle those who are trying to topple both old and new bridges. Twenty-one years ago we struggled with the recognition of difference within the context of commonality. Today we grapple with the recognition of commonality within the context of difference. While *This Bridge Called My Back* displaced whiteness, *this bridge we call home* carries this displacement further. It questions the terms *white* and *women of color* by showing that whiteness may not be applied to all whites, as some possess women-of-color consciousness, just as some women of color bear white consciousness. This book intends to change notions of identity, viewing it as part of a more complex system covering a larger terrain, and demonstrating that the politics of exclusion based on traditional categories diminishes our humanness.

Anzaldúa (2002, p. 2)

Feminism has no end. As Anzaldúa and Keating (2002) noted, "Today categories of race and gender are more permeable and flexible than they were for those of us growing up prior to the 1980s" (p. 2), and yet these fluidities can create their own new marginalizations. No matter how we work toward inclusivity, as they did, including by incorporating emerging new voices (from new regions, newly identified trans* and other women, new formations of cisgendered women, etc.), in the process we all end up "revealing how much has shifted in the last twenty years, but also how little has changed" (p. 3). This is the role of feminist activism, and also importantly the job of feminist scholarship.

Beyond the Waves: Feminisms across the Globe

As we outlined earlier, we are not arguing that feminism is now or was historically bounded by its waves (eras) and certainly do not see them as distinct or appreciably separate. We have provided the preceding overview in order to orient the new feminist scholar in a way that makes linear sense, or that contextualizes a range of feminisms along a kind of timeline. But we wish to stress that we see feminist research (and activism) not as a monodirectional arrow, but rather as a web, a crossword puzzle, or a grid.

Feminisms abound (and have abounded historically) in a weblike way, more than a linear one. These ripples or grids or layers can be read completely differently by altering the reader's perspective. That is, South Sudanese diasporic feminist scholars may not use the same language or theories, or argue for the same pressing concerns as White Scottish sex workers but practice feminist scholarship all the same. Mothers in rural Minnesota may not share the same feminist concerns as urban lawyers or entrepreneurs in Delhi, but they often consider themselves part of the same movement or scholarly discourse. Both the differences *and* the commonalities are equally important and addressed in this book.

Why Is Feminist Scholarship Political?

Feminist scholarship is an inherently political project, and as such it relies upon local contexts, concerns, and relationships. The principles of feminists' projects in diverse locales can be absolutely the same and the particulars continue to proliferate in new and individual ways. For example, Boler's concern with invisible feminist labor applies equally well to the Occupy Wall Street movement and to single mothers' child care pensions. As grounded political scholarship and social movements, then, it makes perfect sense that these feminist projects might look different, yet it can be hard to categorize them in university research and theoretical work that seeks to standardize and categorize ideas and information. The difficulty of working in consistent ways across these multidiversities will be discussed in further detail in Part II: "Feminist Approaches to 'Doing Research.'"

Different Sociocultural, Epistemological, and Ontological Approaches?

As we have noted, there is an increasingly wide range of approaches to the very notion of feminist research, and this book will walk you through some major examples. The most important questions we wish to stimulate in readers' and researchers' minds are the new ways in which feminism may act as a pivot for this new century. There are myriad ways in which feminist theory and research practice has influenced other fields such as critical theory and philosophy, as we have already touched upon. But what might feminism promise ontologically that remains globally emergent?

One brief example may be how feminism has helped create a more nuanced understanding of ontology that goes beyond the postmodern binary between **social constructivism** and objective knowledge:

1. **Social constructivism:** the idea that knowledge and even perception and identity are all formed in relation to others, to the society as a group.
2. **Objective knowledge:** the notion in traditional Western culture and research that some things just exist outside of perception and are there to be "discovered" or "interpreted," a notion that feminist and poststructuralist research rejects.

Feminist scholarship has argued against the distinction between the idea of knowledge or experience as "constructed" and the old-fashioned notion that there is one true or objective "reality" that research aims to uncover. The ways in which this binary are institutionalized, however, are hard to shift and present themselves in both theoretical and everyday lived experiences.

For example, feminist scholarship has at times claimed that **collectivity** (the notion of an equal collection of people in which all have equal power) is a binary opposite of traditional Western cultural hierarchical structures and processes (in which power is distributed from the "top" to the "bottom," unequally). That is, hierarchies can be understood as a differentiated and striated approach to relationships, structures, and processes, as opposed to a more consultative collectivist approach. These two different approaches to social structures have also been aligned with feminist and masculinist ways of being, in which collectives are feminist and hierarchies are masculinist.

This argument often becomes conflated with "women" and "men" and their essentialized gendered ways of doing things, and most poststructuralists would disagree with these kinds of essentialisms (see Chapter 4). Eve Kosofsky Sedgwick claimed that at times in gender activism and research it can be useful to form strategic alliances along more stereotypical or biologically essentializing lines (which she terms **strategic essentializing**). Yet in feminist and other minoritarian movements, the ascendence of trans* and other noncisgender orientations and subjectivities offers further problematizing of such binaries and biologically defined categories.

What Does Critical Theory Have to Do with Feminist Research?

Feminist ontology is a way of approaching the study of knowledge formation that comes from a feminist worldview, and sees things relationally or some say collectively (see Table 2.1). In her essay "Constructing the Ballast: An Ontology for Feminism," Susan Hekman argues that "feminists in particular and critical theorists in general are facing a theoretical and practical crisis" (2008, p. 85), and

> **Critical research approach** is an important overall lens which includes any research that challenges traditional (also known as positivist) research approaches that claim objectivity through scientific enquiry.

she draws upon two pivotal essays that, she claims, have helped establish an emerging feminist paradigm: Donna Haraway's famous "A Manifesto for Cyborgs: Science, Technology, and Socialist Feminism in the 1980s" (also known as the Cyborg Manifesto). In it, Haraway names the cyborg metaphor as representative of a new **feminist ontology** (Stanley & Wise, 2002), one that can replace second-wave feminism's commitment to socialism. Her work has proven, in Hekman's view, that "postmodernism had transformed feminism" (p. 87).

The second text Hekman calls upon is Bruno Latour's "Why Has Critique Run Out of Steam? From Matters of Fact to Matters of Concern" (2004) in the journal *Critical Inquiry*. Latour claims that critical theory has failed and that it too needs a new paradigm (a "second empiricism"), which moves toward a kind of realism (2004, p. 231). Both essays discuss the dangers of a discursive over material focus.

Hekman reminds us, however, that "the linguistic turn has been immensely fruitful for feminism. We have learned much about the social construction of 'woman' and 'reality.' But the loss of the material is too high a price to pay for that gain . . . [and] we need, in Karen Barad's terms, to construct 'a ballast against current tendencies that confuse theorizing with unconstrained play' " (Hekman, 2008, p. 88). Hekman's review is representative of the kinds of sociocultural, epistemological, and ontological considerations of feminism and its role in contemporary emerging critical theory. This is just one brief example of the ways in which feminist scholarship offers keys toward new constructions of meaning, both through language and objects, but other new examples continue to emerge.

New Paradigms for Doing Feminist Work?

One of those is the work of Elizabeth Grosz. She, too, calls for completely new ways of doing and thinking feminism, and in her 2011 text *Becoming Undone,* she revisits Charles Darwin, linking his notion of sexual selection to Deleuze, Irigaray, art, sex, new materialism, and more. In doing so, she not only theorizes the need for a new paradigm in feminist thought, she models it.

In Part II of *Becoming Undone,* "Disturbing Differences: A New Kind of Feminism," Grosz asks readers to see how

> Darwin's, Bergson's, and Deleuze's entwined conceptions of life are explored from a feminist perspective, and some of the most central concepts of contemporary feminism—questions of agency and identity, questions of diversity and intersectionality, questions about feminism's relation to epistemology and ontology—are addressed and in some ways shifted using their insights. (p. 5)

She is not claiming that they are feminist theorists, "only that their work provides an alternative to the traditions of liberal political thought" (p. 5). In doing so, she sets out to explore how a new approach in which human subjects can be contextualized and understood "not only by human constructs, that is, by linguistic and cultural environments, but also by natural and animal geographies and temporalities" (p. 5)—and how these shifts might help us think differently about/through feminist thought. For Grosz, this implies a complete overhaul of how we have been "doing" feminist research, and how we have been doing life.

She sees Irigaray at the center of this need for reassessment of the foundations of feminist practice and thought:

Irigaray is among the few contemporary theorists committed to the creation of a new ontology, one which addresses the forces of becoming, which, in Irigaray's case, must be understood in terms of at least two sets of forces, two kinds of processes, two relations to the world that cannot be generically combined into one. . . . Irigaray's work on sexual difference, arguably the greatest concept within feminist thought, opens up unexpected connections between her concept of sexual difference and Darwin's understanding of sexual selection. (Grosz, 2011, p. 6)

TABLE 2.1. Understanding Feminisms Relationally

	Liberal Feminism (First Wave)	Radical/Cultural Feminism (Second Wave)	Materialist/Socialist Feminism (Second Wave)	Poststructural/ Postmodern Feminism (Third Wave and Beyond)
Source of oppression	Unequal access to/ opportunity within existing institutions	Patriarchy	Economies (capitalist, familial, etc.)	Symbolic order (language/discursive structures/institutions) and the material consequences it creates
Response	Seek equal access/ opportunity	Radical: Create and enact alternatives to patriarchy Cultural: Invert patriarchy, create separatist organizations, experiences, lifestyles	Transform these economies (via communism, socialism, other economies of power)	Break down/into and challenge this symbolic order and the very real material consequences it creates (via deconstruction and other forms of critique/reimagining); question "woman" (a singular, foundational subjectivity) as the foundation of feminist politics
Mode	Equality	Revolutionary, supremacist, separatist	Revolutionary	All modes in various moments
Moments	Women's suffrage, civil rights movement, ERA	Civil rights movement, consciousness-raising groups, separatist events/institutions (women's music festivals, women-owned businesses, etc.), abortion rights	Rise of communism in multiple contexts, civil rights movement and beyond, ERA, debates about public/private split, abortion rights, pornography	Critiques of emphasis on sameness (essentialism) within feminisms, critiques of psychoanalysis (Freud and Lacan), *l'écriture feminine*

Source: Stacy Holman Jones, unpublished teaching materials.

Grosz acknowledges how surprising to some feminists her turn to Darwin may be, but in fact her bricolage approach to combining these unexpected theoretical bedfellows makes perfect 21st-century feminist research sense. If Grosz remains committed to the project of "how new forms of feminist, antiracist, and class theory might be created, and what epistemological forms—what philosophical concepts—may be more appropriate to an ontology of becoming, a philosophy of difference, such as that developed by Deleuze and Guattari" (2011, p. 6), she does so by continuing to unsettle current feminisms with all the tools at her disposal.

By now your eyes may be crossing at the potentially complex ways in which feminist research can be done, but this book offers readers an opportunity to dip your feminist research toe into the water as deeply or as tentatively as is needed—you alone are the judge of which parts of this book will serve you best.

The Activist and Public Nature of Feminist Research

> For positive social change to occur we must imagine
> a reality that differs from what already exists.
> —GLORIA ANZALDÚA (2002, p. 5)

As we have discussed, feminist research and scholarship is intrinsically activist. Beyond its roots in social movement/s and its research-activist sociocultural role, feminism in the 21st century joins participatory action research and other applied research approaches as few other frameworks do. Whether documenting the work of social movements like Occupy Wall Street in Canada, or conducting applied gender research with young people in schools, as Emma Renold and Jessica Ringrose have in the United Kingdom, contemporary feminist research is certainly testing Haraway and Latour's calls to move beyond simple either/or notions like "socially constructed and discursive" versus "real-world interventions."

Theresa Senft and her Hey Girl Global network point to evolving ways in which feminism's ability to bridge multiple worlds and ways of understanding is increasingly also bridging hybrid online/off-line worlds. Some of the most exciting emergent areas of feminist research are in activist and digital realms because the nature of feminist research means it can adapt and change as quickly as social change occurs. Some of the most recent innovations (to be discussed in more detail in Chapter 9) include:

Vlogging and Sex-Positive Camgirls

Digital media and feminist theorist Theresa Senft (2008) has tracked the forms and performances of girls and women online, those both commercial and activist in orientation. This subfield is strongly linked with social media, digital media, and social movement theory. Vlogs, blogs, Twitter, Snapchat, Instagram, and other forms of social media are changing the way feminist scholars do their research, and also the ways in which it is disseminated. Senft's pivotal work has detailed the ways in which marketable online representations remain gendered and sexualized for women, while men and boys are allowed more freedom of interaction as well as representation. This is one of the fastest-growing subfields of gender, sexuality, and feminist research today.

PheMaterialisms (Feminist Posthumanism and New Materialism), Postfeminisms, and Post-Postfeminism

Perhaps the most famous foundational document of posthumanism is Donna Haraway's Cyborg Manifesto (discussed earlier in this chapter, and later Chapters 3 and 4). Yet this was only the beginning. The concurrent shifts in focus within feminist scholarship toward both ecologies/geographies and animal and **nonhuman others** jointly heralded a new era in feminist theoretical work, noted by scholars including Grosz, as the posthuman becomes increasingly intersectional with the work of 21st-century feminist research. Yet sidestepping the term "new materialism," Grosz says she would

> prefer to understand life and matter in terms of their temporal and durational entwinements. Matter and life become, and become undone. They transform and are transformed. This is less a new kind of materialism than it is a new understanding of the forces, both material and immaterial, that direct us to the future. (2011, p. 5)

Karen Barad (2007), Jane Bennett (2009), Iris van der Tuin and Rick Dolphijn (2012), van der Tuin (2015), and Hinton, Treusch, van der Tuin, Dolphijn, and Sauzet (2015) are all contributing to an explosion of feminist (new) materialist scholarship that moves beyond a humanist approach to attending to the lives and affects of things themselves.

Ecofeminism

Globalization, indigenous knowledges, new materialism, and eco-activism intersect in ecofeminism, pushing forward into new considerations of religion and theology, ecologies, gender, and environmental studies. The subfield ecofeminism largely began with Françoise d'Eaubonne, who coined the term in her 1974 treatise *Le feminisme ou la mort [Feminism or Death]*.

Ecofeminism as an area of scholarly (and activist) inquiry gained momentum in the 1980s and '90s, linked to protest movements around environmental consciousness raising. Like other emerging feminisms, its intersectionality is central to its political and epistemological commitments, most recently represented by *Ecofeminism: Feminist Intersections with Other Animals and the Earth* (Adams & Gruen, 2014).

Donna Haraway is widely seen as having both contributed extensively to the field through her cyborg symbology, and also as having promoted ecofeminism as a fiercely divergent approach to enacting a feminist environmentalist agenda (for more on this see Noel Sturgeon's *Ecofeminist Natures: Race, Gender, Feminist Theory and Political Action* [Routledge, 1997/2016]).

CONCLUSION

As we have said, one of the strengths of the current feminist landscape is its diversity and agility. Whether we are looking at trans* and queer feminisms through dense theoretical frames or graphic novelist Alison Bechdel's "Bechdel Test," digital feminisms and their aesthetic and political opportunities, or ecofeminisms and contemporary global activist movements, 21st-century feminist research has something for everyone.

There has never been a better time to be studying or conducting feminist research. Across the following chapters, we offer in-depth ways of approaching some of the key concepts you have encountered in these first two introductory chapters, including theory, epistemology, ontology, paradigms, and a range of established and emerging approaches to feminist research and its social implications. Whether you are a beginning researcher, a student, an expert in your field, or a feminist activist dipping your toes into research waters for the first time, we hope this chapter and the ones to follow will help you break down the components and concepts of feminist research praxis in ways that move you, and the field, forward.

DISCUSSION QUESTIONS

1. Why was Gloria Anzaldúa so pivotal in contemporary feminist research?

2. What are the most important differences between so-called first-wave and second-wave feminism?

3. Define "ontology" and "epistemology," and describe what impact feminism in research contexts has made on these two areas of study?

ACTIVITIES

1. Make a video blog (vlog) or a podcast on the history of feminist research that is 3 minutes or less, explaining why it is important to know and trace our roots.

2. With a partner, design a 3-D model that demonstrates the impact of digital media on the rise of global feminisms and the spread of feminisms beyond the northern hemisphere/Western world. When/where/how did this happen, and what are the benefits of decentering feminist research and activism from the Western world?

3. Interview (and record) someone involved in the cultural events of the 1960–1970s "second-wave feminism," which included and were contextualized by the civil rights movement; the student rebellion of 1968; the assassinations of Martin Luther King, Jr., John F. Kennedy, and Robert Kennedy; consciousness-raising groups; separatist events/organizations (women's music festivals, women-owned businesses, etc.); the abortion rights campaign; and the "free love" movement. Find out if you can how these things were related, what the participants thought they were fighting for, and what eventually occurred? You can represent your findings in the transcript of your interview.

SUGGESTED RESOURCES

Books

Daly, M. (1978). *Gyn/Ecology: The metaethics of radical feminism.* Boston: Beacon Press.

Mary Daly was a founding feminist philosopher, scholar, and theologian, and in this book addresses the timeless practices that perpetuate patriarchy.

Davis, A. (1990). *Women, culture, and politics.* New York: Vintage books.

First published in 1984, Angela Davis's groundbreaking volume links her activist roots with her feminist and antiracist work in the academy, providing a unique perspective on early intersectionality in the academy.

Disch, L., & Hawkesworth, M. (2016). *The Oxford handbook of feminist theory*. New York: Oxford University Press.

An excellent introduction to feminist theory with geographical and methodological diversity.

Smith, B. (1983). *Home girls: A Black feminist anthology*. Latham, NY: Kitchen Table/Women of Color Press.

Barbara Smith and the Kitchen Table Press were both pivotal in bringing feminist scholarship and popular texts to the public, and this early compilation is a classic.

Nussbaum, M. (2006). *Frontiers of justice: Disability, nationality, species membership*. Cambridge, MA: Harvard University Press.

This work of practical philosophy is from renowned feminist philosopher Martha Nussbaum, who has brought emotions into the study of classics and philosophy, among other contributions.

Articles and Chapters

Haraway, D. (2003). Situated knowledges: The science question in feminism and the privilege of partial perspective. In Y. S. Lincoln & N. K. Denzin (Eds.), *Turning points in qualitative research: Tying knots in a handkerchief* (pp. 21–46). Lanham, MD: Rowman & Littlefield.

In this essay, originally published in 1983, Haraway argues against the positivist notion of "objectivity," suggesting that feminist research offers a counternarrative to traditional research approaches.

Tuck, E., & Yang, K. W. (2012). Decolonization is not a metaphor. *Decolonization: Indigeneity, Education and Society, 1*(1), 1–40.

In this groundbreaking essay, Eve Tuck and Wayne Yang caution against appropriating the term "decolonization," explaining that it is not a metaphor for doing just anything to address inequity in schools and societies, but rather a very particular practice and notion that refers specifically to repatriation of stolen land and Indigeneity in a postcolonial world.

🖵 Digital Resources

Feminist Psychologists Talk about . . . Research Methods

www.youtube.com/watch?v=Fm14F3vabhw

A short video in which feminist psychology scholars discuss research methods, including core questions for feminist psychologists about the way psychological research has traditionally been conducted. This snapshot is expanded into individual scholar video profiles at the website Psychology's Feminist Voices at *www.feministvoices.com.*

Films for the Feminist Classroom

http://ffc.twu.edu

Films for the Feminist Classroom (FFC) is hosted by the Department of Women's Studies at Texas Woman's University (it was formerly hosted by the Rutgers-based editorial offices of *Signs: Journal of Women in Culture and Society* and the Rutgers Women's and Gender Studies Department. FFC, an online, open-access journal, publishes film reviews that provide a critical assessment of the value of films as pedagogical tools in the feminist classroom. Special features, such as interviews with filmmakers, reviews of film festivals, and discussions about pedagogy are included to further promote engagement and discussion. FFC serves as a dynamic resource for educators and librarians that enhances feminist curricula, bringing film into the classroom through thought-provoking, relevant, and dynamic content.

CHAPTER 3

Intersectionality, Feminist Epistemology, and Standpoint Feminism Theoretical Frames

> Standpoint theories map how a social and political disadvantage can be turned into an epistemological, scientific, and political advantage.
>
> —SANDRA HARDING (2004, p. 7)

LEARNING OBJECTIVES

- To distinguish clearly between structuralist and poststructuralist approaches to feminist research
- To introduce the major differences between feminist empiricism and standpoint feminism
- To explain and contextualize the history and significance of intersectionality as a concept in feminist research
- To profile and contextualize some of the central feminist researchers who have influenced the development of the field, including Cynthia Dillard in her own words (by video).

Recently, we were on a subway train in New York City, traveling from Brooklyn to a writers' event at Columbia University in Manhattan. Two women sat across from us in the near-empty train: one appeared to be college age and the other around 60. They were talking about feminism and debating its relevance today:

YOUNG WOMAN: I mean, of course I'm pro-woman—I'm a woman after all! But I'm definitely not one of those angry feminists going around with a chip on my shoulder. Nobody cares about that today; we are all just trying to get ahead.

OLDER WOMAN: But that's feminism. That's exactly what feminism is; it's about the influences on whether or not you will be able to get ahead.

YOUNG WOMAN: If you're a woman, fine. But what about men? The guys are also having a hard time getting ahead today; that's what I don't like about it. It's all poor me, poor girls, but the only thing that's changed since the 1970s is that guys don't hold the door open for us anymore.

OLDER WOMAN: That's completely untrue! A lot has changed. Like you can get financing to buy your own house, for example. And you can hold your own door open. Feminism is for men too. Why don't you know this stuff?

YOUNG WOMAN: I know what I need to know. Obviously there is not the same need for feminism now as there was in your day; otherwise everyone would care.

Why Do Feminist Research?

This overheard conversation made us think about *how* we do feminist research, but also *why*. It's not an unusual exchange between people from different generations. One of the reasons we agreed to write this book is for people exactly like that young woman: bright young folks who want to get ahead, want to live the "good life" but don't always know what limits and facilitates that good life they are pursuing.[1] Many, like that young woman,

---

[1] For more on the good life, see Sara Ahmed's discussion in *The Promise of Happiness* (2010), in which she problematizes the contemporary notion of "the good life" as "imagined through the proximity of objects. There is no doubt that the affective repertoire of happiness gives us images of a certain kind of life, a life that has certain things and does certain things. There is no doubt that it is hard to separate images of the good life from the historic privileging of heterosexual conduct, as expressed in romantic love and coupledom, as well as in the idealization of domestic privacy" (p. 90). For more, and more generally on the value and vulnerability of various types of lives in contemporary culture, see Judith Butler's seminal 1988 essay "Performative Acts and Gender Constitution: An Essay in Phenomenology and Feminist Theory" (1988). And on the grievable life, see Butler and Athanasiou's *Dispossession: The Performative in the Political* (2013).

have not necessarily had the opportunity to consider all the influences and obstacles weighing on their own growth into full adulthood, and on their efforts at being seen and heard. This book is for that young woman, both as food for thought and for tools to anticipate navigating the 21st-century world in which she lives. But to understand feminism today, one needs to understand not just where it has come from, but why and how it has changed. To establish the links between the everyday lives, politics, and needs of different eras of feminism and feminist research, let's turn to some feminist foremothers and foundational ideas that have established agendas that still thrive today.

Feminist Foremothers and Their Foundational Ideas

Gloria Steinem, Betty Friedan, and Bella Abzug were among the leaders of the gender equality movement in the 1960s and 1970s. Shirley Chisholm, Betty Friedan, and Muriel Fox made a bold step toward empowering women in 1966 by founding the National Organization for Women in Washington, DC, an organization that would form the cornerstone of the emerging women's movement. In many ways, Gloria Steinem became the spiritual leader of the movement throughout the 1970s, with the kind of White middle-class privilege that placed her front and center as a spokesperson to the "powers that be" for the gender equality the women's movement was fighting for. In 1970, she testified in front of the U.S. Congress as part of the movement to institute the Equal Rights Amendment.

Steinem also cofounded *Ms.* magazine, the first female-run popular magazine (1971) and started the National Women's Political Caucus. Still active at time of this writing at age 83, Steinem—along with Jane Fonda and Robin Morgan—cofounded the Women's Media Center in 2005 to increase women's visibility and influence in the media. Throughout second-wave feminism in the 1960s and 1970s (especially radical feminism), these and other feminist activists engaged in what today might be called acts of "terrorism." Indeed, queer feminist scholar Jack Halberstam (1993) very much describes the strategies (and even uses the language) of "terrorism" in describing the activist work that could find no other forms of expression, but carried a very different meaning than "terrorism" today.

Like the young woman on the subway, back in 1981 Cherrie Moraga and Gloria Anzaldúa (1983) were also thinking about the relevance of the feminist movement and how it seemed to only respond to the needs and concerns of White women. For them, this exciting public attention to the lived experiences of women was passing women of color by. They, too, wondered what it could offer *their* lives, in that time and place, and particular to their own experiences.

They thought it would be good to pull together a book of writings by other women of color, who wanted feminism, but wanted it to address their concerns. *This Bridge Called My Back: Writings by Radical Women of Color,* an edited anthology that went on to define a generation of feminism for women beyond the White Western demographic, was that book. It also exemplified what has come to be known as **intersectionality** (Crenshaw, 1991), or **intersectional feminism,** as it focused not only on the concerns of women but on race, class, disability, and geography.[2]

Some also have called this book the catalyst for the beginning of what have been called **third-world feminisms** or non-Western feminism.[3] These other aspects of their lives could not be disentangled from their womanness, both publicly and privately. In 2002, AnaLouise Keating and Gloria Anzaldúa edited a follow-up anthology called *This Bridge We Call Home: Radical Visions for Transformation,* which made an equally important contribution to feminist research literature and the different ways of seeing and doing this work. Such major milestones in the **herstory** of feminist research and politics are intertwined (as the feminist mantra *the personal is political* has highlighted), and importantly inform today's feminist research work, which has more powerful public impact than ever before.

What Is Feminist Theory?

Feminism and feminist theory are concerned with the social, political, and cultural practices of gender inequity. Much contemporary feminist theory not only sees "gender" as a two-way split between male and female but has become much more expansive in considering what constitutes gender identity, and has come to understand gender as moving along a continuum in

---

[2]Feminist scholar Rosemarie Tong reflects, "Since writing my first introduction to *Feminist Thought* twenty-four years ago, I have become increasingly convinced that feminist thought resists categorization into tidy schools of thought. *Interdisciplinary, intersectional,* and *interlocking* are the kind of adjectives that best describe the way we feminists think" (2014, p. 1).

[3]"Third world" is for some a derogatory and marginalizing term, originally used to refer to developing nations, which also tended to be non-Western nations. However, as Anzaldúa and Moraga pointed out, "third world experiences and living conditions" are an inherent part of all national and regional societies, even the most affluent.

which there are many more gender expressions than the simple (and wholly inadequate) **male–female binary.**

That is why, in this book, we have chosen to use a range of pronouns including nonbinary ones such as he/she/they. This recognition of gender diversities acknowledges the additional gendered inequities besides just the traditionally female. Feminist research then must be understood not only in terms of the act of knowledge construction as a highly subjective activity (commonly known as feminist epistemology; see Chapter 2 for more on this), but also as deeply informed by context (as feminist activism is) or by discipline (in academic work).

Major Fields and Disciplines

Feminist theories are used in a wide range of disciplines. One of its many strengths, feminist research is multiperspectival, and as such it is conducted from numerous distinct epistemological and theoretical perspectives, including but not limited to standpoint theory (Harding, 2012, 1998, 1987; Collins, 2009, 2008); feminist psychology (McHugh, 2014; Harding, 2012); intersectionality (Crenshaw, 1991; Rowe, 2009, 2008, 2005, 2000; Malhotra & Rowe, 2013); poststructuralist queer theory (Halberstam, 2012, 2011, 2005; Sedgwick, 1990); emotion and feminist epistemology (Jaggar, 1983); posthumanism and feminist postmodernism (Haraway, 2014); new materialism (van der Tuin, 2015); postfeminism (Ringrose, 2013; Dobson 2016); critical race and spirituality epistemologies (Dillard, 2012, 2008, 2006; Dillard & Okpalaoka, 2016); double consciousness and intersectionality (Collins, 2009, 2008); global south gender perspectives (Connell, 2014); feminist economics (Waring, 1988); Pasifika feminisms (Teaiwa, 2014a, 2014b; Figiel, 2014); and indigenous/native epistemologies (Tuhiwai Smith, 1999; Tuck, 2009; Rowe & Lindsey, 2003), to name just a few. Figure 3.1 offers a visual aid for understanding what eras resulted in what kinds of feminist theoretical evolutions.

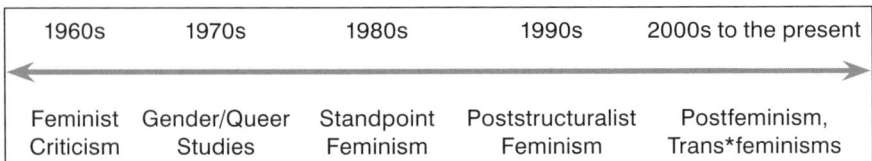

1960s	1970s	1980s	1990s	2000s to the present
Feminist Criticism	Gender/Queer Studies	Standpoint Feminism	Poststructuralist Feminism	Postfeminism, Trans*feminisms

FIGURE 3.1 Timeline of feminist theoretics.

In the 1980s and 1990s, during the last big explosion of feminist scholarship before our current era of what some call "protest feminism," one of the founding thinkers and theorizers of Black feminism was bell hooks (1982, 2000a, 2000b), who brought (and continues to bring) a generation of feminist thinkers to consciousness about the ways in which White or majoritarian feminisms have ignored the specific contributions and concerns of African American women and other women of color in feminist scholarship. She also centers much of her work on the power of education to change both the minds and material conditions (economics) of marginalized people, a project that must go hand-in-hand with **conscientization** (1994), the process of become critically aware of social inequities.

Intersectionality and the Move Away from Whiteness

Any theory section of a feminist research book pays attention to the major conceptual, cultural, and historical foundations upon which feminist research is constructed. It also acknowledges the rapidly proliferating ways of thinking about and doing feminist research. To understand one of the most important transitions from a singular notion of feminist theory to the multiple feminisms we now know there to be, one must understand the history and importance of Kimberle Crenshaw's idea of intersectionality (Crenshaw, 1991). Crenshaw's idea moved feminist scholarship from an area of research activity to a way of doing almost any kind of research—a lens. Let's pause here to look at the historical context from which intersectionality grew.

> **Intersectionality** is a metaphor originally invoked by the African American scholar Kimberle Crenshaw (1991) to describe the way multiple oppressions are experienced, like traffic at an intersection.

As Collins and Bilge tell us, "Intersectionality's history cannot be neatly organized in time periods or geographic locations" (2016, p. 63), and there were many from the late 1960s to the early 1980s who espoused the central ideas of intersectionality without using that word (see Chapter 4 on the Combahee River Collective Statement, for more on this). Collins and Bilge urge us to see beyond the simplistic attribution of the notion (that became an academic field) to one person as is usually done with Kimberle Crenshaw. Rather, they ask us to view the uptake of intersectionality as the result of a "synergy of . . . critical inquiry and critical praxis" (2016, p. 64), a groundswell of need and articulation and lived experience by many, rather than one. This is precisely its strength.

Collins and Bilge remind us that the multiple social movements of civil rights, gay and lesbian rights, women's rights, class and Chicana/Chicano rights, and student uprisings on multiple continents offered a context which *over time* allowed these multiple oppressions to be addressed in an equally multiple manner, in which "African-American women understood that addressing the oppression they faced could not be solved by race-only, or class-only or gender-only or sexuality-only, frameworks" (2016, p. 65).

Others have taken intersectionality even further: Eve Tuck's work on intersectional indigenous perspectives (featured here in depth), but also Patricia Hill Collins's notion of "double consciousness" (1991), Lisa Duggan and Jose Munoz's (2009) dialogue on queer and critical race perspectives, Bird's (2004) work on queer and education intersectionality, and Alexander-Floyd's "post-black feminist intersectionality" (Alexander-Floyd, 2012) highlight the ability of feminist scholarship to acknowledge the multiple perspectives and lived experiences at play in research contexts and knowledge production. These areas of study all to some extent have intersectionality to thank for opening up the ways research engages with feminist ways of seeing.

While foundational feminist scholars like Spivak (1988), Cixous (2003), de Lauretis (1984, 1991), and Irigaray allowed some of us for the first time (like the young woman on the subway) to consider how nonmasculinist perspectives construct the world differently and occupy important theoretical and practical space in our shared worlds, Judith Butler, Jack Halberstam, Cynthia Dillard, Eve Tuck, and other feminists with nondominant identifications continued to push the foundational concepts of feminist thought into more intersectional spaces where the study of women's lived experience is inextricable from other oppressions and marginalizations from which we speak and practice research, namely, what we call **minoritarian perspectives,** including racialized, agist, cis- and other nonbio gender identifications, ablist, regional, cultural, ethnic, socioeconomic, and nonhetero and nonhomonormative perspectives.

Intersectionality has helped complicate the terrain of "feminist studies" by problematizing not only silenced voices in the academy (such as women's) but also problematizing feminist research itself once intersectional theorics highlighted the difficulty of holding many threads of oppression as they are often experienced, in life as well as scholarly research (Carbin & Edenheim, 2013). This attention to a utopian "single voice" (or what Haraway calls a "common language" [1991]) in feminist research and its problematic remarginalizing tendencies has meant that feminist research can continue to expand within the complexities that it addresses.

Intersectionality beyond Gender Binaries

Sure, feminist research (like feminist activism) began by asking such foundational questions as "What is women's experience?" and "Who is a woman?," but it has continued to ask increasingly complex questions that extend this foundational work. From the men who encountered resistance in the 1970s by claiming to be feminists and **feminist allies,** to contemporary **non-cisgendered women** and feminist allies who work across other categories of oppression, feminism has continued to struggle with issues of ownership, revolution, and relevance across a wide (and ever-widening) landscape of communities, individuals, and practices. Intersectionality asks how we can examine oppressions and marginalization rooted in gender without looking at class, race, ablism, and other conditional positionalities.

It helps us, for example, to select and better understand the ways in which critical race theory is enlarged and emboldened by considering the intersection of Blackness with gendered oppressions. It helps us understand the interrelated nature of subjugated knowledge as being multiple and threaded. Nikol G. Alexander-Floyd's social science theorization of intersectionality extends Crenshaw's foundational intersectionality to a "reconstructive liberatory project" that centers on Black women's subjectivity (2012, p. 1) and opens new possibilities for others.

What Is Essentialism?

One danger of an **essentialist approach** to feminist research is assuming that all women and girls speak, think, or want the same. As McHugh has noted, "postmodern feminists view empiricist and standpoint feminists as reverting to essentialist claims" (2014, p. 144). Feminist research is not all about the same things, or con-

> **Essentialism,** in feminist or gender theory, is the idea that women and men have inherently different characteristics, preferences, and behaviors.

ducted in the same ways. Indeed, some recent and rapid advances in gender diversity have suggested that feminist research must be liberated completely from biological notions of "womanness." That is, that feminist and other gender research can now claim to focus more broadly on diverse issues of gender-based inequalities and oppressions, and need not be reduced to a binary or essentialized notion of "male" or "female" at all.

All chapters in this volume—especially this one—provide readers with a feminist theoretical perspective on methodological and practical approaches to this work. This chapter is punctuated by video "snapshots" that spotlight leading feminist scholars in their own words, giving readers a one-on-one engagement with the theories explored here in depth. Feminist research has "posed a serious challenge to the alleged value neutrality of positivistic social science. In an attempt to transform social science, feminists have developed innovative ideas, methods, and critiques" (McHugh, 2014, p. 158). This chapter and these video snapshots highlight the ways in which feminist research is not just for women in 21st-century praxis, but rather for all those doing gender-based research, and from a range of methodological and theoretical approaches.

Two Traditions/Two Streams

This chapter and the one following detail the three main feminist epistemological traditions: **feminist empiricism, standpoint feminism,** and **postmodern/poststructural feminism.** Although we decided in the end to do what many books like this do and separate them for ease of study, in practice they are overlapping and cross-informing. The first two approaches align with an **enlightenment perspective** and **realist epistemology** that values equality, liberation, and rationalism, so they will be the focus for the rest of this chapter.

Chapter 4 picks up where this one leaves off, and addresses the "post-" approaches, which made a significant departure from the empiricist and standpoint approaches, focusing on the **social constructivism of gender** itself. It is important to study them together in order to see how they have built upon one another, borrowing as they go along, yet equally important to distinguish between them and point out the foundational and epistemological differences. Acknowledging that all theoretical research evolutions are important and interconnected as they draw on what has come before, while advancing knowledge to the next stage of innovation, is crucial to good scholarship.

Another way to understand these distinctions is through Teresa Ebert's (1996) famous critique of Judith Butler, which reminded us that there are other ways to characterize these three main epistemological spokes: what many call **feminist empiricism** is for Ebert "equality" feminism (men and women are the same, just have unequal access to the system); **standpoint feminism** she calls "difference" feminism—there is a fundamental difference between men and women and so women's perspectives must be acknowledged and voiced; and lastly there is **"postmodern/poststructuralist"** or ludic feminism, which takes up difference and wants to undermine the stable, coherent subject and say that there is no certainty or **master narrative.**

What Do Different Streams of Thought Have to Do with Me?

The central difference between foundational feminist "humanist" theoretical approaches and more recent "post-" approaches should not be understood in terms of the latter's intent or ability to "correct" some error in humanist feminist approaches, but rather "they offer opportunities for limit-work, work that operates at the boundaries of the possibilities of humanism" (St. Pierre & Pillow, 2000, p. 2).

Post- (postmodernist/poststructuralist) feminist theories then allow us to analyze and critique Cartesian, Hegelian, and positivist epistemologies that

> assume the historical progress of man toward absolute knowledge and freedom; that assume it is possible to measure, represent, predict, and control knowledge of the social world; that assume metaphysics can rise above the level of human activity; that assume a knowing, disinterested, rational subject who can uncover "objective" knowledge; that assume the scientific method is the path to true knowledge. (St. Pierre & Pillow, 2000, p. 6)

How to Use This Chapter

The remainder of this chapter examines, first (in Section One), the foundational feminist theoretical approach—feminist empiricism or "equality" feminism—and finishes (in Section Two) with the other "enlightenment" feminism: standpoint epistemology or "difference" feminisms, which primarily take an essentialist or *dualistic* (**us/them**) approach to feminism as focused on (a traditional understanding of) *women* as opposed to on *men*, and the theoretical approaches that adhere to that epistemology.

Chapter 4 moves on to the poststructuralist approaches to feminist research, focusing on how deconstructing the essentialized feminist perspective by exploring feminist theories that challenge the notion of stable subjects offers new directions for understanding the still-urgent work of feminist research. Each section will outline the foundational strand, then offer a critique or counterpoint that helps readers understand the pros and cons of each approach.

Section One: Foundations

Feminist Empiricism

> **Feminist empiricism** asserts that, with the inclusion of women in all phases of research (including observation and theory formation), gender bias can be eradicated and objective knowledge achieved.

Feminist empiricism can be partly characterized by its methodological (including content) orientation: it is research that collects data about girls'/women's lived experiences, based on testimony about inequality and gender-based oppressions, using primarily traditional research methods such as interviews, observations, and surveys. Feminist empiricism has played a vital foundational role in a range of social science fields such as medicine, law, health studies, international relations, and economics, where it is used to understand and interpret legal and political landscapes, in social work where it is used to understand systems of inequity in service provision, and in medicine and nursing for understanding gender-based health care issues.

Feminist researchers are "cognizant of the impact of power on the research process . . . [and are] concerned with the complex relationship between social power (and inequalities in social power) and the production of knowledge" (McHugh, 2014, p. 146). Thus, feminist **onto-epistemologies** imply new ways of doing research as well as new considerations of what counts as research. Central to feminist research theory is a challenge to the traditional hierarchical means of knowledge production. That is, feminist research and researchers question hierarchies within research teams, within the forms through which we represent data, and within forms of dissemination of research findings such as publishing, public speaking, and online and popular media.

These formal and theoretical concerns are tied to the ways in which feminist theories question the notion of validity itself. The notion of **validity,** a cornerstone of quantitative measurement and much scientific research, has been challenged by feminist postmodern and poststructuralist theorists like Alison Jaggar, who researches feminist research, objectivity, and emotion.[4] In this chapter we provide an in-depth look at some of these theoretical or conceptual lenses.

---

[4] The notion of validity in research draws from the positivist concept of objectivity, the goal of avoiding bias in research practices, a concept that many qualitative researchers (and poststructuralists) find not only impossible but also objectionable, given what they believe is the subjective nature of all knowledge.

Feminist Health Scholarship

Feminist research in medicine, nursing, health, and well-being continues to expand and offer important ways into understanding the sociocultural and biological experiences of women and health in medicalized contexts. Sue V. Rosser has made major contributions into family and preventive medicine, but also into (feminist) science more generally. Her work continues to question why women in science are still somehow controversial (2014), and why they continue to struggle gaining professional recognition and promotion. Her work spans a wide range of science-related challenges to the limitation of women, including in the academic areas of medicine, biology, sexuality, and in health leadership. As with many other feminist scholars, Rosser continues to argue that feminism in science and health is not a "woman's issue" but rather a topic of concern for all of society.

Feminist Geography

In 1993, Gillian Rose published the pioneering text *Feminism and Geography: The Limits of Geographical Knowledge,* in which she claimed that "feminist geographers have long argued that the domination of the discipline by men has serious consequences both for what counts as legitimate geographical knowledge and who can produce such knowledge" (p. 2). According to Rose, these consequences, as in other social sciences, have included creating a bias in geographical research and knowledge creation that favors what appeals to men (thus alienating women from both the discourse and the field), as well as contributing to ongoing and even growing discrimination against women geographers by men in the field.

While **feminist geography** began this way (as a feminist lens on the field of geography), it has evolved since then toward more diverse ideas about what constitutes a "feminist geography," including research on geographies of the body and identity, space and place-based studies, human geography, and feminist methodologies.[5]

Ally Scholarship

Another contribution of standpoint feminist theory is the growth of "ally" scholarship, or companion work to primarily feminist research (think, for example, of critical race theory and its ally scholarship arm, "whiteness studies"). All social movements (and the scholarship that examines them)

---

[5] For more on feminist geographies, see McDowell (2013), Bondi (2002), Moss and Al-Hindi (2008), Johnson (2000), and Nelson and Seager (2008).

require the support and participation of a range of allies who don't necessarily come from the same community or share the same identification, yet share many of the same values.

The very notion of "allies" has, at times, come under attack within the queer and gender movements, but second- and third-wave feminism has used allyship to great effect. While leaders like Gloria Steinem used her public visibility to speak out against the United States's involvement in the Vietnam War, feminists of color were pointing out the need for second-wave feminism to be more inclusive of non-White communities, concerns, and agendas. This turn to broader activist platforms, but also the power of ally advocacy, can be attributed to second-wave feminism and its coming of age in regard to racism and Western-ism.

Today allyship is characteristic of feminism as its critique expands to address masculinism, racism, classism, Islamophobia and other expressions of religious intolerance, cultural appropriation, and the shared project of equality for all. Both Jack Halberstam and Gloria Steinem have talked about the need for more plain speaking in feminist scholarship and more popular dissemination of that work. Yet in *Gaga Feminism*, Halberstam attempted to do just that, an experiment that was, Halberstam has said, only partially successful (see the section on Halberstam later this chapter). One thing is certain: feminist theory, as with feminist and other gender scholarship and activism, still grapples with questions of belonging, strategic essentializing, and increasing diversities. In Section Two and in Chapter 4, some of these productive splinterings are signposted for readers.

Critiques of Feminist Empiricism

Critics of feminist empiricism point to its association with positivist (more traditional, scientific, logical) methods and epistemologies, but feminist empiricists argue that it is exactly for this reason that empiricism is best suited to respond to gender bias in scientific or more positivist contexts. Critics say there is no way to adequately fight this men-and-women-are-equal debate from the inside, using the same explanations and methods that have been used to oppress and exclude women in the first place. This critique of feminist empiricism is often leveled by standpoint feminists (among others), who support their view with quotes like the famous Audre Lorde rallying cry, "The master's tools will never dismantle the master's house," but feminist empiricists wholeheartedly disagree.

Section Two:
Differentiation and Standpoint Feminism

As discussed in the opening to this chapter, **Latinx**[6] scholars Cherri Moraga and Gloria Anzaldúa's *This Bridge Called My Back* (1983) has extended "third-wave feminisms" beyond the Black/White dichotomy into more nuanced and intersectional discussions and alliances between a range of feminist scholars of color, as well as what Gloria Ladson-Billings (2000) has called "culturally relevant pedagogy," and Elizabeth McKinlay (McKinlay, Gan, Buntting, & Jones, 2015) has called "culturally responsive" science education for indigenous, Maori, and ethnic minority students in Australia. For additional recent scholarship on diasporic feminist perspectives, see, for example, Rajan and Desai (2013), Rodriguez, Tsikata, and Ampofo (2015), Ahmad (2010), and Harris (2012a, 2012b, 2012c, 2012d, 2016a, 2016b, 2016c, 2017).

It is equally important to note the differences between critical scholars from "the Americas," which often get conflated. Generally, "American" refers to those from or working within the United States; "North American" usually refers to those from Canada, with "Central American" and "South American" being distinctive subgroups from "Latin America."

In writing about non-White American scholarship, it is important to distinguish between Latinx, African American, Native American, Asian American, and other specific groups and perspectives (who are often grouped together). This is important due to the very distinct and diverse political projects and perspectives that are emerging from each community; it is also important to note that there is no singular "African American" or "Black feminist" perspective, even within the United States. While this seems obvious, it is still a frequent error made by non-Black scholars, and even when done inadvertently contributes to systems of oppression and exclusion that feminist scholarship is actively working against.

It is important to note that **"global feminisms," diasporic feminisms,** and third-world feminisms are not all the same: indeed, as postcolonial feminist scholarship has shown, non-American or European feminist scholarship is not all constructed as an "alternative" to global north epistemologies. Australian sociologist Raewyn Connell (1987, 2014), in theorizing a

---

[6] "Latinx" is the contemporary preferred gender-neutral adjective to describe those from a Latin American ethnic, cultural, or national background.

> **Global feminisms,** also known as world feminism, international feminism, third-world feminisms, and diasporic feminisms, have grown out of and are still influenced by (and influence) postcolonial theory. They primarily address nondominant, non-White, non-Western perspectives and issues.

distinctive theoretical framework for the **global south,** made the point that even this half of the globe cannot be chunked in a singular subjectivity that is always positioned in opposition to Euro-American scholarship, using Euro-American theory.

In *Southern Theory,* Connell articulated the need for a range of epistemological approaches to doing scholarship. Yet many Euro-American scholars continue to group "global south" into one group, a group that always theorizes in contradistinction to their own work. Imagine grouping Sydney, Australia, Dhaka, Bangladesh, and Rio de Janeiro, Brazil, into the same "global south" grouping. It would be as absurd as grouping New York City, Nuuk, Greenland, and Aleppo, Syria, together and saying they are the "global north" with a shared unitary perspective. Yet it happens all the time.

As feminist research centers on the particularity and individuality of cultural and social constructedness, it is extremely difficult to do justice to the great range of important feminist research theoretical innovations and traditions in a chapter like this one, particularly in the postempirical era. That is why we have chosen to offer some "essentializing" categories that nonetheless offer readers an overview and suggestions about where to go for further reading.

Standpoint Epistemology (Feminist Standpoint Theory)

> **Standpoint feminism** or **feminist standpoint theory** argues that knowledge stems from social position, rejects the idea of objective knowledge, and seeks to be transparent about the particular perspectives (or standpoints) from which researchers view the world and their work.

Generally considered to have begun with Nancy Hartsock's (1983) theoretic on the need for feminist standpoint-specific scholarship, standpoint feminism is a social science theoretical approach that is not specific to any particular content area but advocates for women's perspectives as important and distinct from men's. Some postmodern feminists, though, have critiqued standpoint feminism as still returning to an essentialized view of "women," as though there is a stable and identifiable perspective to be identified

and differentiated, yet this was still a major step away from feminist empiricism.

Both standpoint feminism and feminist empiricism played a major
role in moving from traditional **positivist attachments** (largely White western male notions of truth and knowledge production), based on so-called
evidence-bases and "objective" reasoning, to a more multiple and **postpositivist** view of research knowledge production. In their own ways, both
standpoint feminism and feminist empiricism helped to break down singular, **hegemonic notions** of knowledge creation and contributed to the
deconstruction of positivism and the notion of objective truth.

As Naples and Gurr have noted (2014), standpoint theoretical and
methodological approaches were instrumental in recentering nonmasculinist and lived women's experiences in order to problematize the limitations
of positivism and what was previously considered validity in research theoretics, methods, and areas of inquiry. One of the things that makes contemporary feminist research so powerful is that, as Linda Tuhiwai Smith
notes, "The critique of positivism by feminist theorists, ethnic minorities
and indigenous peoples has emerged from the experience of people who
have been studied, researched, written about, and defined by social scientists" (1999, p. 169). Perhaps most central to this charge is the work alter-
nately known as African American feminisms, Black feminism, and women
of color feminism.

Black Feminist Epistemologies

Many feminists cite Sojourner Truth's famous 1851 speech "Ain't I a
Woman?" as a beginning of Black feminism in the United States, a precur-
sor to Kimberle Crenshaw's articulation of intersectionality, both of which
articulate the inextricable nature of race, class, and gender. But feminism
moved into scholarship later than it found voice in popular politics, with
Mary Jane Patterson becoming the first Black woman in the United States
to gain a college degree in 1862 and the first three doctoral degrees awarded
to African American women not coming until 1921 (Georginna Simpson,
Sadie Tanner Mossell Alexander, and Eva Beatrice Dykes).

While there are many foremothers of Black feminist scholarship, no
one is arguably as central as bell hooks. Since bell hooks (1982, 1994,
2000a, 2000b) first led a more **Africanist** view of feminism in America,
Africanist and Black feminisms have proliferated. Patricia Hill Collins,
Gloria Joseph, Elizabeth Higginbotham, Robin Boylorn, and Bettina Love,
to name just a few, have advanced the study of Black feminist thought in
the academy. The next section, and our first video "snapshot," focuses on

the work of Professor Cynthia Dillard and her articulation of "endarkened feminist epistemologies," bringing together African and African American ways of knowledge construction.

Endarkened Feminist Epistemology

Cynthia Dillard (2016, 2008, 2006, 2000; Dillard & Okpalaoka, 2011) has advanced the study of Black feminist theory in part by proposing and developing the concept of an **endarkened feminist epistemology**, which addresses the intersection of identity, difference, and the politics of representation, and which has influenced qualitative research more generally. Her work has crossed educational, racialized, and gendered boundaries, enriching multiple disciplines as it goes. It is Black feminism with a focus on spirituality and African heritages.

Dillard describes her work as a "conscious choice to engage alternative cultural discourses other than postmodern discourse, in keeping with the spirit of an African ethos and frame of reference" (2006, p. 120), and notes the continuing power and relevance of standpoint theory. In the video provided, Dillard discusses the power of her paradigm for feminist scholars of color, but also identifies some ways in which endarkened feminist epistemology can be put into practice by other (non-African/African American) feminist scholars.

Feminist Science Scholarship

Another area of importance for feminist standpoint theory is in the discipline of science. Sandra Harding's *Is Science Multicultural? Postcolonialisms, Feminism, and Epistemologies* (1998) was a breakthrough text for feminist standpoint epistemology. Pinnick, for example, claims that Harding,

> presents the strongest case for an epistemologically relativist, feminist critique of science by using various interpretations of T. Kuhn's *The Structure of Scientific Revolutions* (1970) and WVO Quine's underdetermination thesis, the Strong Programme in the sociology of scientific knowledge, and general themes within the feminist critique of modern society. Her writings represent a forceful expansion of feminist theory into well-developed and mature areas of epistemology, and her works are cited widely in cognate fields, especially in the social studies of science. (Pinnick, Koertge, & Almeder, 2003, p. 21)

Pasifika Feminisms

There is a growing body of critical feminist research that is self-characterized by its geolocation within the South Pacific, and which therefore is included in the standpoint section for the purposes of this chapter (although, as with other fixed "categories," this does not preclude scholars using poststructuralist or other intersecting theoretical approaches). **Pasifika** scholars— Samoan, Fijian, Hawaiian, and others—track non-Western, nonpositivist ways of knowing, such as the Samoan system of "fa" (Iosefo, 2016), and suggest proliferating approaches to knowledge production. They include Enloe (2014), Evans (1994), Freeman (1999), Fresno-Calleja (2014), Jenkins and Pihama (2001), McNicholas (2004), Mohanram (1996), Tupuola (2004, 1998), Wilson (2013), and Iosefo (2016).

Sia Figiel (2014), a Samoan performance poet, has written and performed works about how she and her female relatives rehearsed feminisms in their childhood "girl circles," where they dreamed of their female futures, their interconnected lives, their villages, and men. While grouping "Pasifika" scholars together does exert a degree of essentialism, we note that Pasifika is regionally distinct and specific from "Asian" or the "Pacific Rim," which typically describes those from east Asia and/or the north of the Asian region.

Asian Feminisms

Once again, "Asian feminisms" is an umbrella term that enacts what Gayatri Spivak has called a "strategic essentializing" role for helping to understand some patterns in feminist research. Of course, feminisms from various nations and regions of the Pacific—like all other feminisms—vary widely. Yet for the purposes of this text, and due to limited space, we must include Asian feminisms as a regional grouping in order to highlight their considerable contributions, while acknowledging the insufficiency of a summary section of this kind.

Some influential feminist scholars from this region include postcolonial and feminist filmmaker and scholar Trinh T. Minh-ha, whose exploration of "subaltern" and "inappropriate/d others" (Minh-ha, 2009, 1987) in both her films and critical scholarship have led those who wish to address racism and misogyny through practice-led research methods. Her name has come to be synonymous with Vietnamese critical race reflexivity and postcolonial scholarship, inviting "minoritarian" women and raced others to critically gaze (and turn filmic lenses) back on White Western culture and interrogate its gendered, aesthetic, and scholarly practices.

Like Minh-ha, contemporary Vietnamese scholar Lan P. Duong (2012) takes a comprehensive look at Vietnamese films and literature, noting the ways in which so many Asian cultural and national bodies of work are intersectional, as is their geographical positioning. Traditional and modern, family and public, the critical and rapidly changing contexts of many Asian feminist scholars, activists, and artists are reflected in their work.

But perhaps more than in any other 21st-century Asian nation, women's roles in China have been transforming at a breakneck pace and, as a result, have provided the impetus for some of the most innovative feminist research on the globe. Social changes in areas such as the role of unmarried women and women's rights in modern China and the rise of feminist theory have all been "entangled in China's political, cultural and social transformations" (Ko & Zheng, 2006, p. 463). China's relatively recent economic and cultural contact with the West has had a huge impact on Chinese women and their demand for human rights (Wu, 2011, p. 16).

Critiques of Standpoint Feminism

Critics of standpoint feminist (often postmodern or poststructuralist feminists) cite three main criticisms of the approach: (1) it is erroneous to argue that if knowledge can be "legitimately" produced from a female point of view (replacing the dominant male point of view), then equality will necessarily follow; (2) perpetuating a dualistic (binary) approach is no longer a helpful way of separating the world or honoring difference; and (3) even standpoint feminism remains largely dominated by White, Western, middle-class women. Sandra Harding (2004), commonly held as a foundational standpoint feminist scholar regarding women and science, argues that there is an essentially "male" and "female" approach to science and other fields of research, and that women's approaches should be brought to the center in these fields. Patricia Hill Collins, a foundational Black standpoint feminist, believes there is an essential "Black" feminist standpoint that should also be more highly valued. By separating people (not practices) into these us/them oppositions, some claim, standpoint feminists are still arguing philosophically that there is a singular "truth" or an essential kind of "character/perspective" to each of these categories, which postmodernist, poststructuralist, and queer theorists disavow completely. For them, *subjectivities* (perspectives, practices) replace *identities* (which are fixed and essentializing). In Chapter 4 we will address these "post-" theoretical perspectives in more detail.

CONCLUSION

In Chapter 3, we have identified the main differences between "primary feminist theoretics" and poststructuralist ones, and unpacked some of the core scholarship and approaches of the first stream. The breadth of both theory chapters also reflects the incredibly large and rich body of feminist literature and discourses available to 21st-century feminist researchers today. From our earliest feminist theorists up to and continuing through postfeminist, new materialist, and digital feminist researchers today, there is no limit to the ways in which research can employ feminist epistemologies to advance not only theoretical innovation but also methodological approaches.

DISCUSSION QUESTIONS

1. Name one foundational feminist scholar and her main contribution to furthering feminist research or theory.

2. Discuss intersectionality and why you think it's so important to feminist research theorizing.

3. Discuss some differences between standpoint and empirical feminist approaches.

ACTIVITIES

1. Research the origins and different perspectives of one standpoint and one empirical feminist scholar of the 21st century and contrast their views.

2. Create a mind map of the second-wave feminist political movement versus the scholarly field of feminist studies.

3. Research a non-Western feminist scholar working in feminist health scholarship and describe what makes this feminism distinct from Euro-American health feminisms.

4. Make a short video or visual artifact detailing the ways in which "global feminisms" have advanced the overall global feminist research project.

SUGGESTED RESOURCES

📖 *Books*

Alcoff, L. M. (2006). *Visible identities: Race, gender, and the self.* Oxford, UK: Oxford University Press.

An important text that critiques intersectionality because of its potential essentializing aspects, yet values the expansion of feminism that intersectionality has made possible.

Anzaldúa, G., & Keating, A. (Eds.). (2013). *This bridge we call home: Radical visions for transformation.* New York: Routledge.

The 20-year sequel to the ground-breaking anthology *This Bridge Called My Back* similarly calls for a recommitment to women-of-color feminist principles, practices, and relationships, newly imagined for the 21st century.

Baksh, R., & Harcourt, W. (2015). *The Oxford handbook of transnational feminist movements.* New York: Oxford University Press.

A valuable text for its overview of historical, epistemological, and geographical diversity in feminisms.

Evans-Winters, V. E., & Love, B. L. (2015). *Black feminism in education: Black women speak back up and out.* New York: Peter Lang.

Two leading "next-gen" Black feminist scholars on racism in education.

Fraser, N. (1989). *Unruly practices: Power, gender and discourse in contemporary critical theory.* Minneapolis: University of Minnesota Press.

A classic text on the intersection of feminist and other critical theories.

hooks, b. (2015). *Feminism is for everybody: Passionate politics.* New York: Routledge.

An accessible and powerful introduction to feminist and race scholarship. A foundational scholar of the feminist academic and popular movement reminds us once again that the personal is political.

Mann, S. (2012). *Doing feminist theory: From modernity to postmodernity.* New York: Oxford University Press.

A great overview of second-wave feminist scholarship.

Articles and Chapters

Crenshaw, K. (1991). Mapping the margins: Intersectionality, identity politics, and violence against women of color. *Stanford Law Review, 43*(6), 1241–1299.

From the originator of the term "intersectionality," this essay is an excellent and concise introduction to the concept.

Davis, A. (1996). Gender, class, and multiculturalism: Rethinking "race" politics. In A. R. Gordon & C. Newfield (Eds.), *Mapping multiculturalism* (pp. 40–48). Minneapolis: University of Minnesota Press.

Famed activist Angela Davis offers her views on multiculturalism.

Lorde, A. (1997). The uses of anger. *Women's Studies Quarterly, 25*(1/2), 278–285.

A foundational text from a founding feminist poet and scholar.

💻 Digital Resources

Black American Feminisms: A Multidisciplinary Bibliography
http://blackfeminism.library.ucsb.edu/introduction.html

This online bibliography of interdisciplinary Black American feminist thought stretches from the 19th century to the modern era, including those who did not explicitly refer to themselves as feminists but who were doing feminist work. A valuable resource.

Lean In Circles
http://leanincircles.org/chapter/singapore#circles

Lean In Circles, small groups meeting for gender support and community, are an outgrowth of Sandberg's best seller *Lean In*. These are in Singapore.

Women's March 2017
www.genderandeducation.com/issues/womens-march-2017

Gender and Education Association blog post from Emilie Lawrence on the Women's Marches, social media, and intersectionality.

CHAPTER 4

Postmodern/Poststructuralist Theoretical Frames to Feminist Research

> While the third wave says, "We've got a hell of a lot of work to do!,"
> postfeminism says, "Go buy some Manolo Blahniks and stop your whining."
> —ALISON PIEPMEIER (2007, p. 143)

LEARNING OBJECTIVES

- To demonstrate the differences between postmodernist and poststructuralist feminist theories
- To explore the major contributions of feminist psychology and feminist sociology scholarship
- To highlight emerging feminist epistemologies, including videos from Eve Tuck and Aimee Carrillo Rowe.

What Is Different about the "Posts"?

This chapter picks up where Chapter 3 left off, having set out the differences between the foundational main strands or streams of feminist theoretical work, feminist empiricism, and standpoint "difference" feminisms. This chapter is devoted entirely to exploring **postmodernist and poststructuralist feminisms** (or the "posts"). As we noted in the previous chapter, while we decided to break these traditions down into two separate chapters for clarity, in practice they are overlapping and cross-informing. The first two approaches align with an Enlightenment perspective and realist

60

"empirical" knowledge construction that values equality, liberation, and rationalism, and believes truth or information is out there to be "collected." Chapter 4 focuses on social constructivism of gender, and the major leap of thought into what is considered a more unstable or flexible notion of knowledge. In gender terms, this means that there is no one essential "truth" out there to be observed and collected, but rather that gender is a socially constructed event that has no beginning, no end, and no one singular truth. As noted, it is important to study them together in order to see how they have built upon one another, yet also to be able to compare their distinctions from one another. Postmodern/poststructuralist or ludic feminism takes up difference and wants to undermine the stable, coherent subject, rejecting any "master narrative" or essentializing truth. To review, the "post-" approaches should not be interpreted as a correction to empirical or standpoint feminisms (the humanist feminist approaches) but rather as extending this foundational work beyond its original limits (see Table 4.1).

"Post- What?"

This chapter unpacks the "turn" in feminist research beyond an acknowledgment of **multiplicity,** the limitations of essentialism and a one-truth

TABLE 4.1. DIFFERENCES BETWEEN MODERNISM (ENLIGHTENMENT) AND POSTMODERNIST FEMINISM

Modernism	Postmodernism
Posits a stable and unified "self."	A self is a socially constructed thing, and is always changeable.
The self can reason to find reliable and valid knowledge.	The self is always biased and "subjective," affected by the conditions within which it is perceiving and operating.
Reason is trustworthy.	All knowledge is affective, perceptual, and subjective.
Reason allows us to "know" things in an objective way.	No knowledge or thinking process is objective or wholly reliable or unbiased.
Knowledge can be objective and universal.	Knowledge is not always subjective, culturally situated, and interpersonally constituted.
Language represents what our reasonable mind perceives: it is simply "reporting" what is observed.	Language constructs meaning by social conventions, education, and other social conditions. Nothing exists outside of language.

approach, and moves feminist theory into a challenge to stable and static identity itself. Feminist theory does this differently in postmodern and post-structuralist approaches, but both challenge traditional **positivist** (fixed) notions of a given research topic or body of knowledge.

When we say "postmodern feminism" or "feminist poststructur-alist research," we mean bringing together a recognition of multiplicity, an acknowledgment of the various perspectives and lived experiences of women and our allies. Postmodern and poststructuralist feminist theories recognize that feminism is not only concerned with a single topic, perspec-tive, or politic, and they suggest in their multiplicity the kinds of intersect-ing threads that characterize intersectionality in feminism, the kinds of multiple oppressions and multiple concerns that make up much of feminist research.

In particular, postmodern feminist research explores the power of "multiple relative truths of personal construction" (Frost & Elichaoff, 2014, p. 43). It most often takes into consideration a **sociocultural or socially constructivist** approach to subjectivity; that is, postmodernism is more con-cerned with individual perspectives (subjectivities) than a fixed notion of identity ("man," "woman," etc.). Like postmodernism, poststructuralism questions the notion of the group itself, preferring to explore the individual and intersubjective (or interpersonal) dynamics between people and within social groups, rather than make categorical statements or analyses of those groups themselves.

Thus, both postmodernism and poststructuralism are **anti-essential-izing approaches,** in which neither approach tries to get to the heart of an "essential" idea of what it means to be a woman or any other "type." Instead, critical theoretical approaches like these prefer to focus on the ways in which an individual experiences being what they self-identify as "woman" or anything else—they focus on the co-constructed experiences of individuals in an effort to gain deeper insight into the relationships and dynamics of perception.

Who Are the Foundational "Post-" Scholars?

An overview of feminist critical theorists and their most pivotal concepts and game-changing theories includes Judith Butler's performativity of gender (1993, 1990a); postmodernist Luce Irigaray's approach to wom-en's commodity value (1985); Gayatri Spivak's critique of the "subaltern" and representations by largely White, Western scholarship (1988; Spivak & Grosz, 1990); Teresa de Lauretis's articulation of "queer theory" and critique of Foucault's elision of the female body in his analyses of corporeality (1984, 1991); Eve Kosofsky Sedgwick's development of modern queer theory (1990); and Joan Scott's feminist history scholarship (2011).

In many ways, postmodernist and poststructuralist feminism jumps off from the notion of intersectionality explored in the previous chapter. In order to explore more performative notions of a nonunified feminist "self," feminist scholars first benefited from exploring the multiple oppressions under which they suffered, the multiple perspectives which they embodied, and the multiple communities with which they needed solidarity in order to fight these oppressions.

A Defining Moment: The Combahee River Collective Statement

This multiplicity was typified by the Combahee River Collective Statement (Collective, 1977), a key early text of intersectionality, primarily authored by Barbara Smith, Demita Frazier, and Beverly Smith, which articulated the notion of multiple and interlocking oppressions of Black lesbian feminists around race, sexuality, and gender. These women were activists in the National Black Feminist Organization, a group that separated from the middle-class White concerns of the mainstream feminist movement at that time (think National Organization for Women). Yet they felt that the pervasive lesbian oppression and class oppression within even this group left them feeling like outsiders, and they cowrote the Statement to address these inextricable multilayered lives they were living.

While contemporary criticisms of intersectionality often concern the "identity politics" aspect of the approach (which some, including Alcoff [2006], find overly essentializing), Collins and Bilge (2016) remind us that "Contemporary renditions of identity politics generally miss the fact that the identity politics articulated in the Statement are collective and structural . . . a collective space that accounts for the particularities of location," and that "systematic analysis is central to the CRC's understanding of the compound nature of the oppression they grapple with. . . . The analysis is not only systemic . . . but also integrated" (p. 63).

So feminist theories, like other theoretical innovations, are built upon the conceptual and political work that has gone before; intersectionality is built upon the intellectual and activist work of the CRC Statement and lived activisms of Chicana, African American, and other global feminists and feminist thinkers, which found expression not only in the academy but in film, literature, and all cultural and creative practices and artifacts.

Giving Everyone a Chance to Speak

Intersectionality can also be seen in Spivak's famous question "Can the subaltern speak?" which advanced not only so-called third-world (non-Western) feminisms but also brought us back to Audre Lorde's caution against **epistemic violence** (Spivak, 1988, p. 280) more generally. The history of intersectionality highlights the need for nondominant voices to be heard more often, more widely, and in more nuanced ways—especially by the White feminists who were supposed to be comrades. Yet what does postmodernist and poststructuralist feminism do that these previous theories did not? Crucially, it not only suggests ways forward into greater diversities of perspective, but also continues to break down the very notion of **binary gender** itself.

Feminist poststructuralism, for example, importantly draws on the bodies of literature of postmodernism, psychoanalysis, and **sociocultural theory,** and—as Linda Tuhiwai Smith notes—"recent poststructural and **psychoanalytical feminist theorists** have argued against the claims made by earlier generations of feminists that women as a group were different" (1999, p. 73).

Extending **20th-century Continental philosophy,** postmodernism and poststructuralism challenged "traditional biological essentialism and binaries that dictated gender characteristics and roles and questioned the notion that all women were the same" (Hesse-Biber, 2013a, p. 10). Indeed, poststructuralism in particular takes issue with a static category of "women" itself. Thus the influence of critical theory on feminist research has not only moved it away from lingering notions of **positivism,** but focuses on the interrelatedness of oppressions more broadly, and toward more **gender-fluid** and expansive notions of **gender-informed sociality** overall.

The vast range of theoretical approaches in contemporary feminist research celebrates and demonstrates the diversity of what gender and feminist studies' commitments are and can be, liberated as they increasingly are from biological determinism and the constraints of binary categories of "woman" and "man." Today, feminist research highlights the intersectional axes of fighting continued inequality and oppression not only within communities of oppression, but also in solidarity across categories as well.

The Power of Language

Language is at the center of constructing identity. If you think about it, it makes perfect sense: when you tell a friend or family member the story of what happened to you last night at a party, you yourself are participating in constructing their knowledge of that party. Whether your version of events is somehow "true" or not is irrelevant; what matters is that in your story-telling, and based on the relationship you share when the telling occurs, "the party" gets constructed in their mind. Gender, some postmodernists and poststructuralists would argue, is similarly constructed interpersonally, through language.

Julia Kristeva (1981) as well as Hélène Cixous (2003), Luce Irigaray (1985), and others all consider "language as responsible for creating repressive structures by equating biological gender with femininity and masculinity" (Frost & Elichaoff, 2014, p. 45). This focus on language "is based on the premise that there is an inextricable link between language (or knowledge, expressed through language)" and power.

Feminist postmodernist (e.g., Lather, 1991) and poststructuralist approaches position themselves against feminist empiricism and standpoint epistemology by "exploring the ways in which language serves to create and reinforce the essentialist views of women as different from men," (Frost & Elichaoff, 2014, p. 45) rather than the much broader project of exploring the multiplicity of women's lived experiences, or gender inequity more broadly. For a closer look, first let's turn to postmodernist feminism.

Postmodernist Feminism

Feminist scholar Rosemarie Tong summarizes the essence of postmodernist research as pursuing a truth that can be defined as "whatever power proclaims it to be . . . science is no more objective than politics or ethics, both of which are subjective, contextual, historical, contingent, and almost always deployed to serve self-interest" (2013, p. 194).

By doing so, she notes the central position of language in postmodernist knowledge construction as serving a function that is not necessarily "represent[ing] reality, because there is no reality for it to signify. On the contrary, language constructs reality—a relating that depends on words for its existence" (Tong, 2013, p. 194). We begin an examination of postmodernist feminism with this orientation, a rejection of **objectivity, static identity,** a recognition of subjectivity, and the role of language in constructing meaning, not reporting reality. For feminist researchers, these orientations are aligned with a challenge to traditional patriarchal texts and ways of researching.

Moving beyond Biological Determinism in Gender Orientation

Feminist writer Simone de Beauvoir first urged women to define ourselves for ourselves (not by men), and to do so outside of the "male/female dyad," thus throwing down the basis for much of the postmodern and poststructuralist feminist thought to follow. Postmodern feminism incorporates postmodernist and poststructuralist theory with feminist approaches, and in so doing goes beyond earlier binarized modernist dichotomies in doing feminist research. It seeks equal rights for all genders, not just **cisgender** women and girls, and it is inherently intersectional.

Because language is always at the center of postmodern feminist theory, **discourse analysis** is a common analytic tool coupled with this theoretic, across diverse fields of study. The combination of feminist theory with postmodernism has opened both theoretic frameworks out by questioning many assumptions that were previously left unexamined (see Table 4.2).

Performativity of Sex, Sexuality, and Gender

> **Gender fluidity** is an umbrella term that refutes binary (male/female or masculine/feminine) distinctions, and spans a range of gender identifications including, for example, nonbinary, multigender, agender, transgender, and more. This spectrum is also sometimes denoted by the key term trans*.

Judith Butler has contributed to feminist and gender theory in multiple areas, but we focus here on her work on **gender fluidity**, its relationship to (but distinction from) sex, and her famous development of the term **performativity** in relation to bodies and gender. Extending John Searle's speech-act theory, Butler tells us that gender is a performative act, both **illocutionary** and **corporeal**,[1] an act that performs itself into being in a social context, rather than an act that expresses some essential truth that preexisted the act (e.g., "He was somehow a *boy* before he began to act like a boy").

---

[1] For Searle and John L. Austin, *illocution* represents the meaning or intention of the speech act or the act of speaking itself, or of the speaker's intent (i.e., to pursue, to save, to advise), a different aspect of the speech act than *locution* (what is said), or *perlocution* (what eventuates). Butler uses *illocution* to draw attention to what the speaker is intending to *do in the act of speaking*. It is not static, as gender and identity are equally not static or fixed in a postmodern and poststructural conceptual approach, and they do not have meaning in and of themselves.

TABLE 4.2. Some Well-Known Postmodern Feminist Theorists	
Jacques Derrida	Derrida's rejection of a single truth establishes a core postmodern feminist view that all is constructed with language.
Hélène Cixous	Foundational postmodern feminist, built on Derrida, and rejects what she called the binary nature of men's writing (men's writing is filled with binary oppositions), suggesting women's is not.
Luce Irigaray	Psychoanalytic approach, resisting Freudian theoretic, reclaiming women from the abject margins, yet her famous statement "mime the mimes men have imposed on women" has been used to suggest women should be hyperfeminized in order to transcend patriarchal oppressions.
Julia Kristeva	Unlinks biological "man" from the notion of masculinity and bio females from the "feminine." Rejects all gender essentialisms.
Judith Butler	Performativity of gender, sex/sexuality/gender, bridges postmodernism and poststructuralism.

I Am a Boy If I Say I Am

The act of performing "boy," for example, is part of a set of social codes and circumstances (including biology) that help or force people to think of all individuals in binary gender ways. Butler helped us see that these social codes extend back to the beginning of human society, and so preexisted the particular "performativity of gender" of any boy, girl or gender-diverse person alive today. For Butler, all ways of "performing gender" are co-constructed by the individual and his/her/their group, and these ways of "doing gender" make sense based on already-existing **social codes.**

A large part of Butler's argument is social justice oriented: if all gender identities are performative and **socially constructed,** and there is no essentializing or "natural" gender truth, then there is no reason to oppress sexually or gender-diverse performances of self. Butler is also famous for helping think about sex and gender as different and distinct. **Sex** is determined by biological characteristics, although this, too, is not as straightforward as history would have us believe—take, for example, people who are born with sexual characteristics of both male and female, who are now known as **intersex** but used to be called **hermaphrodite** or **androgynous.** Just along this one continuum alone, there are many diverse expressions of sex identification.

So Biology Has Nothing to Do with It?

Butler helped distinguish between these biological characteristics and a person's gender, which does not always correspond with their biological sex as has been previously thought. For Butler, gender is a set of ritualized repetitions or performances that express a person's chosen gender identification, which is often neither male nor female, but can also be unfixed or fluid. **Sexuality,** on the other hand, describes a person's sexual interest, orientation, and attractions.

Further, Butler argues that "gender cannot be understood as a *role* which either expresses or disguises an interior 'self,' whether that 'self' is conceived as sexed or not. As performance which is performative, gender is an 'act,' broadly construed, which constructs the social fiction of its own psychological interiority" (Butler, 1990b, p. 279). She tells us that "performativity is neither free play nor theatrical self-presentation; nor can it be simply equated with performance" (1993, p. 95).

Of course her gender theorizing goes much deeper than this. But, in short, suffice it to say that Butler untangles aspects of performance just as thoroughly as she does gender and bodies. For a snapshot of the differences between postmodernist and poststructuralist feminisms, see Table 4.3.

TABLE 4.3. Differences between Postmodern Feminist Theory and Poststructuralist Feminism

Postmodernist feminism	Poststructuralist feminism
Language constructs meaning by social conventions, education, and other social conditions. Nothing exists outside of language.	Signaled by a "linguistic turn," particularly per Foucault.
Language is slippery but a tool of the "real," and external to the research activities.	Discourse is constitutive, rather than descriptive, and therefore feminist scholarship is not tied to patriarchal research histories.
A self is a socially constructed thing, and is always changeable.	Even bodies are discursively (linguistically) realized.
Gender and sexuality are determined, natural conditions open to desconstructing.	Characterized by the rise of the subject and the becoming of gendered subjects.
The self is always biased and subjective based on the conditions within which one is perceiving and operating.	Increasingly openly rejects humanism (human-centered analyses).
Remains human-centered but focuses on the affective, perceptual, and individual realms.	Turns away from the individual subject, anti-neoliberalism, and anti-capitalism.
Knowledge is always subjective, culturally situated, and interpersonally constituted.	Rejects realist/empirical goal to understand experience and describe it.

Note: For more on the distinctions between postmodern, poststructural, and critical theories as deployed by feminist researchers, see Gannon and Davies (2012).

While stressing the "forced reiteration of norms" (1993, p. 94), she cautions that "performativity cannot be understood outside of a process of iterability, a regularized and constrained repetition of norms," a repetition that is neither a singular event nor "performed *by* a subject; this repetition is what enables a subject" (1993, p. 95), and also what creates the conditions in time and space for this subject to perform itself into being (always in relation to others).

Recognizing Gender

Butler (here and elsewhere) goes on to say how her theory of gender is "constituted in social discourse" and that "genders, then, can be neither true nor false, neither real nor apparent. And yet, one is compelled to live in a world in which genders constitute univocal signifiers, in which gender is stabilized, polarized, rendered discrete and intractable" (1990b, p. 279), and the intensity with which society demands this compliance with two static genders, and punishes those who perform something other than these two options, is for Butler even more evidence that the fragility and performativity of gender is fluid and unfixed.

Clearly Butler's "view of gender does not pose as a comprehensive theory about what gender is or the manner of its construction, and neither does it prescribe an explicit feminist political program" (1990b, p. 280), but a **Butlerian notion of gender** has become central to 21st-century feminist research. Her commitment to linking scholarship and culture, to holding gender research accountable to the real conditions of people's lives, has reminded us for nearly 30 years now that "any theory of gender constitution has political presuppositions and implications, and [that] it is impossible to separate a theory of gender from a **political philosophy of feminism**" (1990b, p. 280).

Lastly, it is important to note that Butler underlines Gayatri Spivak's view of gender as relying on a **strategic or operational essentialism** in order to advance a feminist political program. This does not mean, as some have claimed, that Spivak believes in an essentializing view of gender, only recognizes that the way gender continues to function socially and culturally is often essentialized and so must be fought at times along essentializing lines, for efficacy and solidarity.[2] She reminds us of the impossibility of finding an "essence, a nature, or a shared cultural reality" of womanness (Butler, 1990b, p. 280).

---

[2] For more on this, see the subsection on ally work in Chapter 3.

Critiques of Butler's Theory of Gender

1. Martha Nussbaum critiqued Judith Butler's "dark impossibility" of gender equality (and also of jargon-heavy poststructuralist theory, for which Butler is widely critiqued), by calling it "hip defeatism" that will help no one but oppressors (Nussbaum, 1999).

2. Butler exemplifies a persistent association between these theories and a **biological essentialism**[1] with no clear core theoretic that unites different approaches, making identifying a central philosophy difficult.

3. But the main objection leveled against postmodern feminism is what some call obtuse, jargonistic, elite, incomprehensible, or intentionally dense language, given that one of its central analytics is a rejection of so-called male binarized writing, making some of this body of literature difficult to access.

[1]The real or perceived reduction of gender possibilities to biological (or cis-) sex.

Mostly, she encourages us to remain critically reflective in doing feminist work so that we do not slide into reessentializing or falsely binarized notions of "woman" or "man" or indeed any two opposing positions along a gender continuum, but rather work toward more nuanced agendas of understanding the way gender works in social, economic, and interpersonal ways.

The Long Legacy of Colonialism: Alive and Well in Feminist Studies

📹 VIDEO PROFILE

Eve Tuck
www.guilford.com/leavy-harris

Eve Tuck's impact in **decolonizing** and **native scholarship** cannot be underestimated. She is well known for expanding the fields of **settler colonialism,** and indigenous/Native ways of knowing, from a North American perspective. Tuck and Yang's (2012) pivotal essay "Decolonization Is Not a Metaphor" has quickly become a classic go-to text for understanding the intersectional and **critical race theory** concerns of settler colonialism and decolonization scholarship, and the ways in which these inform so many other areas of study.

The works of other Native and indigenous scholars of note include Arvin, Tuck, and Morrill (2013); Iosefo (2016); Teaiwa (2014a, 2014b); and Chilisa (2012). More recently, Tuck has been exploring the political and ecological implications of **place-based methods** and **native feminisms** (see Tuck & McKenzie, 2015, among others).

Tuck's work innovates in contributing what she has called "Native feminist theories." Tuck has argued that the United States is a settler colonial nation-state and that settler colonialism is a gendered process. She has also proposed five central challenges that Native feminist theories pose to gender and women's studies—including a focus on intersectionality in placing contemporary colonialism and indigenous consciousness within feminist studies.

> **Settler colonialism and native feminisms:** Settler colonialism refers to the legacy of our violent colonial past and its current manifestations, and to the belief that formerly colonized countries such as the United States and Australia, as well as most of Africa, South America, and Asia, are characterized by imperialism and the need to make more ethical social contracts going forward.

Her articulation of the "five obligations" for indigenous scholarship implicates nonnative scholars and educators as well as native ones. Her work has found a wide audience because it speaks to the particular contribution of Native feminist theories, theoretics tied to sustainability, new materialisms, and concern with both human and more-than-human areas of study and political orientations. Like the recent Dakota Access Pipeline protests in the United States, Tuck's work bridges native and wider communities' concerns with ecologies, and with intercultural and social justice work. The intersection of these areas of concern with feminisms (which by Tuck's own definition include issues of gender and sexuality diversity, race, class, etc.) is at the forefront of 21st-century scholarship.

> **Critical race theory (CRT)** is a theoretical framework in the social sciences that focuses on the application of critical theory to culture and social relations and acknowledges the micro- and macroaggressions, inequities, and legacies of institutional racism, historically and currently.

Some decolonizing feminist scholars (such as African and Indian scholars) point out other readings of decolonizing scholarship missing from Tuck's conflation of a land-policing focus and the critique of decolonization. For example, some decolonizing methodologies (Tuhiwai Smith, 1999) point to non-land-based critiques of colonialism, such as in India, where land reallocation is no longer the most pressing threat to native communities and cultures. These scholars point out that decolonizing agendas are different in every community, and that an insistence on land-centered critiques actually serves to "police the field" in unhelpful ways.

Some have warned that Tuck and others who are held up as representatives of any field (e.g., Halberstam in gender studies) risk creating new hegemonies by asserting a (default) singular decolonizing agenda which holds up that way as the only way, where everyone else is "doing it wrong." Tuck (together with Yang) famously addressed this question and its pitfalls in "Decolonization Is Not a Metaphor" (2012). Decolonizing scholars argue that people have been colonized in different ways; for example, India has a colonizing history but its people do not have the same repatriation issues or agenda as indigenous or Native Americans.

Feminist Psychology Scholarship

One of the most significant areas of postmodernist feminist research is in the field of psychology. Michelle Fine (1992), Deborah Tolman (2009), Valerie Walkerdine (see Walkerdine, 1984, 1997), Rebecca Campbell (2002; Campbell, Shaw, & Fehler-Cabral, 2015), and Deborah Britzman (2011) have all made significant contributions to feminist research in the area of psychology. Britzman and Fine work within the field of education, Tolman in social welfare, and Walkerdine in psychology, while Campbell researches family- and gender-based violence. Britzman uses psychoanalytic theory, while Fine identifies as a social psychologist, and her research focuses on social inequities. Campbell uses a community psychology lens to conduct rape and sexual assault research.

Both Tolman and Walkerdine are developmental psychologists concerned with the ways in which adolescent girls navigate relationships, gender roles, and sexuality. Valerie Walkerdine has made a significant contribution to feminist scholarship in a range of areas, including popular culture (1997), mathematics (2012), and, especially, developmental psychology (1984), in a ground-breaking chapter that was instrumental in the critical retheorization of gendered psychology, social theory, and educational practice and research. Using Foucault and psychoanalytic theory, Walkerdine (2001) helps us understand popular culture and the sociocultural sexual anxieties about girls and women drawing on a psychoanalytic frame.

Tolman does research in the areas of girlhood, pleasure, and adolescent sexuality. In *Dilemmas of Desire,* she uses a psychological analytic as well as a social constructivist approach to understanding adolescent girls' sexual desire. One of the contributions of Tolman's significant body of work is in bringing girls' voices to research in the field of psychology, providing opportunities to understand girls' sexuality from a psychological perspective, but through their own voices. Her work has been influential in providing a counternarrative to what she believed was still a largely male-dominated field in the 1980s, when she began her work, yet she claims feminist approaches can still make a significant impact in the field.

Michelle Fine's major contribution to educational psychology has had an impact in a range of subfields, including critical race studies, urban education, and whiteness studies. Her coedited book *Off White* (2004) contains many excellent contributions that address not only psychological approaches to the study of gender, but innovations in feminist methods more generally. Contributors Hurtado and Stewart reinforce the point that feminist social scientists have, since the 1970s, "made a case for the need for new methods and approaches by showing that the apparently, or supposedly, 'neutral' studies of sex differences were riddled with bias and sexism" (2012, p. 316). Michelle's close collaboration with Lois Weis has produced a number of intersectional texts that address the interconnectedness of race, gender, class, and psychology. They have contributed groundbreaking work in the area of participatory action research design but have also done important synthesizing work around the important differences yet common goals of White feminists and feminists of color (Bhavnani, 2001), subjectivity/objectivity, scientific and constructivist forms of knowledge (Haraway, 1988), and other topics. For example, in applying Bhavnani's "three criteria for 'feminist objectivity': inscription, micropolitics and difference" (in *working method,* p. 99), Fine and Weis extend the possibilities of feminist intersectionality, psychology, and social policy scholarship.

These feminist scholars draw on a range of psychological lenses to advance feminist understandings from rigid biological deterministic approaches to the more flexible, performative, and constructed nature of gender expressions.

Critiques of Postmodern Feminism

Each new "strand" of feminist theoretical advancement seems to grow out of critiques of the ones that have gone before. For postmodern feminism, its critiques include attention to its discursive nature and, as some perceive, its inability to address real-world conditions of gender inequity. Fraser and Nicholson note differences and critiques even between postmodernism and feminism: "Postmodernists have focused primarily on the philosophy side of the problem . . . [while] for feminists, on the other hand, the question of philosophy has always been subordinate to an interest in social criticism" (1990, p. 20). That is, "a postmodernist reflection on feminist theory reveals disabling vestiges of essentialism while a feminist reflection on postmodernism reveals androcentrism and political naivete" (p. 20). So while critics of postmodernist feminism often side with the "too philosophical" side of Fraser and Nicholson's observation above, others find in it the perfect fusion of both.

Feminist economist Marilyn Waring (1988, 2014) has argued about the radical implications of "counting" women's work (across domestic to volunteer spheres) and the negative impact of the exclusion of women's work from national income accounts, particularly in developing nations (1988). But this is not only an economically oriented consideration among feminist scholars. Valuing women's work in capitalist social structures is a question that has been addressed through a range of fields and epistemological approaches.

One feminist scholar who has attended to women's work and contexts is Patti Lather, perhaps best known for her book *Troubling the Angels* (Lather & Smithies, 1997). This and its follow-up, *Getting Lost* (Lather, 2007) both detail the ways in which her deep ethnographic study of women living with HIV/AIDS became an exemplar for feminist methods, and the contexts in which "feminist methodologies" are required and more appropriate than others. This powerful contribution has placed Lather as an important feminist researcher who celebrates the difficulties and contingencies of reflexive qualitative research through a feminist conceptual lens, using feminist methods.

The Postmodern Turn

The postmodern critique of science and epistemology has been much disputed in feminist studies. The encounter between feminism and postmodern philosophy has often been storm tossed. But the skepticism about traditional science and knowledge production, which is shared equally by many feminist theorists and postmodern philosophers, has also generated a lot of synergy . . . the postmodern turn toward anti-epistemological, anti-foundational, self-reflexive and deconstructive stances has been in consonance with feminist ideas and has inspired feminists to criticize and expose problems in feminist empiricism and standpoint epistemology in order to create space for alternative ways to do Feminist Studies. A significant moment in the postmodern turn in feminist epistemological thought was Judith Butler's head-on attack on the category "women" . . . Butler's problematization of the notion of "women" implies a radical critique of both feminist empiricism and standpoint epistemology. Seen through a Butlerian lens, both these epistemologies display a naïve relationship to the notion "women."

Lykke (2010, p. 125)

Chicana Indigenous Feminisms

Aimee Carrillo Rowe's scholarship has long contributed to the area of **transracial and transcultural feminist alliances** (see Carrillo Rowe, 2008), as well as the tensions and opportunities of **transcultural migration.**

Carrillo Rowe defines her own current feminist practice and scholarship as intertwined with and characteristic of the broad diversity of contemporary 21st-century feminisms. As an evolving project across both her own lifetime and across the history of global feminism, Carrillo Rowe calls her work an "ongoing search for empowerment."

Chicana Indigenous Feminisms

[Feminist work] can shift over the course of one's life and over the course of what sites of community and struggle we participate in, and of course it also depends on your social location, your identity and where you are in the globe. And who you are there with. To me, it's always been about healing, it's always been a spiritual practice, and that's taken me in different directions over the 25 years that I've identified as a feminist. Some of those different directions are I feel like in my early work I was trying to discover who I am as a Chicana, as a queer Chicana, as a woman of color, as a person of mixed race heritage and as a cisgender woman. What does it mean to be a queer woman of color walking in a body that could presumably pass as white straight? And so that was my first book, my first pretty intensive exploration into feminism. And what I came up with in that iteration of what was feminist for me then was it had to do with alliances and belonging. Like where do we place our bodies and our emotional ties and our commitments, and how those commitments are political. Currently the work that I'm doing comes out of my spiritual practice as a spirit dancer. I dance in sun-moon dances and I do other kinds of spiritual ceremony that comes out of a Native American tradition. So that work has led me to think of the relationship between being Chicana, and Chicana relationships to Indigenous ancestry and Indigenous spirituality. But not in an unproblematic way. So how do nonnative people who are invested in native spiritualities and learning from native people do that in a respectful way that actually joins with native struggles for sovereignty, recognition, land, visibility? Decolonization? So then that brings me to my current iteration of feminism, which has to do with how do I be in alliance with indigenous people and recognize the ways in which I am and am not indigenous as a queer Chicana.

Interviewed by Anne Harris on December 12, 2015,
in Carrillo Rowe's home in Los Angeles. Unpublished video interview.

For Carrillo Rowe, like so many of the other contemporary feminist theorists and practitioners discussed in this book, feminism is a way of life that goes far beyond theory practices and has become central to her spirituality, her lifestyle, and her way of being in the world.

Maori Feminist Knowledges

Indigenous New Zealander scholars are creating a body of research that highlights the particular ways of knowing that emerge from their Maori cultural heritage. Among these are—most prominently—Linda Tuhiwai Smith, author of the core text *Decolonizing Methodologies: Research and Indigenous Peoples* (1999), which has had a profound impact on most subsequent indigenous research, regardless of the region from which it comes. Reprinted nine times in the past 17 years, not only does Smith's volume address the colonial histories and habits from which indigenous peoples are emerging and also continuing to live, but crucially she sets out alternative ways of knowing in contrast to the centrality of Western and Cartesian thought and knowledge production.

   She argues a persuasive case against not only the pattern of Western imperialism that colonized land and people, but also the devastating effects of "colonizing knowledges," a process that continues today. The "formations of western research," Smith charges, are still clearly evident in today's research culture, despite the mitigating influences of Marxism and Western feminism (held to account by Western women of color). Smith has shown how "gendering contemporary indigenous debates occurs inside indigenous communities and while it is debated in other contexts, such as in Western feminist debates, indigenous women hold an analysis of colonialism as a central tenet" (p. 152). She has also noted how not only feminism, but also critical approaches more widely, "have greatly influenced the social sciences" (p. 9), another sign of the spreading influence of diverse feminisms on the ways of doing and understanding research.

Poststructural Feminism

Much of the poststructuralist critical lens has changed the ways in which a range of feminist scholarly approaches are done. They are not all interdependent, but they have certainly continued to inform and expand one another. Elizabeth St. Pierre has argued that "feminism is a highly contested term, as is poststructuralism, so it is impossible to produce a comfortable synthesis" (2000, p. 477) of the two, yet both offer compatible critical theoretical

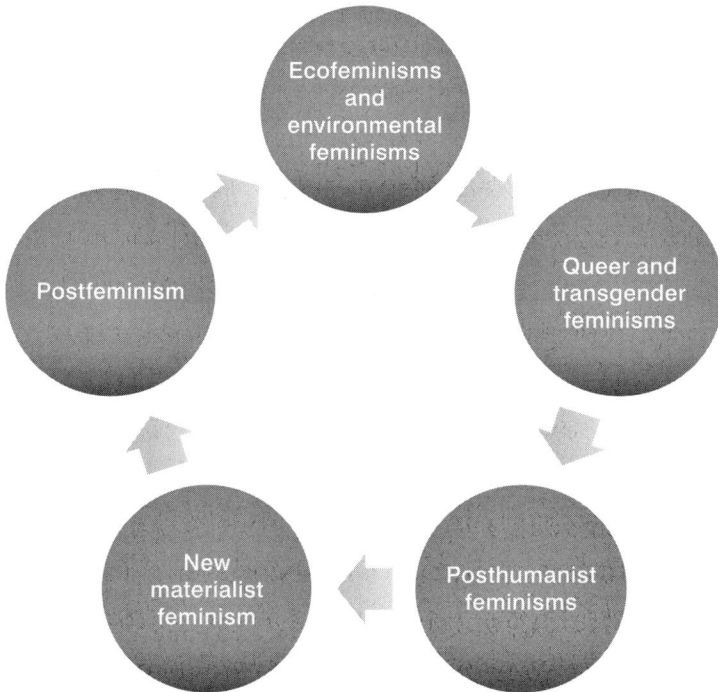

FIGURE 4.1 Types of poststructuralist feminist theoretical frameworks.

lenses through which to view any number of disciplinary pursuits. Rather than considering 21st-century poststructuralist feminisms as a finite set of concepts that guide research practices, these feminist frameworks encourage a **rhizomatic** approach[3] that understands them all working together and co-evolving at the same time (see Figure 4.1). Poststructural feminists "are troubled by the very category "woman" and work to keep that category unstable and undefined" (St. Pierre & Pillow, 2000, p. 7).

The Crisis of Representation

Well-known poststructural feminist education scholars Elizabeth St. Pierre and Wanda Pillow describe how from the "ruins" of postmodernism's "crises of representation and legitimation" which "troubles all those things we

---

[3]Rhizomatic approaches to research draw from ideas described by Gilles Deleuze and Felix Guattari in an influential text of theirs called *A Thousand Plateaus: Capitalism and Schizophrenia* (1980). They (and others) have borrowed the botanical image of the rhizome, which references the ways plants and roots shoot out in many directions as they grow.

assumed were solid, substantial, and whole" (2000, p. 1) throughout the last half of the twentieth century, "feminists have found possibilities for different worlds that might, perhaps, not be so cruel to so many people . . . produce different knowledge and produce knowledge differently" (2000, p. 1) in **poststructuralism**. More than this, they suggest, "the two theories/ movements work similarly and differently to trouble foundational ontologies, methodologies, and epistemologies" (p. 2) in ways that have the potential to change theoretical but also practical work and lived experience.

A persistent concern of feminist poststructural theory is "the process of **subjectification** and the **discursive regimes** through which we become gendered subjects. In this way, it breaks with theoretical frameworks in which gender and sexuality are understood as inevitable, as *determined* through social structures, cognition, or biology" (Gannon & Davies, 2012, p. 73) but also rejects any kind of essentialism that attributes the experiences or perspectives of women to a kind of natural or biological notion of what being a woman "is."

Lastly, they and other poststructural feminists widely agree that "the question for poststructural feminism, then, becomes that of **agency** and

TABLE 4.4. Theorists Pivotal to Poststructuralist Feminist Theory
Michel Foucault
Barely mentions women or gender directly at all, yet his conceptual work on power, the body, and sexuality has greatly impacted poststructuralist feminist thought.
Judith Butler
Philosopher and gender theorist primarily known for her theories of performativity and her challenge to traditional feminism's definitions of what constitutes "female" (like that of Halberstam).
Gayatri Chakravorty Spivak
Postcolonial feminist theorist who famously asked "Can the **subaltern** speak?" (1988), thus turning, along with Trinh T. Minh-ha and others, the ethnographic gaze of the academy from non-Western subjects back onto itself. Also known for "strategic essentialism."
Eve Kosofsky Sedgwick
Pioneer of queer theory. Sedgwick famously made the distinction between gender and sexuality, and debunks the binaries of male/female as well as gay/straight.
Donna Haraway
Formulated cyborg theory, which led to the contemporary emergence of posthumanism, new materialism, and some forms of environmental feminisms and spirituality. Haraway pioneered new understandings of the link between technology, social codes, affect, and feminist theory.

what possibilities there are for action" (p. 73). It is however important to note that they and other scholars do not suggest that these two theoretical frameworks must work synthetically, but rather "beside each other" (see Figure 4.1 and Table 4.4).

Feminist Sociology

Feminist sociological theory is concerned with gender in relation to power. That is, with the social construction of gender as it intersects with power relations and larger sociocultural institutions, codes, and practices. It primarily expresses this focus in research contexts through engagement with race, culture, and socioeconomic and gender/sexuality diversity. Feminist sociology looks at the systematic oppression of women by men globally, including social practices like heteronormativity and patriarchy.

A good place to start reading feminist sociology may be "Bridging Feminist Theory and Research Methodology" by J. S. Chafetz (2004), which examines feminist theory in the social sciences, and more specifically in sociology. Despite the existence of many influential poststructuralist sociologists, in this essay Chafetz argues that the defining features of sociology are nevertheless mostly empirical. In order to change social inequalities, Chafetz argues, testable evidence-based data must be produced and interpreted, a widely accepted social scientific approach.

Yet here comes the contradiction: possibly the most widely cited article in the field of sociology is West and Zimmerman's 1987 article "Doing Gender," which holds that empirical research is structurally insufficient to measure the sociological—and social—practices and theories of gender. Today, there are methodologically and conceptually diverse applications of feminist lenses to sociological research.

Kum-kum Bhavnani (2001; Bhavnani & Coulson, 1997) and Jessica Ringrose (2013, 2007) are both prominent feminist scholars who use a sociological lens to examine the social patterns of feminist study. Bhavnani's work is situated within feminist studies, cultural studies, and critical race theory, while Ringrose is an education scholar who primarily explores postfeminist perspectives in young women's sexuality and social lives (covered in more detail later in this chapter under postfeminism). Readers who are interested in broader sociological feminist research can also explore visual sociological feminist research, digital media in feminist sociology, and more.

Cyborg Feminism and the Posthuman

Setting the stage not only for feminist philosophy in education, Donna Haraway's *Cyborg Manifesto* (first published in 1984, and then in a well-known 1991 collection of essays) also foreshadowed the theoretical frames of posthumanism and new materialism through her concept of the cyborg, also known as *cyborg feminism* or *posthuman cyborg feminism*.

Haraway's cyborg blends questions of postgender biology, science fiction and futurism, and animals and nature. Haraway is a foundational figure in feminist studies, and her work stands alongside Rosi Braidotti's "nomadic subject" (2011), Eve Kosofsky Sedgwick and Judith Butler's notions of queer (Butler, 1993, 1990a, 1990b; Sedgwick, 1990), and Trinh Minh-ha's "subaltern" and "inappropriate/d others" (Minh-ha, 2009, 1987). As Lykke (2010) has noted, Haraway's adaptation of the notion of the cyborg has radical implications for feminism and feminist scholarship:

> Haraway suggests the cyborg figuration as a possible ally for feminists and other radicals who want to fight the dualisms and hierarchies of modern society. Haraway stresses that the cyborg should not be considered as an innocent partner . . . the cyborg can be considered as a figuration that breaks down a range of dualisms on which modern technoscience and power differentials of present-day society are based. As a fusion of body and technology, the cyborg challenges the borders between nature and culture—and hence also the borders between biological sex and sociocultural gender. The cyborg makes it explicit that concepts such as "nature," "body," "sex" and so on are not universally given, but changeable, ethnospecific constructions . . . the cyborg may radically delegitimize all kinds of gender-conservatism, which argues for biology and nature as steady, fixed and unchangeable phenomena. According to Haraway, this makes it apt as a feminist figuration, and her interpretation has been influential in Feminist Studies. (pp. 39–40)

Perhaps Haraway's cyborg became the feminist studies cult trope it did due to its link to the core notion of a nonfixed, nonessentialized gender and its relation to biological sex characteristics, a relationship that had, until that time, been conflated in the sex/gender categories of mostly "male" or "female." No matter what the reason, Haraway's feminist cyborg has had a lasting impact on feminist research.

Trans* Feminisms

The more recent emergence of trans* (transgender) and genderqueer feminisms (Halberstam, 2012; Stryker, 2009; Stryker & Whittle, 2013; Serano, 2016a, 2016b; Scott-Dixon, 2006; Dicker, 2016) ably demonstrates that more biologically determined definitions of "girls" and "women," as well as more traditionally framed notions of feminism, no longer offer sufficient scope or specificity for feminist research today. There is much debate in feminist scholarship regarding the "mainstreaming" of trans* and genderqueer identities. Some argue that the increased visibility has negative effects, including as a failure of a broad movement to stay diverse, exchanging assimilation into the mainstream for a proud transgender political and activist history. Others argue that this "thin end of the gender wedge" means the door is pried further open for less simple gender identifications. For some, the rage and resistance that typified both the queer (LGBTIQ) and gender diversity movements seems to be gone, and with it a sense of community, purpose, and commitment to changing the status quo.

Julia Serano, for example, is one transgender female feminist (and a research biologist) who argues for the importance of breaking down biological or cisgender notions of gender when discussing feminisms. In her introduction to the second edition of her important work, *Whipping Girl*, she lays out how and why her work questions the "commonsense" notion of nature versus nurture when examining gender, and her concerns about her own experiences of being further marginalized in both feminist and queer activist communities. She details not only how much things have changed, but also how much work still needs to be done for the equality and well-being of transgender people, including feminists (Serano, 2016b).

Serano's story and her scholarly approach to her trans* experience exemplify a number of intersectional issues core to trans* feminisms and to nondominant feminist research in general. For example, she explains intersectionality in her particular context by addressing the 1990s and 2000s developments in feminist and queer theory as "portraying gender as something that we "do' rather than something that we 'are'" (p. 5), which she and many others find only partially sufficient. While she acknowledges that much has changed in media representations of trans* women and voices, she laments that, particularly in feminist circles, there is still so much conflict and misunderstanding when exploring the diverse feminisms and gender expressions that typify trans* feminisms. Yet she also tracks an important trans* contribution to feminist research.

Yet these very perspectives have caused discomfort for thousands of lesbian feminists (and others) who have been socially ostracized and marginalized for being "masculine women," a gender expression that is fairly universally read as "aggressive," "angry," or at least unwanted in the mainstream. These kinds of tensions persist even (and sometimes especially) within feminist conceptual and methodological considerations and enactments in this area of study and activism.

Trans* Feminisms

At the risk of overgeneralizing, feminism circa the '70s and '80s was largely disdainful of femininity, portraying it as a set of artificial behaviors that women were coerced into achieving in order to appease men. By the '90s, this view was increasingly challenged by third-wave feminism and the femme movement [and, I would add, by postfeminism]. While I was certainly influenced by these latter movements, I was often disappointed by how they only tended to defend certain 're-appropriations' of femininity. For instance, they would praise riot grrrl fashions, or femmes who are paired with butches, for being nontraditionally feminine and/or for re-working femininity toward feminist or queer ends. This, of course, implied that traditional and/or heterosexual expressions of femininity remain suspect . . . the premise that femininity is inherently artificial and only exists for men's benefit struck me as not only false but patently sexist . . . the wholesale condemning of femininity is one of the more unfortunate missteps in the history of feminism.

Serano (2016a, p. 6)

Thus, Serano's (as well as Stryker and others') scholarship concerning gender, **cissexual privilege** (having transitioned from male to female) and the exclusion of trans* women's politics from many feminist organizations and events are important and pivotal scholarly contributions toward understanding trans* feminisms today.

Genderqueer Diversity Theory: Jack Halberstam

Halberstam's work on female masculinity, drag, gender, and queer sexualities over the past 25 years has influenced many fields, feminist research among them (2012, 2011, 2005, 1998, 1993). With the rise of transgender studies in particular, Halberstam's contribution to queer theory and gender and trans* scholarship has meant that feminist and masculinist studies have by necessity moved away from cisgender (born or biological gender identity) identifications and into more gender-fluid approaches to these two growing fields.

Halberstam has—in a series of groundbreaking works—continued to challenge simple "his" and "her" gender identities and focused instead upon the performance of gender identities, including his/her/their own. Halberstam for a long time refused to choose a binarized his or her gender identity and pronoun, continuing to use his/her/their scholarship and profile as a way of reminding readers that gender identifications can now be fluid, multiple, or "gender creative" and ever changing. One small example of how Halberstam did this was by never correcting anyone's use of any pronouns to describe her/him/them. In more recent times (post-2017), Halberstam is currently represented by male pronouns, yet his scholarship and personal commentary in this respect remain an important provocation for considerations of nonbinary gender expressions. Halberstam's research on gender has also importantly intersected with other (broader) analyses of social codes and power relations under Western capitalism and global consumer culture.

Halberstam's long-term project regarding gender fluidity and what he calls "floating gender pronouns" as a flexible intervention into gender essentializing influenced the thinking of many regarding the role of feminism as a field of study, theoretically, methodologically, and politically. Halberstam has noted the importance of Roxanne Gay's text *Bad Feminism* (2014) as a "game-changer" moment in feminist theory in which the feminist scholarly discourse successfully "crossed over" and reached a popular audience. For Halberstam, the politics and theory of queer feminisms are inherently linked, which his work reflects and which he attributes to having come of age with the political activism and feminist sensibilities of Andrea Dworkin and Catherine McKinnon during the height of second-wave 1970s feminism in Minneapolis, where he studied.

Halberstam Research Snapshot: Feminist Rage and "Imagined Violence"

In a 1993 essay on Prabitha Parmar's film *A Place of Rage,* Halberstam argues that "rage is a political space opened up by the representation in art, poetry, in narrative, in popular film, of unsanctioned violences committed by subordinate groups upon powerful white men" (p. 191), and explores the relationship between **imagined violence** and enacted violence. While today's era of small- and large-scale terrorist acts suggests that real violence seems to be escalating, the political space of **feminist rage** seems to be shrinking. The kind of feminist rage that characterized second-wave feminism (think bra burning and large-scale pro-choice marches, etc.) is no longer popular or even, some would argue, an effective way of galvanizing public opinion and fighting for social intervention. Even in affect studies—an emerging field defined by its attention to emotions and intensities of experience—both rage and feminism seem to be in short supply.

The notion of feminist rage and an increasing numbness to both real and imagined violence is exemplified by a recent Christmas card photo circulating on Facebook. In it, a white American family of five is portrayed like this: the mother and two daughters' mouths are taped and their wrists bound with a string of Christmas lights, while the father and son smile on, thumbs up, with a sign that reads "Peace on Earth." The power of this image, which Halberstam discussed in that 1993 essay, seems as relevant today as the rage this photo unleashed online about the relationship between imagined and real domestic violence.

Popular culture images like these provoke the question: has anything changed at all for gender equality, either imagined or "real," in the 22 years since that essay was first published? Halberstam wrote that "we have to be able to imagine violence and our violence needs to be imaginable because the power of fantasy is not to represent but to destabilize the real" (1993, p. 199). Halberstam's large and important body of work offers readers both popular cultural and poststructural ways of exploring the explosion of gender proliferations, as well as "paradigm proliferations" (Lather, 2008a) for understanding what feminism has to offer 21st-century researchers.

Girlhood Studies

Another area of feminist inquiry that typifies 21st-century research praxis is that known as **girlhood studies**. There is significant crossover in girlhood studies with postfeminism and also youth studies, yet it remains distinct in its focus on the ways contemporary girls and young women respond to gender politics and navigate new landscapes of gendered presentation including the digital world, and the ways social media has changed young women's understanding of themselves, but also changed the ways they are popularly portrayed by nongirls and men. Some significant contributors to this field of study include Jessica Ringrose, Marnina Gonick, Emma Renold, and Lisa Weems (see, e.g., Ringrose & Renold, 2016; Gonick, 2004; Gonick, Renold, Ringrose, & Weems, 2009). Youth studies scholar Anita Harris's (2004) *All about the Girl* focuses on the important subgenre of girlhood studies within the field of youth studies and addresses additional intersectional concerns of recent contemporary feminism, including rape culture and digital media. Both Michelle Fine's foreword to the book and Harris's introduction offer useful overviews of important turns in 21st-century girlhood and feminist research.

A number of edited volumes such as *Girlhood: A Global History* (Helgren & Vasconcellos, 2010) demonstrate the wide scope of girlhood studies (this volume, for example, traces girlhood studies since 1750), and have offered welcome and comprehensive histories of research that focus on girls and girlhood, but it's worth noting that there are still considerable limitations in the ways girlhood is categorized.

Primarily, girlhood is still largely conceived of in traditional cisgendered ways and categorized and studied in terms of regional, cultural, and ethnic identifications, girls and education, interpersonal constructions and communications, and digital media/activism.

Postfeminism

The scholarly area of **postfeminism** is not far from Serano's discussion of femme or feminine gender expressions. Yet the nuances here—confusing as they sometimes are—are important to the evolution of 21st-century feminist research. Some scholarship suggests that postfeminists and third-wave feminists believe different things, with postfeminists believing that

> **Postfeminism** "broadly encompasses a set of assumptions, widely disseminated within popular media forms, having to do with the 'pastness' of feminism, and whether that supposed pastness is merely noted, mourned, or celebrated" (Tasker & Negra, 2007, p. 2).

there is no longer a need for traditional feminism as expressed in third-wave feminisms.

Some claim that postfeminism is rather an expansion or extension of second-wave feminism. However, many leading feminist scholars, including Rosalyn Gill and Jessica Ringrose, have worked against this polarization. It is important to note, however, that all of these are important evolutions of feminist research, which in itself indicates its vitality and relevance. Such debates also point to the pervasiveness of diverse and at times vicious expressions of **backlash**[4] that have continued to plague the feminist project throughout history.

Rosalyn Gill (Gill, 2016; Gill & Scharff, 2011) and Angela McRobbie (2004, 2008) have led the field of postfeminism, followed by an explosion of work in this area in the second decade of the 21st-century. Education and cultural studies scholars Jessica Ringrose, Emma Renold (Renold & Ringrose, 2011), and Amy Dobson (2016) have published widely on the topic, as have Projansky (2007), Tasker and Negra (2007), and Jackson, Vares, and Gill (2012). In an overview of third-wave feminism and postfeminism, McRobbie offers,

> Feminism is aged and made to seem redundant. Feminism is thus cast into the shadows, where at best it can expect to have some afterlife, and

---

[4]Backlash is generally considered to be a kind of pushback against most political movements or movements for social change. Feminist backlash has been particularly well documented, though, due to the relentless and almost universal resistance to equal rights for women. In 1991, Pulitzer Prize-winning author Susan Faludi argued that the media fuel these misogynistic trends, in a book called *Backlash: The undeclared war against American women*, which continues to be relevant in today's debates over postfeminism and non-Western feminisms globally.

where at worst it might be regarded ambivalently by those young women
who must in more public venues stake a distance from it, for the sake of
social and sexual recognition. (2004, p. 3)

McRobbie also notes that "postfeminism is, for me at this stage, an
enabling concept for the examination of a number of intersecting but also
conflicting currents . . . broadly, I am arguing that for feminism to be
taken into account, it has to be understood as having already passed away"
(2004, p. 3).[5] She takes 1990 as a turning point which marks "the moment
of definitive self-critique in feminist theory" at which

> the representational claims of second-wave feminism come to be
> fully interrogated by postcolonialist feminists like Spivak, Trinh, and
> Mohanty, among others, and by feminist theorists like Butler and Har-
> away who inaugurate the radical denaturalizing of the postfeminist body
> (Spivak 1988; Trinh 1989; Mohanty 1995; Butler 1990a; Haraway 1991)
> [in which] there is a shift away from feminist interest in centralized power
> blocs (e.g., the state, patriarchy, law) to more dispersed sites, events, and
> instances of power conceptualized as flows and specific convergences
> and consolidations of talk, discourse, attentions. (pp. 4–5)

She concisely summarizes why young female students (like the one in
the opening of Chapter 3) decline the invitation to celebrate their female
elders' feminist identifications, a shift throughout the 1990s and early
2000s that some have described as the failure of feminism and women's
studies courses in higher education. These distantiations and disengage-
ments from feminism, McRobbie says, "have consolidated into something
closer to repudiation than ambivalence, and it is this vehemently denun-
ciatory stance which is manifest across the field of popular gender debate.
This is the cultural space of postfeminism" (2004, p. 6).

Many postfeminist scholars, including Gill and Scharff (2011), have
identified a need for the links between neoliberalism and postfeminism
as "mutually reinforcing discourses or logics and how neo-liberalism is
'gendered,'" particularly the ways in which "both discourses thrive on a
current of individualism and free choice, arguing women are to a greater
extent than men figured in the dynamics of change, transformation and
self-regulation invoked through neoliberalism" (Ringrose, 2013, p. 4). Set
within education contexts, this link establishes worrisome measures for
what constitutes female success.

---

[5]Note that McRobbie has adapted this chapter from a lecture she gave at Yale University
in October 2002, and some like Halberstam might claim that much has changed in social
feminisms, especially those expressed and performed in online/social media, in the intervening 14 years.

In education, these links and patterns emerge as a kind of "moral panic" (shared group anxieties), which Ringrose calls "postfeminist panics" about girlhood, a way to make transparent "the power of some educational discourses to grip the public imagination and individual psyches and enliven controversy and fear over the 'gender order'" (Connell, 1987; Ringrose, 2013, p. 5). Postfeminist scholar Rosalind Gill has argued that while postfeminism has become a central term of feminist critique in recent years, it is often used in fuzzy or shifting ways. Yet three clear distinctions remain:

1. Postfeminism has been positioned as a "new feminism," implying an epistemological break with earlier feminisms, aligning it with postmodernism or poststructuralism (Genz, 2006);

2. Postfeminism is conflated with third-wave feminism (Gamble, 2001);

3. Postfeminism has been described as a "media-generated 'backlash' discourse that blames feminism and women's gains for social ills, generating new forms of 'retrosexism' or 'new sexism,' that suggest men are the victims of political correctness, affirmative action, etc." (Ringrose, 2013, p. 5).

Angela McRobbie on Postfeminism

McRobbie (2008) asserts postfeminism as a kind of focus for critical analysis rather than a new theoretical orientation, whereas Ringrose, using "the notion of 'post' to signal different spaces and moments," understands postfeminism as "a 'sensibility' or set of dominant discoursees that infuse and shape the zeitgeist of contemporary culture" (Ringrose, 2013, p. 6).

McRobbie (2004, 2008) describes postfeminism as "a set of defensive gender discourses and politics in our contemporary era, that position feminism as having achieved its aims and as therefore now not only obsolete but regressive and backward, which suggests that women have unlimited choice and options to 'succeed'" (Ringrose, 2013, p. 65). For more on postfeminism see also Banet-Weiser (2007); Gonick (2004); Banyard (2010); Baker (2008); Gonick, Renold, Ringrose, and Weems (2009); Ringrose and Renold (2016); and Griffin (2011).

One contribution postfeminism in all its forms continues to make, however, is a confrontation of the Marxist foundations upon which feminist theories have been built, upending the inherent consumer culture critique and asking in new ways what women-identified subjects might be, or indeed want. Yet this axis forms its most widespread **critique** as well.

As Tasker and Negra note, "it is important to note that postfeminism absolutely rejects lesbianism in all but its most guy-friendly forms, that is, divested of potentially feminist associations and invested with sexualized glamour" (2007, p. 21), an extension of McRobbie's famous observation that the "new female subject is, despite her freedom, called upon to be silent, to withhold critique, to count as a modern, sophisticated girl" (McRobbie, 2007, p. 34).

While the postfeminist subject has potentially unprecedented "voice" and "power" in online/off-line contemporary worlds, critics continue to argue that the form of this power is more limited and heteronormative than before the advent of even first-wave feminism.

Critiques of Poststructural Feminism

1. That "poststructural feminist theory is more concerned with language and discourse than with working to improve the everyday oppressions women suffer" (St. Pierre & Pillow, 2000, p. 8). In particular, Martha Nussbaum's critique of Judith Butler highlighted a more general concern with jargonism and inaccessibility of the language of poststructuralist feminism.

2. That a focus on the fluidity of subjectivity shifts the methodological but also epistemological project of standpoint and postmodern feminism, which is still unrealized.

CONCLUSION

In this chapter we have explored postmodernist and poststructuralist feminist theory, building on its foundations in humanist feminist theory, in order to explore the great variance and range of feminist conceptual and theoretical frameworks available, and to demonstrate how they can be largely understood as flowing in two main streams.

The breadth of both theory chapters also reflects the incredibly large and rich body of feminist literature and discourses available to 21st-century feminist researchers today, and we acknowledge that even these cannot be exhaustive explorations due to the exciting and constantly evolving nature of this field. In Part II, "Feminist Approaches to 'Doing Research,'" we discuss the ways in which these and other feminist theories inform the methods that you might choose to conduct feminist research, and the ethical issues each implies.

DISCUSSION QUESTIONS

1. Brainstorm (on paper or with a friend) the core differences between post-modernist and poststructuralist feminism.

2. Why is it important to hear from feminists from different parts of the globe, if we are living in a global culture?

3. Discuss the usefulness of working in "gender studies" or "feminist studies," considering that much of this chapter detailed the reasons for not adhering to static ideas of "women" and "men."

ACTIVITIES

1. Research the origins and different perspectives of one "postfeminist" and one "feminist" scholar of the 21st century and contrast their views.

2. Create a mind map of native feminisms from at least three parts of the globe and compare/contrast them.

3. Research a regionally specific body of feminist scholarship not from the global north and share your findings about what makes this feminism distinct from Euro-American feminisms (e.g., Central or South American feminism, Middle Eastern feminisms, Russian feminism).

4. Using one of the videos provided as an example, make a feminist "manifesta" in the same "in her own words" style, proposing a new feminist theory of your own.

SUGGESTED RESOURCES

Books

Carson, R. (1962). *Silent spring.* Boston: Houghton Mifflin.

This classic text warns of the poisoning of the earth and its inhabitants, and the relationship between these practices and patriarchy.

Collins, P. H., & Bilge, S. (2016). *Intersectionality.* Cambridge, UK: Polity Press.

A comprehensive introduction to the concept of intersectionality, its ascendency, and its praxis in popular and scholarly culture.

Combahee River Collective. (1986). *The Combahee River Collective statement: Black feminist organizing in the seventies and eighties.* New York: Kitchen Table/Women of Color Press.

The Combahee River Collective was a Black feminist lesbian organization, active in Boston from approximately 1974 to 1980, that was at the forefront of bringing attention to the fact that the second-wave feminist movement was largely White and middle-class, and was overall not inclusive of the different concerns of women of color. Barbara Smith, who became instrumental in raising lesbian issues even within the Black feminist movement, was central to the CRC and later cofounder of Kitchen Table Press.

Datara, C. (2011). *Ecofeminism revisited: Introduction to the discourse*. Jaipur, India: Rawat Publications.

A great introduction to ecofeminism from a non-Western, non-Northern States perspective, avoiding the biological determinism that some have argued against.

Dobson, A. S. (2015). *Postfeminist digital cultures: Femininity, social media, and self-representation*. New York: Palgrave.

A clear, yet complex, treatment of postfeminism within digital cultures and online/off-line performances of gender.

Fine, M. (1997). *Off white: Readings on race, power and society*. New York: Routledge.

A core text on whiteness studies and the need for intersectionality scholarship in any feminist (or other) critical considerations of equality and social practices.

Gamble, S. (Ed.). (2004). *The Routledge companion to feminism and postfeminism*. London: Routledge.

A great introduction to the differences/overlaps between these different identifications and theoretics.

Grosz, E., with Cheah, P. (1998). *Irigaray and the political future of sexual difference*. Baltimore: John Hopkins University Press.

A close analysis of Irigaray's writings on sexual difference.

Phoca, S., & Wright, R. (1999). *Introducing postfeminism*. New York: Icon Books.

An excellent introduction to postfeminism overall.

Rai, S. M. (2008). *The gender politics of development: Essays in hope and despair*. London: Zed Books.

Offers important alternative gender perspectives on nation building, globalization, global governance, and the politics of development.

Ress, M. J. (2006). *Ecofeminism in Latin America*. Maryknoll, NY: Orbix Books.

A cogent argument for the connections between diasporic subjectivities and ecofeminist custodianship of the earth.

Singh, K. D. (2004). *Feminism and postfeminism: The context of modern Indian women poets writing in English.* New Delhi: Sarup & Sons.

Postfeminism from beyond the "center."

Smith, D. E. (1987). *The everyday world as problematic: A feminist sociology.* Boston: Northeastern University Press.

An introduction to some core concepts of feminist sociology.

Sprague J., & Zimmerman M. K. (1993). Overcoming dualisms: A feminist agenda for sociological methodology. In P. England (Ed.), *Theory on gender: Feminism on theory* (pp. 225–280). New York: Aldine de Gruyter.

A valuable core text on the sociology of feminism.

Sturgeon, N. (2008). *Environmentalism in popular culture: Gender, race, sexuality, and the politics of the natural.* Tucson: University of Arizona Press.

Linking popular culture and the intersectional nature of the eco-movements.

Tasker, Y., & Negra, D. (Eds.). (2007). *Interrogating postfeminism: Gender and the politics of popular culture.* Durham, NC: Duke University Press.

An accessible and cogent critique of postfeminism.

Wilkinson, S., & Kitzinger, C. (Eds.). (1993). *Heterosexuality: A feminism and psychology reader.* London: SAGE.

A foundational volume for feminist psychologists.

Articles and Chapters

Alaimo, S. (1994, Spring). Cyborg and ecofeminist interventions: Challenges for an environmental feminism. *Feminist Studies, 20*(1), 133–152.

A Haraway scholar addresses environmental feminism.

Butler, J. (1997). Subjection, resistance, resignification: Between Freud and Foucault. In *The psychic life of power: Theories in subjection* (pp. 83–105). Stanford, CA: Stanford University Press.

A core essay from the poststructuralist gender guru herself.

Colebrook, C. (2013). Modernism without women: The refusal of becoming-woman (and post-feminism). *Deleuze Studies, 7*(4), 427–455.

An excellent introduction to postfeminism.

Deleuze, G. (2005). What can a body do? In *Expressionism in philosophy: Spinoza* (pp. 217–234). Brooklyn, NY: Zone Books.

A core poststructuralist essay on the body as performance and affect.

DeVault, M. L. (1996). Talking back to sociology: Distinctive contributions of feminist methodology. *Annual Review of Sociology, 22,* 29–50.

A foundational essay on feminism in sociology.

Dzodan, F. (2011). My feminism will be intersectional or it will be bullshit. *Tiger Beatdown, 10.* Retrieved from *http://tigerbeatdown.com/2011/10/10/my-feminism-will-be-intersectional-or-it-will-be-bullshit.*

Essay on the inescapability of intersectionality in minoritarian subjects and others.

Fraser, N., & Nicholson, L. J. (1990). Social criticism without philosophy: An encounter between feminism and postmodernism. In L. J. Nicholson (Ed.), *Feminism/postmodernism* (pp. 19–38). New York: Routledge.

I have mentioned postmodernism and feminism, which are the focus of the chapter.

Harris, A. (2010). "I Ain't No Girl": Representation and reconstruction of the "Found Girls" of Sudan. *Race/Ethnicity, 4*(1), 41–63.

A redress of the gendered exclusion of South Sudanese girls and young women from the popular construction of refugee identities.

Linstead, S., & Pullen, A. (2006). Gender as multiplicity: Desire, displacement, difference and dispersion. *Human Relations, 59*(9), 1287–1310.

A Deleuzian treatment of gender as a site of intersecting practices.

Lord, B. (2011). "Disempowered by nature": Spinoza on the political capabilities of women. *British Journal for the History of Philosophy, 19*(6), 1085–1106.

A sophisticated analysis of Spinoza's commentary of women and women's agency.

PART II

Feminist Approaches to "Doing Research"

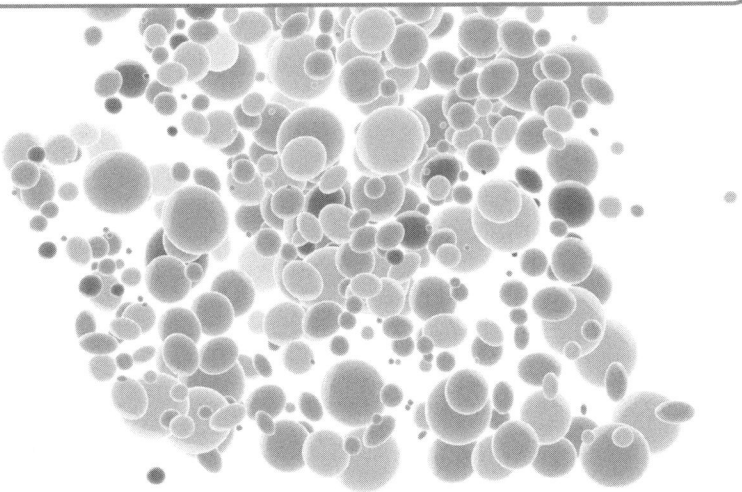

CHAPTER 5

Feminist Ethics

> Voices from the past were interspersed with those of my
> participants, and at times, I also heard my own.
> —ROBERTA P. GARDNER (2015, p. 124)

LEARNING OBJECTIVES

- To explain what ethics are
- To provide a historical overview of ethics in research, including the effects of the social justice movements
- To learn about cultivating and implementing feminist ethics in practice during all phases of research from topic selection to the dissemination of research findings

---

Feminist research requires us to balance embodied standpoints, commitments to social and political justice, and respect for the dignity of all those affected by our research practice. It requires us to listen to ourselves, our participants, our data, and the needs of those communities in which we are enmeshed as well as the broader feminist community we aim to serve. This is necessarily a political, activist undertaking. Even when using methods that value "objectivity," the act of feminist research is value laden, not value free. Even when feminist researchers create knowledge for the sake of knowledge, as opposed to making direct attempts to apply that research to some real-world situation, the enterprise still aims to chronicle, document, and revise the historical record. Feminist research is always *engaged*. These complex and dynamic commitments infiltrate both the feminist understanding and practice of **ethics**.

Feminist researchers have long been at the forefront of discussions regarding ethical research practice and have contributed immeasurably to our understanding and practice of ethics. Samantha Brennan (1999) has gone so far as to suggest there is now a "blurring" between ethics and feminist ethics.

Ethics as Moral Reasoning

The word "ethics" comes from the Greek word *ethos,* which means "character." Ethics is about morality—making determinations about what is right and wrong. The history of theorizing morality and how, in fact, we determine right from wrong has itself been shaped by androcentric (male-centered) bias, which feminists have sought to correct.

Psychologist Lawrence Kohlberg, a key figure in the literature on moral development, created a prominent theory about how people reason through ethical choices (Colby & Kohlberg, 1987; Kohlberg, 1981).[1] He posited there are six stages of moral development operating on three levels: (1) preconventional, (2) conventional, and (3) postconventional. He theorized that at the latter two levels people make choices based on rules and principles. He assumes this applied universally to people and made no room for gender or other differences. Women consistently scored lower on moral decision making according to Kohlberg's system. This was because women emphasized maintaining and building relationships over uniformly applying abstract principles. Based on his classifications, which were grounded in male ways of rationalizing, women were deemed inferior at moral reasoning. The criterion was not based on female ways of rationalizing. This illustrates the need for feminist researchers to investigate a host of topics, including ethics. Today, feminist ethics has grown into a distinct topic in philosophy (Bell, 2014; Brennan, 1999; Tong & Williams, 2009).

Feminist psychologist Carol Gilligan (1982, 1995) contributed greatly to our understanding of ethical decision making by exposing the gender differences Kohlberg failed to account for. Gilligan asserted women's decision making is *relational* and thus based on value for relationships over universal principles. Gilligan modeled a relational understanding of ethics that challenged binary thinking. The binaries on which research had historically been based—objective/subjective, absolute/relative, abstract/concrete, universal/particular, cognitive/affective, principle/relationship—all

---

[1] Kohlberg was influenced by Jean Piaget's work.

inevitably privileged one side of the binary. Those privileged sides of common binaries are identified in bold:

objective/subjective
absolute/relative
abstract/concrete
universal/particular
cognitive/affective
principle/relationship

Now consider this common binary:

male/female

When looking at all of these polarizations and which sides of the binaries are privileged (in the first position), a pattern emerges as to what is viewed as superior. These binaries uniformly privilege male ways of reasoning. It is the other, undervalued sides of these binaries that represent female ways of knowing. Those sides are identified here in bold:

objective/**subjective**
absolute/**relative**
abstract/**concrete**
universal/**particular**
cognitive/**affective**
principle/**relationship**

To be clear, we do not wish to further essentialist thinking that assumes males only think in one way and females in another. Nor do we wish to normalize a male/female binary, which is also problematic. However, as gender is socially constructed and we develop different perspectives that are based on our positionality within gendered societies, there is evidence to suggest that males and females may approach ethical problems differently. Further, feminist scholars do not aim to privilege either side of these binaries, but rather expose their inherent fallacy. By challenging dualistic thinking, feminist researchers have expanded our understanding of what morality is and how individuals engage in questions of "right" and "wrong" in actual situations.

The dismantling of dualistic thinking has prompted new ways for feminists to conceptualize morality. Margaret Urban Walker (2007) suggests morality is located in "practices of responsibility" in which there are "shared understandings about who gets to do what to whom and who is supposed to do what for whom" (p. 16). Nel Noddings (1984, 2003) developed the concept "an ethics of care," which is grounded in relationships and activities (Bell, 2014) and has also been written about by others (e.g., see: Edwards & Mauthner, 2002; Ellis, 2007; Held, 2006). What these perspectives have in common is a *situational* and *relational* view of morality.

A Historical Glance at Ethics in Research Practice

> **Ethics:** Ethics is an area in which our ideas about morality merge with our practices (e.g., research procedures, regulations).

Understandings about morality, which are constructed and constantly evolving, impact how we conceptualize and practice research. Ethics is an area in which philosophy and praxis merge (Leavy, 2017). There is an ethical substructure that impacts the entire research process (Hesse-Biber & Leavy, 2011; Leavy, 2011a; Leavy, 2017). We each bring a philosophical values system to the research experience, which, in turn, shapes decisions we make about how to carry out research (the level of praxis). Neither do our community standards or individual values regarding ethical practice develop in a vacuum. Both the discovery of the history of abuses in biomedical research and the cumulative effects of the justice movements have shaped contemporary ethical practice.

The Exploitation of Research Subjects

Sadly, there is a long history of biomedical abuses and the exploitation of human research subjects. In World War II brutal experiments were conducted on prisoners in concentration camps that often resulted in death or mutilation. For example, gruesome experiments were conducted on homosexual prisoners to "cure" them of their so-called sexual deviance. As a result of these war crimes, the Nuremberg Code (1949) was established, outlining rules for experiments involving human beings. For example, voluntary participation became established as a standard. While the Nuremberg Code was not a law, it was a significant first step in prompting the medical community to regulate itself. In 1964 the Declaration of Helsinki was created, which, together with the Nuremberg Code, forms the basis for federal codes regarding the treatment of human participants in medical research.

Unfortunately biomedical abuses have not been exclusive to times of war, nor has the United States remained immune from such violations. The Tuskegee Syphilis Experiment, which occurred from 1932 to 1972, is the most well-known case of unethical biomedical research in North America. In 1932 the U.S. Public Health Service began working with the Tuskegee Institute. They recruited 600 poor, African American men in Alabama, 399 who had syphilis prior to enrollment and 201 who did not. What makes this experiment unconscionable is that the men did not know they had syphilis and were not treated for it. They were instead told that they had "bad blood" and were being treated for that. By 1947 penicillin was the legitimized treatment for syphilis, but the researchers still withheld it from the unknowing research subjects. Many of the men in the study died of syphilis and related complications, many infected their wives, and some had children born with congenital syphilis. The experiment was only stopped in 1972 when the truth was leaked to the press. Although only made known publicly in recent years, from 1946 to 1948 the U.S. Public Health Service conducted even more unethical experiments in Guatemala on prisoners and patients in mental health facilities. They purposely infected 696 people with syphilis and in some instances, gonorrhea, and then treated them with antibiotics.

Racism, and more specifically, stereotypes about African American men being sexually promiscuous, permeated Tuskegee. The men in the study were not regarded as medical patients, or even as human beings, thus absolving the doctors involved of treating them to the best of their abilities. They were deemed only as research "subjects" available for the exploitation of the researchers. As a result of Tuskegee the research community developed a new set of principles or values regarding the rights of human participants in research studies. Participants began to be viewed as people first, with the right to know the nature of the study they are participating in, including possible risks and benefits, and to voluntarily choose whether or not to participate. The term "research subject" has also been called into serious question. Today, most researchers use the words respondents, participants, or collaborators. Feminist researchers, in particular, tend to use the words "participants" or "collaborators." Further, over time a **principle of mutuality,** of research benefiting both the researchers and participants (Loftin, Barnett, Bunn, & Sullivan, 2005), has become important to many practitioners, particularly feminists. This harkens back to the earlier discussion of the feminist challenge to binaries and why many feminist researchers reject the objective/subjective and researcher/researched dichotomies that served to create otherness and privilege researchers.

These core values were put into ethical praxis with the development of various codes and regulations regarding research. The Tuskegee Syphilis Experiment precipitated the Belmont Report (1979), which led to the development of the National Commission for the Protection of Human Subjects. It also led to federal laws regarding **Institutional Review Boards (IRBs)** and the protection of human beings in research.

Institutional Review Boards, Regulation, and the Protection of Research Participants

IRBs were established in universities in order to ensure that ethical standards are adhered to, and to determine and regulate morality in research practice. As a result of the historical abuses reviewed in the last section, *first do no harm* became the primary principle governing the protection of research participants. Adapted from the biomedical community, this principle states that no harm should come to research participants. This protection is extended to the settings in which research occurs in cases where you are conducting research in real-world environments such as the participant's community. IRBs dictate **procedural ethics** (Ellis, 2007).

Prior to beginning any data collection, including contacting potential research participants, you must seek permission from your IRB. This process involves creating a proposal for review and approval. It is not uncommon to have to revise and resubmit your proposal, often multiple times. Consult with your university website regarding the specific requirements for your IRB; however, generally they require you to detail the purpose of the study, the benefits of doing the research, the intended outcomes, the population you are interested in, your proposed sampling strategy (how you will select participants), the possible risks to participants (which may include physical, psychological, and/or emotional harm), benefits to participants, and your plan to garner informed consent (which means that participants understand what their participation will entail, the possible risks and benefits, and that their participation is voluntary, can be discontinued at any time without recourse, and is confidential, and their anonymity will be protected).

While IRBs have been the best system we have been able to devise to protect research participants, it is by no means perfect. Some researchers note there has been a noticeable shift from a focus on morality to a focus on **regulation,** which has serious implications for feminist researchers (Miller & Boulton, 2007, as cited in Bell, 2014). In her review of feminist ethics,

Linda Bell (2014) offers an example of how the shift to a discourse of regulation has changed the ethics landscape for feminist researchers.

Feminist researchers Christine Halse and Anne Honey (2005) wanted to do research with Australian women engaged in "self-starvation," a broad label that did not satisfy their IRB. They encountered numerous problems over labeling and thus defining the group they were interested in sampling. They did not feel comfortable labeling participants as anorexic if they did not self-define as such and noted a host of potential ethical problems in doing so. In short, they felt such a label would compromise their feminist ethics as they attempted to work with a vulnerable population. However, the institutional ethics committee reviewing their proposal was working within a set of strict guidelines that didn't make space for the broad and inclusive labeling of their sample. Bell writes: "[they] had to engage not only with the challenge of obtaining a suitable sample that need not restrict their feminist ideals, but also with the challenge of an ethics committee whose officers could not see the relevance of their arguments (2014, p. 85)." After going back and forth with the ethics committee, they ended up compromising and defining their sample as "girls who have received a medical diagnosis of anorexia nervosa" (Halse & Honey, 2005, p. 2147). However, this "solution" impacted who they were able to recruit as participants and left them feeling as if they had compromised their morals. They write: "our positioning as actively complicit in perpetuating this story undermined our ethical and moral responsibility to our participants and had troubling moral implications for our desired identities as ethical feminist researchers (Halse & Honey, 2005, pp. 2147–2148, as quoted in Bell, 2014, p. 89).

The preceding illustrates the challenges feminist researchers can have as they confront review boards that have the power to deny or approve their research (Bell, 2014). Any researcher can face challenges in their attempts to obtain IRB approval. However, given the ideals that many feminist researchers are committed to, coupled with a predilection for working with vulnerable populations and studying sensitive topics, feminist researchers may be particularly disadvantaged if IRBs focus on linear "rule following" and "box checking" overtakes their focus on working ethically with research participants. Halse and Honey have continued to explore this topic and suggest that one set of regulatory standards and the discourse that accompanies it has "infiltrated different disciplinary traditions and research methods" with disregard for those differences (2007, p. 340). They note that the prevailing "discourse of ethical research" has had "colonizing effects" in which feminist and particularly qualitative researchers are disadvantaged (2007, p. 340). Similarly, Elizabeth Chin (2013) has noted that feminist ethnographers are often judged more harshly by IRBs. She suggests feminist researchers should challenge how IRBs operate. In her view, IRBs should employ feminist principles in order to carry out their work, operating in an open, dialogical, and collaborative manner (Chin interview in Davis & Craven, 2016, p. 100).

The Effects of the Social Justice Movements

> **Power-sharing:** One way in which feminists account for power in the research process is to create methodologies based on power-sharing with research participants.

The social justice movements of the 1960s and 1970s—the civil rights, women's, gay rights, and labor movements—reflected and created significant shifts in our cultural values. Not only have feminists been involved in all of these movements, but both the general and feminist research landscapes have changed as a result. A common effect of the social justice movements was a reexamination of power within the research process. The goal was twofold: to stop the production of knowledge that continued to be complicit in the oppression of minority groups and to engage in the production of knowledge that carries the potential to do some social good. Different segments of the research community began to reconsider why we undertake research, who should be included, what topics are valuable to study, and the uses to which research might be put. All researchers have been impacted by these ideas, but they have shaped feminist researchers' values system in specific ways.[2]

Feminist educationalist Judith Preissle (2007, p. 515) notes that feminism itself is a "moral and ethical framework" that guides the research practice. The justice movements further articulated values *within that framework*, including inclusivity, addressing inequalities and injustices, societal betterment, and agendas opposing sexism, racism, homophobia, and classism. Further, the justice movements illuminated the potential for feminist research to become a major vehicle for identity politics and correspondingly, social change, including influencing public opinion and policy.

Across the research landscape at large, inclusivity centered on including underrepresented groups in research. This often meant seeking out

---

[2] We do not intend to homogenize feminist researchers, nor the value system from which individual feminist practitioners are operating. However, just as a focus on the lives of girls and women is a constant across the feminist research landscape, so too are some of the ways in which feminist research practice has been influenced by the justice movements although there are many variations there.

White women, people of color, and sexual minorities for inclusion as these groups had formerly been rendered invisible in research or included in ways that reinforced stereotypes. However, research practices ranging from the kinds of questions asked to the **methodologies** employed often remained the same. Many of these attempts simply added women to preexisting research agendas. Inclusivity has been more complicated for feminist researchers, who already always placed the concerns and experiences of **girls and women** at the center of research practices. In addition to prioritizing the concerns, situations, and experiences of girls and women, feminists have sought to ask *new* research questions, ask old questions in *new* ways, build *new* methodological strategies, and include underrepresented groups. As noted in Part I of this text, feminists of color and queer theorists posed serious challenges to the historically White, middle-class, heterosexual concerns that dominated feminist research practice. Feminist researchers more broadly began to consider issues of intersectionality—combining opposition to sexist/classist/homophobic/racist/ableist agendas, as well as indigenous perspectives. Feminist researchers also explored the origins of many of our methodological practices, which have been exclusionary.

With a renewed understanding that social research can be an important vehicle for identity politics, social change, and influence on public policy, issues of audience also received greater attention. This issue will be discussed in depth in Part III of this text.

Reflexivity

Through a reexamination of power in the research process, **reflexivity** has become a guiding concept in feminist research. Feminist postmodern, poststructural, and postcolonial theories have contributed to our understanding of reflexivity (Carroll, 2013; Doucet, 2008). Reflexivity addresses how power comes to bear on the research process and how we reflect on our own position within the research endeavor. Feminist researcher Katherine Carroll (2013, pp. 550–551) writes: "being reflexive requires the researcher to situate her personal, political, intellectual, theoretical and autobiographical selves during all stages of research (Doucet, 2008), and interactional process of growing self-awareness that occurs in relation to the environment and seeing the self from the perspective of others (Rosenberg, 1990; Turner & Stets, 2005)." Throughout the research process we must ask ourselves how our role is shaped by our personal experiences and characteristics (Brisolara & Seigart, 2007). Our own presence in the research process, as embodied actors enmeshed in social contexts, influences our methodological decisions and the knowledge we create (Stuart & Whitmore,

2006). Reflexivity requires us to be mindful of the **context of discovery,** which is where we account for our own role in the research process as embodied social actors. This is about personal accountability and an awareness of the complex role of power in research practice. Therefore, the context of discovery is not only about "*what* we have discovered, but *how* we have discovered it" (Etherington, 2007, p. 601).

> **Feminist epistemologies:** Concerns surrounding how power shapes the research process encourage many feminist researchers to work from epistemological positions that place researchers and participants on the same plane.

Being reflexive in our research practice means paying attention to how power influences our attitudes and behaviors, and our own role in shaping the research experience. Reflexivity also requires us to pay attention to *difference* and how differences in status characteristics and experiences guide research projects from topic selection all the way through to data interpretation (Hesse-Biber & Leavy, 2007). These differences must be acknowledged, explored, and embraced, as they cannot be disavowed (Hesse-Biber & Leavy, 2007). There are related issues of hierarchy and authority. Many feminist researchers reject a hierarchical relationship between researchers and participants. There are a range of power-sensitive or power-attentive approaches one can adopt (Haraway, 1991; Pfohl, 2007).

Another way that we engage in reflexive practice is to be attentive to issues of **voice.** This term is typically used to talk about the ability to speak and is implicitly political (Hertz, 1997; Motzafi-Haller, 1997; Wyatt, 2006). Who is seen as an authority? Who has the right to speak on behalf of others? The issue of speaking for those with whom we share differences or who may be members of marginalized or oppressed groups, often referred to as "others" in the social science literature, is an ethical quagmire. As we have learned from the social justice movements, it is important to seek out the perspectives of those who have historically been marginalized for active inclusion in the knowledge-building process. However, when doing so we must be very mindful of the ways in which we attempt to speak for others or represent the experiences and perspectives of others. In our attempts to be inclusive we don't want to inadvertently colonize the stories and experiences of others. In this regard, it is important to be cognizant of these issues and to carefully reflect on how we position ourselves and others in representations of our research.

There is also an important issue of "emotional reflexivity," which will be discussed in the section on balancing roles and relationships during data generation.

Ethics in Research Practice

Ethical issues come to bear during all phases of research design and execution, including data generation, analysis, interpretation, representation, and dissemination.

Topic Selection

Ethical considerations begin with topic selection. Researchers initially come to a topic because of some combination of personal interests, experiences, and values, previous research experience, and/or opportunities (such as funding or invitations to collaborate). There are a range of pragmatic issues to consider in order to ensure the topic is researchable, such as access to participants, funding, available time, and emotional readiness for the project. This last issue is not self-explanatory and carries real significance for feminist researchers, so we will elaborate.

Research carries psychological and emotional aspects that need to be considered during topic selection. As feminist research is necessarily conducted on a topic deemed justice related, it is likely to have deep personal or political meaning for the researcher. Further, feminist researchers often study sensitive topics (Dickson-Swift, 2008). These are topics that may be highly personal for participants, making them feel vulnerable. Taking on these kinds of topics inevitably requires "emotional labour" (Hochschild, 2003) on the part of the researcher. This emotional labor becomes "part of the job" of conducting the research (Hochschild, 2003). **Emotional labor** refers to self-disclosures, demonstrations of empathy and support, and other ways in which the researcher's emotions are called upon in order to facilitate the project (Carroll, 2013). Therefore, many research topics aren't merely sensitive for the participants, but the process also calls on the emotions of, and deeply affects, the researcher. Research environments can be "fraught with emotional landmines" (Boler, 1997, p. 255). This issue is elaborated later in the section on trust, rapport, and emotional reflexivity.

When you are considering a topic to investigate, take a personal inventory and ask yourself these questions: Will this topic make your participants vulnerable in ways that require you to be vulnerable? Is the topic something you have personally experienced, and if so, how will that impact the research? Is this a sensitive topic for you, and if so, do you feel emotionally capable of carrying out the research? Having personal experience with a topic can be an asset, so we in no way intend to suggest the topic cannot be personal or sensitive for you. However, it's important to get real with yourself and do an honest gut check about your relationship to the topic and the potential emotional aspects of delving deeper into it and whether or not that is something you feel able and willing to take on.

Beyond pragmatic and personal issues it is also vital to consider the **significance, value, or worth** of a project. While all researchers should contemplate the value of studying a particular topic, this is paramount for feminists, whose work is necessarily a part of a larger enterprise that is implicitly and explicitly value based.

> **Girls and women:** Topic selection involves a reckoning with the objectives of feminism that centers on improving the lives of girls and women across differences.

To begin, does this topic align with your feminist values system? What is the social justice imperative to learning more about this topic? Is it important, in relative terms, to learn more about this topic? How will learning about this topic address an identified social need, promote new learning, or prompt social change? How will learning about this topic benefit the lives of girls and women? The value of the topic may also be connected to timeliness. Who are the potential beneficiaries of this knowledge? Do current events or "the current political, economic, and social climates" make it important to study this topic at this time (Adler & Clark, 2011, p. 81)? Is there a need for researchers to learn more about this topic in order to advocate on behalf of girls/women? Can the research be applied in some real-world setting in order to make the world better for girls/women? As feminism is a politicized position from which to conduct research, changes in the political or public policy landscape may serve as an impetus for research. For example, at a time when federal funding to Planned Parenthood is being threatened, feminist researchers may be incentivized to conduct research relating to women's health, reproductive rights, and specifically those whom Planned Parenthood serves. Or, as another example, at a time when marriage equality is being debated or threatened in a specific country, feminist researchers in that country may be motivated to conduct research regarding the individual and societal impact of marriage inequality. Further, depending on the feminist framework from which you are working, you may have additional concerns in selecting a worthy topic. For example, Cynthia Dillard's (2008) "endarkened feminist epistemology," reviewed in Chapter 3, is predicated upon conducting research on behalf of Black people (and to advance the Black global community). Similarly, when working from an indigenous theoretical standpoint, research proceeds based on the perspectives and needs of indigenous peoples (Tuhiwai Smith, 2002, 2012). These are just a couple of examples of how one's theoretical and philosophical framework impacts the ethics of topic selection.

Finally, you must ensure there are no potential **conflicts of interest**. For instance, if your research is funded, make sure that the funder's agenda does not compete with your own feminist agenda. There should be no pressure or monetary gain for deriving certain outcomes or research findings.

Informed Consent

Once you have received formal IRB approval to carry out your proposed research you need to obtain informed consent from the research participants. Bear in mind that you begin to form a relationship with participants and set the tone for what that relationship will be at initial contact. All contact with potential research participants should be respectful. You may begin by providing potential participants an **invitation or recruitment letter**. While you don't want to overwhelm people, the letter should outline the basics of the study (Leavy, 2011b, p. 35):

- Identification of yourself as the researcher and your interest in the topic and qualifications (if there is more than one researcher, each one should be identified)
- The purpose of the study
- Why or how they have been selected as a potential participant
- What their participation would entail including the time commitment
- Information about how and when follow-up to this letter will occur
- Contact information for the principal investigator or whoever they should contact if they have questions or concerns

Here is a sample invitation/recruitment letter (reprinted with changes from Leavy, 2011b, pp. 35–36):

Dear Jane Smith,

My name is Patricia Leavy, and I am a sociology professor at Stonehill College, where I have taught for 10 years. I am writing to you because I am conducting an oral history interview study about the experience of divorce for stay-at-home mothers. Through my recruitment process, your name was mentioned as someone who might be interested in participating.

Should you choose to participate, your participation is completely voluntary and you are free to change your mind and stop your participation at any time. Your identity will be kept strictly confidential. It is my hope to publish this study as an academic journal article; however, I will not use your name or any other identifying information.

Your participation would mean that I would set up two or three interview sessions with you, lasting 60–90 minutes each. I would work around your schedule. The interviews could be held in my office, your home, or another quiet location of your choosing. I will provide light refreshments and reimburse you for any travel expenses.

I am very interested in the issues women face regarding marriage, parenting, and work. I myself have been divorced and raised my daughter as a single parent for many years. I think you have valuable knowledge to share that could benefit others. It is my hope that the interview experience would be personally rewarding for you, as well.

I can be reached at (phone) or (e-mail) to answer any questions you may have. I will follow up in 1–2 weeks with a phone call to see if you're interested in learning more (unless, of course, I hear from you first). Thank you.

Sincerely,
Patricia Leavy, PhD

Once you have individuals interested in participation, you will need to obtain their written **informed consent**. Check the website for your academic institution for their guidelines and samples they may provide. There are also many discipline-specific examples available online. Generally, your written informed consent request should include the following (Leavy, 2011b, pp. 36–37):

- Title of the research project
- Identification of the principal investigator (and any other researchers) with contact information
- Basic information, including the purpose of the project and the research methods/procedures
- The intended outcomes of the project (including plans for publication)
- Details about what participation entails, including the time commitment
- Possible risks of participation
- Possible benefits of participation
- The voluntary nature of participation including the participant's right to withdraw at any time
- The participant's right to ask questions

- The steps that will be taken to ensure confidentiality and privacy
- Compensation for participation (even if there is none this should be stated)
- Contact information for the principal investigator or whoever the participant should contact if they have questions or concerns
- A space for the principal investigator and participant's signatures with dates

Here is a sample informed consent letter:

Informed Consent

Title: Oral History Project on Divorce for Stay-At-Home Mothers

Principal Investigator and Contact Information: Dr. Patricia Leavy (contact information)

Purpose of the Study:

The purpose of this study is to learn about the experience of divorce for stay-at-home-mothers from their own perspective. The study aims to produce new knowledge about how divorce impacts the identity of stay-at-home mothers, practical matters such as daily routine, financial issues, and any other points of interest to the participants.

Intended Outcomes of the Study:

The study is intended to contribute to our understanding of the lives of stay-at-home mothers and the impact of divorce on those women. The knowledge gained from the study will contribute to the literature on marriage and family, gender, and identity in the social sciences. The results of the study will be published as an article in a peer-reviewed academic journal, shared in professional conference presentations, and may be published in other forms (such as a book chapter in an edited volume).

Procedures and What Participation Entails:

This study relies on the method of oral history interview, a highly in-depth form of interview in which participants can share their experiences and stories. You will be asked to set up an initial interview expected to last 60–90 minutes. The interview will be scheduled around your scheduling needs. You can elect to have the interview conducted in the principal investigator's office located at (address), in your home, or in another quiet location of your choosing. You may bring a family photo album or any other pictures or objects you wish to share and discuss. During the interview you will be asked a series of open-ended questions about your marriage, divorce, and your life as a stay-at-home mother before and after your divorce. You will be able to speak for as long as you like, and there aren't right or wrong responses. The goal is to share your experience. With your permission, the interview session will be audiotaped so that it can later be transcribed accurately. You will be provided with light refreshments during your interview. After the initial interview there will be an e-mail follow-up within 2 weeks and you will be asked to schedule a second interview (same location and procedure as already described). The second interview is an opportunity to elaborate or explain previous comments and answer new questions that have arisen as a result of your first interview. A third interview session may be requested within 2 weeks after your second interview, if clarifications are needed.

Confidentiality:

Your participation is strictly confidential, your identity will be kept anonymous and you will be assigned a pseudonym (a fictitious name) in any resulting publications or presentations. The audiotapes will be destroyed after they are transcribed and the interview transcripts will only bear your assigned pseudonym. Likewise, any people you mention in your interview will also be assigned pseudonyms. Details that are so specific they might alert readers to your identity will not be used.

Participant Rights and Compensation:

Your participation in this study is strictly voluntary and can be withdrawn at any time without consequence. You also have the right to ask questions at any point during the study. Your time and experiences are greatly valued. While you will not be compensated for your participation, you will be reimbursed for any travel expenses. Please be aware that possible risks of your participation include emotional or psychological distress, brought about by talking about your divorce, children, and identity. Should you experience any distress, please let the principal investigator know. Please be aware that possible benefits you may experience as a result of your participation include having your voice heard and feeling empowered by sharing your experience with the knowledge it may help others.

If you have any questions or concerns about participating in this study, please contact Dr. Patricia Leavy at (e-mail) or (phone).

If you agree to participate in the study, please sign and date this form below and return it to (include information). Once I have received your signed informed consent letter, I will e-mail you to set up an interview time. Thank you.

_____   _____

Participant Signature   Date

In practice, informed consent can be very messy. This is an area in which procedural ethics bumps up against situational and relational ethical issues, which come to bear after you have begun data generation. Situational ethics refers to "ethics in practice" (Ellis, 2007, p. 4). (Situational and relational ethics will be discussed further in the section on balancing roles and relationships during data generation.) The procedural aspect of obtaining informed consent is straightforward. However, once that informed consent has been attained, there are two additional issues to be aware of: process consent and unanticipated experiences.

While informed consent must be obtained prior to beginning research in order to satisfy your IRB, in a project in which participation extends over a period of time, it is appropriate to **process consent** at multiple stages (Adams, Holman Jones, & Ellis, 2015).[3] This means that you designate times to check in with research participants and review consent issues, including the voluntary nature of the study and their right to withdraw. This also provides an opportunity to see how they are doing—if they are experiencing any discomfort, stress, or unanticipated burden from their participation. Likewise this is also a time during which you may hear about the positive benefits of their participation.

A part of obtaining informed consent is detailing all of the possible risks and benefits of participation in the research project. However, despite your best efforts at imagining the likely risks and benefits, no one can anticipate every possible way a participant might be affected, nor can you entirely anticipate every way you as the researcher might be affected. Therefore, it is important to acknowledge that despite your best efforts to foreshadow how the process will unfold, a participant might have unanticipated experiences. Joanna Zylinksa (2005) explains that there is a "surprise element" in social research. R. S. Parker (1990) writes that ethical uncertainty "does not indicate a failure of rule-and-principle-based reasoning; rather, it is a reminder of its limits (p. 36, as quoted in Adams, 2008, p. 178). Tony Adams (2008) summarizes these concerns beautifully:

> Working with ethics involves realizing that we do not know how others will respond to and/or interpret our work. It's acknowledging that we can never definitively know who we harm or help with our communicative practices. And ethics involves the simultaneous welcoming and valuing of endless questions, never knowing whether our decisions are "right" or "wrong." (p. 179)

---

[3]In a short-term study, such as a quantitative survey project or qualitative in-depth interview project where data is collected at one designated time, you don't need to process consent.

These are all issues that emerge once you have begun working with your research participants. It is also important to note that from your initial contact, it can be important to set expectations regarding the nature of your relationships. This may be a mutual process in which you set some boundaries and allow the participants the opportunity to do the same. It is also advisable to begin to set expectations regarding what happens to your relationship at the end of the project. Will you continue to have contact? If friendships are forged, are they sustainable outside of the context of research? What, if any, help do the participants anticipate receiving from you after data generation?

Beyond these issues there is an even murkier quagmire yet to be reconciled in the research community: *those beyond our participants who may be affected by the research.* Many governing ethics policies extend protection not only to primary research participants but also to others who may be impacted by the research (Halse & Honey, 2007). While general codes ask us to consider seriously how other individuals and communities may be affected by research, our standardized practices of informed consent do not include these "peripheral" people. Halse and Honey write:

> By delimiting the "research participants" to the research subjects/objects, the protocols for ethics review occlude from view the many others who are implicated in and (possibly) affected by the research in different ways and at different times, including various individuals, stakeholders, and Others connected with the research projects, research site/s, and/or research "subjects." (2007, p. 342)

They offer their own example of research with anorexic girls, discussed earlier, and note how many others were impacted by their research, including doctors, nurses, clinic staff, relatives of the girls, nonparticipants in the clinic, and others. How can we protect, respect, and ensure we "do no harm" to the greater web of people affected by our research, as mandated by ethical codes, when the regulations we created to enact those codes narrowly focus on the direct "subjects" from who we "collect" data?

Balancing Roles and Relationships during Data Generation

A distinguishing feature of feminist research practice is the emphasis placed on relationships, both between the researcher and participants and the relationship the researcher has with herself during the process. Feminist researchers attend to **relational ethics**. Carolyn Ellis defines relational ethics as follows:

> Relational ethics recognizes and values mutual respect, dignity, and connectedness between the researcher and research, and between researchers and the communities in which they live and work. . . . Act from our hearts and minds, to acknowledge our interpersonal bonds to others. (2007, p. 4)

To begin to understand the complexity of relational ethics it's important to understand that feminists have multiple roles in the research process. Depending on the nature of your project and the level of interaction your methodology entails, your roles may include any combination of the following: methodologist, facilitator, educator, collaborator and activist or advocate (Whitmore, 2014), and friend (see Figure 5.1).

Balancing these roles, attending to the needs of your participants, and developing ethically minded and appropriate relationships per your methodology are the cornerstones of good ethical practice during data generation. What these roles mean in practice becomes clear when reviewing research relationships.

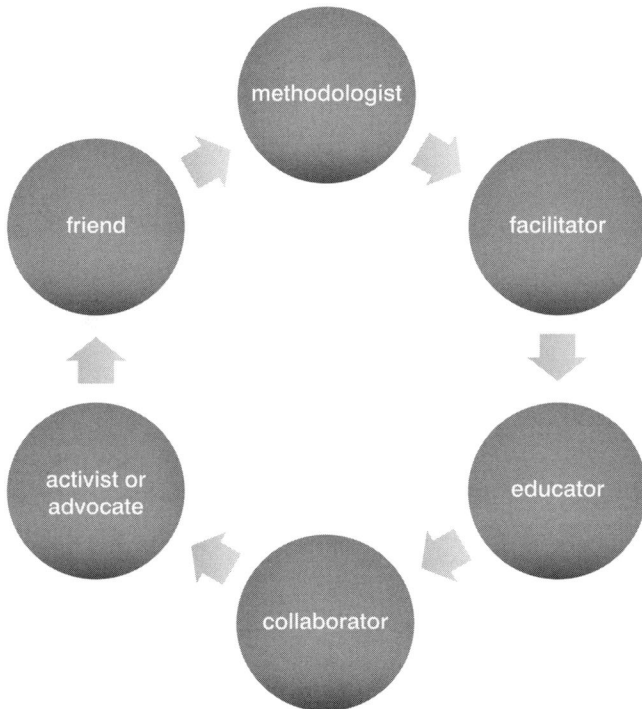

FIGURE 5.1 Researcher roles.

When you're using a research approach that requires you to work closely with participants to unearth data, key ethical issues include building trust and developing rapport. As you attend to these issues, you are in fact building relationships and negotiating your own multiple roles.

Trust, Rapport, and Emotional Reflexivity

Building trust and rapport with participants varies depending on the methodology in a particular study and the level and depth of interaction the methodology demands between the researcher and participants. Building trust and rapport requires researchers to use respectful and culturally appropriate language, explore their insider–outsider statuses, engage in active listening, and, at times, engage in emotional labor such as sharing their own personal experiences and demonstrating empathy and support.

Feminist values regarding **inclusivity** and respecting the dignity of research participants also come to bear during the process of data generation. **Language** is a central issue. While we review participants' use of language shortly in the discussion of active listening, for now we focus on our use of language as researchers.

From the outset, we need to think about how we employ language in all communication and interaction with research participants—both written and verbal communication. With respect to the written word, as we develop our topic, instrumentation for the project (such as a questionnaire or interview guide), and later represent our research for audiences, our use of language must be considered. Likewise, we need to carefully consider the language we use in our interactions with the research participants so that we don't offend or disrespect anyone and in order to cultivate mutually beneficial relationships. In feminist research language is "inclusive, avoids jargon, and is sensitive to differing forms of expression, experiences and perspectives" (Whitmore, 2014, p. 65). Feminists aim to use **culturally sensitive terminology** with respect to status characteristics and other differences. It is important to be culturally competent and employ cultural sensitivity in all dealings with research participants and collaborators (Leavy, 2011a; Loftin et al., 2005) and in the documentation of the process. This means when you are conducting research on or with individuals with whom you have social or cultural differences, such as race, ethnicity, religion, social class, or education, it is important to be mindful of these differences, including different cultural understandings or experiences and commonly used expressions and other ways of communicating. In cross-cultural research "many subtleties" may occur, requiring rigorous attention to developing cultural competence (Whitmore, 2014, p. 65). Some strategies for discovering what language is appropriate with your participants include (Leavy, 2017):

- Literature reviews
- Pilot studies
- Initial immersion into the research setting/field
- Community advisory boards (comprised of various stakeholders in the population you are interested in)

As a result of the historical atrocities reviewed earlier, as well as the values to emerge from the justice movements, some researchers achieve cultural sensitivity by engaging their research participants as full collaborators in the process, which is commonplace in community-based participatory research (reviewed in the next chapter). Celia B. Fisher (2000) suggests feminist researchers should involve participants in all aspects of ethical decision making.

An issue that was touched on earlier is that of *difference*—the differences we may have from our participants. Likewise we may share similarities. **Insider–outsider statuses** are those characteristics you do and do not share with the participants, such as gender, race, age, education, and so forth. Feminist ethics require us to take serious stock of the ways in which we are similar to and dissimilar from our participants so that we can develop respect and trust across those similarities and differences. Audre Lorde (1984) complicated notions of insider–outsider with the term "outsider-within." For example, we may conduct research in a low-income neighborhood similar to the one we came from, so we share some common experiential knowledge with our participants. However, we are now highly educated with a doctorate degree, work in a university environment, and live in a middle-class neighborhood. Our present-day lives do not resemble the lives of our participants, and we share considerable differences. We are not simply insiders anymore; we are outsiders with unique insider knowledge, and thus may be uniquely positioned to understand and empathize with participants with whom we now also share distinct differences.

Active listening is a basic requirement for building trust and rapport with the research participants. Researchers show an active interest in the participants' experiences and stories through deep listening, using appropriate body language and facial expressions, and signaling that they care about the participants' experiences. In the context of a feminist framework showing this kind of interest requires deep and multilevel listening.

Marjorie L. DeVault and Glenda Gross (2007) advocate "radical, active listening." This approach to listening requires "a fully engaged relationship" in which you listen for "gaps and silences" and "pauses and patterns" as you attempt to put what you are hearing into a context (Hesse-Biber & Piatelli, 2007, pp. 149–150). A radical, active approach to listening is compassionate and acknowledges that sometimes our participants can't find suitable language to express their feelings (DeVault & Gross, 2007). Language itself is not gender neutral and reflects male bias (Richardson, 1981). The need to listen deeply to what is said, how it is said, what is said in silences, and what perhaps cannot be said is thus heightened when we work with female research participants. Feminist oral historians Kathryn Anderson and Dana C. Jack note that women's stories are often told from two perspectives, "one framed in concepts and values that reflect men's dominant position in the culture, and one informed by the more immediate realities of a woman's personal experience" (1991, p. 11). When there are no available concepts to reflect their experience, women may "mute their own thoughts and feelings when they try to describe their lives" using the "prevailing concepts and conventions" (1991, p. 11). Anderson and Jack suggest in order to accurately hear women's perspectives "we have to learn to listen in stereo, receiving both the dominant and muted channels . . . and tuning into them carefully to understand the relationship between them" (1991, p. 11).

Sometimes in field research, and community-based research, researchers go beyond active listening into participation by engaging in the activities of the participants. For example, feminist researcher Patti Lather (2000) infamously got into a hot tub with her research participants in order to bond with them and facilitate a research project. Many qualitative researchers advocate "friendship as a method" to garner data and "acknowledge our interpersonal bonds to others" (Adams et al., 2015, pp. 60–61).

Another way that feminist researchers may attempt to build trust and rapport is through sharing personal information and demonstrating empathy. These practices speak to what an "ethics of care" looks like in research practice. This may begin as a personal reflective process. Feminist researcher Venus E. Evans-Winters suggests that in Black feminist research "the researcher often begins with reflection on her lived experiences and brings those insights into the research process" (2015, p. 135). The sharing is often extended into relationships with research participants. Feminist researchers often engage in "self-disclosure, acts of reciprocity and caring . . . showing emotion and empathy or being supportive" (Carroll, 2013, p. 548, citing Dickson-Swift, 2008; Dickson-Swift, James, & Kippen, 2009; Oakley, 1981; Roberts & Sanders, 2005; Sampson et al., 2008).

These acts of "emotional labor" are often required in order to conduct effective research on sensitive topics (Carroll, 2013). This illustrates how a researcher's emotional resources may be tapped in order to build trust with participants and facilitate the research project.

For example, Katherine Carroll (2013) experienced this firsthand when she conducted 20 interviews with female in vitro fertilization (IVF) patients. During the course of the interviews a variety of highly personal topics emerged. Carroll needed to use nonhierarchical, power-sharing, "sensitive research methods" in order to build trust with her participants. This required her to tap into her own reserves of emotion in order to support the participants. In her write-up she interweaves excerpts from her interviews with the IVF patients and excerpts from her own reflexive diary, "which show that emotion is not simply bracketed off while doing sensitive research" (Carroll, 2013, p. 548).

> **Methodologies:** In Katherine Carroll's research we can see how epistemology and methods come together in the development of feminist methodologies.

Sometimes our process of building trust and rapport in the context of sensitive research can push our emotions beyond what we have anticipated. Feminist scholar Cynthia Dillard explains that some stories we encounter from our participants can open up wounds and even "break our hearts" (2012, p. 124). An outstanding example comes from Roberta P. Gardner's (2015) focus group study with Black mothers and children about race and their personal experiences. The participants all lived in a low-income apartment community in the South. Gardner explains that she was prepared to bear witness to the participants' lives but she didn't realize the extent to which she would have to be a witness to herself. This issue emerged when a few of the women started discussing the gang rape of a local woman:

> You heard about ol' girl getting gang raped?
> Yeah, it was like five or six dudes.
> They know they were wrong.
> But come on, she should've known better than to be around them.
>   What do you expect?
> *One of the women glanced my way.*
> You know, she's a loose neighborhood chick.
> Around here, that's what happens when you loose and stupid.
> What happened to the guys that did it?
> Nothing.
> They still around. (Interview, June, 2012).
> (Gardner, 2015, p. 122).

The women's words impacted Gardner deeply, opening old wounds. By staying silent she felt she was being forced to be complicit in promulgating the idea that the woman was responsible for her own rape. Further, she felt complicit in maintaining "the code of silence" the women adhered to in order to cope with the realities of gendered violence in their neighborhood (p. 122). Gardner understood the reality of the environment the women lived in based on her own upbringing. She knew the "mask of a strong Black girl" they were taught to wear in order to navigate the physical dangers and emotional trauma of gendered violence in their neighborhood (pp. 124–125). Their responses to the gang rape reminded her of what it was like when her sister was raped by two men in a public park and she overheard comments "on the back of school buses, in the girls restroom, at the beauty shop . . . on [her] neighborhood street corner" that her sister "should've known better. . . . And that she just should've never gone to that park" (pp. 122–124).

Gardner had to privately break down, in tears, and listen to her own spirit in order to find a way through the research. She did so in order to become "a silence breaker" with the aim of healing herself and "the collective wounds" of her participants (pp. 123–126). In her efforts she developed "a methodology of surrender" that was grounded in "a radical subjectivity stance" based on the principles of love, compassion, and mutuality (p. 127). This is one way in which we can enact an "ethics of care" in highly sensitive research contexts, in which the pain of others taps into our own pain.

Earlier in this chapter we reviewed reflexivity as an outgrowth of the social justice movements. In the examples of Carroll's research with IVF patients and Gardner's research with Black women and children, we see the necessity and complexity of situating oneself in the research process in order to build trust, rapport, and mutuality, and to generate meaningful data. Carroll explains that **emotional reflexivity** can become a source of understanding and analysis in our research (2013, p. 551). We cannot disavow our mental or bodily experiences, including our emotions, as they are tools for conducting effective research on sensitive topics (Carroll, 2013, p. 558). In Chapter 3 we reviewed standpoint and intersectionality theories in fairly abstract ways, but now we can draw links to the ethical practice of feminist research. We must embrace and own our position within the process. For example, Gardner viewed herself as an

> **Reflexivity:** Paying attention to our emotions and other bodily responses is a way of enacting reflexivity during the research process.

"outsider-within" (Lorde, 1984), and it was through embracing that status that she was able to develop her methodology of surrender and develop ethical relationships with her research participants. Citing Elizabeth Dutro (2008), Gardner notes that "we are all positioned and challenged by our wounds" (2015, p. 127). Similarly, Jennifer Griffiths (2009) suggests that unearthing traumatic stories "exposes the vulnerability of listening" (p. 2). Because we are always embodied actors, even when our participants' stories do not bump up against our own, if we are engaged in practices of emotional reflexivity, even active listening alone and the supportive stance it requires can expose our own "vulnerabilities" (Carroll, 2013; Holmes, 2010; Sampson, Bloor, & Fincham, 2008).

Completion of Data Generation

Your ethical responsibilities toward the participants do not end once you have finished data collection. Always remember, these are people whose lives you have disrupted (to some extent) in order to garner valuable information for your research agenda. Depending on the kind of research project you are engaged in, you may build a **debriefing phase** into the research design (Babbie, 2013). This allows you an opportunity to garner feedback from the participants about their experience. Depending on the nature of the project, you may present them with a brief questionnaire, conduct a small focus group, or have a private in-person conversation. In some instances, what you learn during this debriefing phase may cause you to make modifications to the project moving forward or to report on areas you would suggest changing in future research. The debriefing phase is particularly important when the study has investigated sensitive subject matter or presented the research in a form likely to cause an emotional response.

You should also have **resources** for your participants, if appropriate to the topic. For example, if your study focused on eating disorders or body image issues, provide participants with a list of online resources, information about support groups, therapists, and nutritionists, and other professionals who specialize in this area in their community.

It is also courteous to send your participants a letter or e-mail thanking them for their participation. This demonstrates that you value their time and knowledge and may also provide closure for your interactions with them. As noted earlier, there are cases where your relationships with participants continue on after data collection. For example, they may be assisting with the analysis, interpretation, and/or representation of the research findings. Further, you may have developed friendships that will extend beyond the research. Nevertheless, at either the completion of data collection or the completion of their formal participation in the project (such as assisting with representing the research findings) it is customary to send a thank-you letter. Here is a sample letter illustrating the bare bones of what you may include; obviously if this has been highly relational research, as is often the case in feminist research, you may send a much more personalized and detailed letter.

Dear X,

Thank you for your participation in this study (title). Your participation was vital to learning about (topic). I greatly appreciate your time. I will be in touch to pass on my final report on the research study, which I hope to have published in (X amount of time). If you have any follow-up questions or concerns, please contact me at (phone) or (e-mail). Thank you again for your participation.

Sincerely,
Patricia Leavy, PhD

Regardless of whether you have any personal relationship with the participants, it is ethical practice to share your research findings with them. This is discussed shortly in the section on dissemination.

Nonliving Data

Ethical issues still apply in studies involving the collection and analysis of nonliving data such as statistical data, census data, historical or archival data, and other forms of document/textual/visual/audiovisual data. While the issues specific to nonliving data will be discussed at greater length in Chapter 7, here are some of the ethical issues you need to consider during practice (Leavy, 2017):

- Verify the origin of the data.
- Pay attention to any biases or problems with how the data was collected or archived.
- Pay attention to your procedure for dealing with the data.
- Pay attention to anomalies or discrepancies in the data and make sure to report on them accurately.
- Avoid omitting that which refutes your hypothesis or assumptions.

Analysis and Interpretation

The data do not speak for themselves. We have to speak for them.
—W. PAUL VOGT, ELAINE R. VOGT, DIANNE C. GARDNER,
AND LYNNE M. HAEFFELE (2014, p. 2)

What do our data reveal? What do our data mean? How can we derive meaning out of the research experience? Whether we have collected data through surveys, interviews, field observations, or any other method, we need to make sense of what we have learned. While specific data analysis and interpretation strategies vary by method and will be reviewed in Chapters 6 and 7, the processes of sorting any kind of data and imbuing them with meaning requires careful attention to ethics. This is heightened for feminist researchers, who prioritize both respect for research participants *and* contributing to the larger project of feminism.

There are numerous cases where participants have claimed that the researchers "got the story wrong" (Halse & Honey, 2007, p. 338, citing Johnson, 2002). Researchers at all career levels have been confronted with these challenges. Renowned anthropologist Margaret Mead was accused of misinterpretations in her book *Coming of Age in Samoa* (Halse & Honey, 2007, citing Johnson, 2002). Katherine Borland (1991) provides an outstanding illustration of the kind of "interpretive conflict" feminist researchers are vulnerable to.

Borland conducted an oral history project with her grandmother Beatrice. During an interview Beatrice vividly recounted an early experience at the racetrack with her father. She went through a rigorous process to select a horse she thought would win the race. Her father tried to persuade her to change horses, but she insisted on sticking with her choice. Her father begrudgingly placed the bet for her and her horse won. Notwithstanding her win, he again encouraged her to change her horse when she raised her next bet and selected her horse. She won again, which dumbfounded her father. Borland later interpreted this story from her feminist perspective, framing the horserace as a "masculine sphere" and her grandmother's experience as a "female struggle for autonomy" (p. 67). When Beatrice read what Borland wrote, she protested, "That's not what I said." Borland was forced to confront the different ways she and her participant made sense out of the same story.

Part of the conflict evident in Borland's research is that feminist researchers are balancing multiple, complex, and at times competing roles (see Figure 5.1). What does it mean to be an **ally**, activist, or advocate? How do we balance being a methodologist and being a collaborator or in some cases, a friend? How do we educate broad audiences about the

Ally: Becoming an ally can be a difficult process because as feminists we may think we "know the best way to proceed." Being an ally necessitates prioritizing the perspectives of those whom we wish to support.

implications in our research in ways that advance feminism? How can we be an effective facilitator of the stories of others and an effective methodologist analyzing those very stories?

Some of the strategies feminist researchers use to negotiate the process of meaning making with their participants include:

- Sharing data at multiple stages with participants and garnering feedback
- Allowing participants to make corrections/revisions to the data at one or more stages (e.g., correcting statements they made in interview transcripts)
- Working collaboratively with participants during data analysis and interpretation (common in community-based participatory research)
- Noting interpretive conflicts in the final representation(s) and discussing those different interpretations in detail
- Co-sharing the research data (e.g., allowing participants and collaborators to create their own representations of the research data, separate from the researcher's representation of the research)

Representation and Dissemination

As you represent your research findings you will have several ethical considerations. The primary considerations have to do with disclosure of the methodology, the format of the representation, and how you shape the information you present.

Disclosing the methodology involves answering the questions: what did you aim to do and how did you do it (Leavy, 2011b, p. 70)? Disclosing the methodology is sometimes referred to as the **context of justification.** This is where you explain and justify your research design procedures and the methods you employed. Methodological transparency is important so that those who are exposed to your research can understand the process by which you formed your conclusions.

Research may be represented in many different **formats.** Historically research findings were almost exclusively represented as peer-reviewed research articles, reports, or books. Most research studies still result in published peer-reviewed journal articles. However, given the growth in community-based research, the development of emergent methods such arts-based practices, and the goals of feminist research to contribute to social good for girls and women, many feminist researchers represent their projects in other formats. In some instances one research project is represented in multiple formats in an attempt to reach different stakeholders or to emphasize different dimensions of the data. The format you select inevitably impacts who has access to the research findings and that alone makes it an ethical decision. In other words, the format of your research representation is inextricably bound to issues of **audience and dissemination,** which are necessarily bound up with feminist principles of activism and advocacy. Here are some of the ways researchers represent their projects (Leavy, 2011a, 2017):

- Peer-reviewed journal articles
- Research reports
- Conference presentations
- Books
- Brochures/informational pamphlets
- Popular media including op-eds, blogs, vlogs, and podcasts
- Websites
- Artistic forms (in all mediums)

Finally, consider the **content** that you share and how you shape that content. Obviously the form in which you are representing your findings will impact certain considerations. Above all, be honest and truthful. With that said, you have a lot of latitude. You will need to consider what data are included and what, if any, are omitted. As a part of this you will need to make ethical decisions about how to deal with unexpected findings, outliers, or anomalies. Sometimes there is a wealth of data and you simply aren't able to include or reference it all. For example, if you have conducted in-depth group interviews with 25 people you may only quote the exact words of a few people in your research write-up. How do you select which quotes to use? Are they representative of the wealth of data you have collected? How will you contextualize the quotes you selected?

As noted earlier, pay careful attention to language, choosing your words carefully. Use forthright, simple, and clear language whenever possible. Try to avoid unnecessary jargon, and if discipline-specific jargon is needed, define terms so that someone outside of your discipline could follow along. Naturally, also avoid any disrespectful or degrading language and show attentiveness to cultural differences as appropriate to your topic. Soliciting feedback on drafts of the write-up, from participants, members of the audiences we aim to reach, peers, and/or colleagues may be helpful for gauging our use of clear language.

> **Representation:** What you say, how you say it, in what form, and to whom are all ethical decisions.

When working with human participants, strive to sensitively portray people and their situations (Cole & Knowles, 2001). Avoid reifying stereotypes. There are a range of choices you will make that are bound to ethical practice. For example, in a field research or interview study you may quote excerpts from your participants' interview transcripts in your final write-up. When people speak they may stutter, trip over their words, say things like "um" or "uh" or "like," repeat words, and so forth. You'll need to decide how to best represent what your participants have told you. Sometimes researchers beautify transcript excerpts, which means they clean up some of the language to put the participant in the best light. In other cases the researchers do not beautify the transcript excerpts because they may feel it misrepresents or homogenizes the voices of their participants (making them all sound alike). These issues are particularly pronounced when cultural differences are at play. For example, if you are talking with people of a lower socioeconomic or educational background, is it ethical to correct their grammar in quoted transcripts?

Dissemination refers to sharing or distributing your research. As the famous saying goes, "The candle is not there to illuminate itself" (Nowab Jan-Fishan Khan, 19th century). There is an ethical mandate for all researchers, and feminists in particular, to share their findings with others. There are two major questions to answer (Leavy, 2017):

1. With whom do I plan to share the research findings?
2. How can I reach my intended audience(s)?

First, share your findings with your research participants. Historically, social scientists often failed to share the results of their research with participants. Even researchers with the best of intentions can fall into thinking that justifies failing to share the products of research with our participants. For example, Carolyn Ellis, who is now one of the qualitative research community's most vocal advocates of ethics in research practice, writes candidly about mistakes she made in the beginning of her career. As a part of her undergraduate and then later her graduate research, she conducted a study called "Fisher Folk: Two Communities on Chesapeake Bay" comparing two isolated fishing communities. Among the choices she winces at now, her social class biases about those in her study facilitated the idea that she could write whatever she wished because the participants would never see it. She writes:

> It embarrasses me now; however, at the time I sometimes found myself thinking that because most of the people with whom I interacted couldn't read, they would never see what I had written anyway and, if they did, they wouldn't understand the sociological and theoretical story I was trying to tell. (Ellis, 2007, p. 8)

It is important to consider how to share your research findings with your participants. When you engage in this process you inevitably also think about the content of your representations, which facilitates the process of sensitively portraying people and their circumstances. Set expectations up front about how the findings will be made available. For example, this could be covered in the invitation letter and/or informed consent document.

Second, researchers typically share their research findings with their academic research community or communities. It is important that other researchers interested in the subject matter or methodology have access to the research findings. By sharing the research findings within our academic communities we are able to build a repository of knowledge on a topic. Other researchers are able to cite your work in their literature reviews, replicate your study, expand on your study by going in a new direction or using a different population, adapt the methodology, or learn from the limitations of your study. Typically, researchers publish their studies in peer-reviewed journals and present their research at appropriate conferences.

Third, feminist researchers need to decide if they will try to share their research findings with other relevant stakeholders outside of the research academy. In recent years there has been more pressure to share research findings beyond the academy, making research relevant in the real world. This is part of a push toward public scholarship. You will need to make decisions about the audiences you aim to reach and the best way of doing so.

Once you have identified the stakeholders you wish to reach and your goal in doing so, you can determine the best course of action. You may do any of the following, which is by no means an exhaustive list (Leavy, 2011a, 2017):

- Produce popular writings such as op-eds or blogs
- Create a website (which may or may not have an interactive feature for those who log on)
- Appear on local radio or television
- Create and distribute flyers or pamphlets in relevant community spaces

- Offer public lectures in community-accessible spaces
- Share art in venues stakeholders are able to reach (whether it is visual art displayed in a gallery space or library or a performance put on in community theaters or spaces relevant to your topic, from hospitals to schools)

Finally, in some kinds of projects it is also appropriate to **archive** your raw data and/or final research representation. For example, it is common practice in feminist oral history interviews to deposit the transcripts in an appropriate repository. For feminists working with people historically excluded from formal research, it's vital to find ways to document, chronicle, and preserve for the historical record.

CONCLUSION

Ethics is an area in which our ideas and practices merge. Feminists have challenged how the philosophical underpinnings of research practice have privileged male ways of thinking and, in doing so, reconceptualized what research may look like and for what purposes it may be undertaken. This includes our own multiple roles in the process. It's not necessarily about what we do, although it can be, but it is necessarily about *how* we do it, and *why* we do it. Feminist researchers prioritize mutuality, respect, and inclusivity in the research process. Feminist researchers also take seriously issues of power, particularly during data generation and dissemination. We also consider how our research relates to a larger agenda of social justice. To what use or uses will the findings be put? How can we facilitate that process? Keep these issues in mind as you read the next two chapters on methods.

DISCUSSION QUESTIONS

1. How have feminist researchers challenged male-centered conceptions of morality?
2. Why is reflexivity important in feminist practice? What are some of the ways feminist researchers enact reflexivity?
3. How can feminist researchers build inclusivity into their projects?
4. What are the ethical considerations underlying the representation of and dissemination of research findings?

ACTIVITIES

1. Consult your university website's IRB page and download their informed consent requirements. Write a sample recruitment letter and a sample informed consent letter for a project you are interested in conducting.

2. Select a peer-reviewed journal article written by s feminist researcher or research team about any kind of study (ideally pick something in your subject area that is of interest to you). Detail the ethical issues in their study (up to two paragraphs). In their article, have they adequately discussed all of these issues? Justify your conclusion with examples from the article on what they did well and/or what they could elaborate on (up to two paragraphs).

SUGGESTED RESOURCES

📖 *Book Chapters*

Chin, A. (2013). The neoliberal institutional review board, or why just fixing the rules won't help feminist (activist) ethnographers. In C. Craven & D. Davis (Eds.), *Feminist activist ethnography: Counterpoints to neoliberalism in North America* (pp. 201–216). Langham, MD: Lexington Books.

Traianou, A. (2014). The centrality of ethics in qualitative research. In P. Leavy (Ed.), *The Oxford handbook of qualitative research* (pp. 62–77). New York: Oxford University Press.

📱 Select North American Professional Organizations with Online Ethics Codes[4]

Academy of Criminal Justice Sciences (ACJS)

American Anthropological Association (AAA)

American Counseling Association (ACA)

American Educational Research Association (AERA)

American Evaluation Association (AEA)

American Folklore Society (AFS)

American Nurses Association (ANA)

American Political Science Association (APSA)

American Psychological Association (APA)

American Sociological Association (ASA)

National Association of Social Workers (NASW)

National Women's Studies Association (NWSA)

---

[4]Please search online for organizations in other regions.

CHAPTER 6

Feminist Methods for
Working Directly with Participants

In order to learn to listen, we need to attend more
to the narrator than to our own agendas.
—KATHRYN ANDERSON AND DANA JACK (1991, p. 12)

LEARNING OBJECTIVES

- To introduce you to the different approaches to research feminists use,
  including quantitative, qualitative, and community-based participatory
  approaches, and the strengths of each approach

- To learn how to design and carry out a research project using survey
  research, interviews (in-depth, focus group, oral history), ethnography,
  and community-based participatory or participatory action research

- To provide a discussion of the impact of digital technologies on
  emergent feminist research practices, including DIY oral history and
  digital ethnography

There are numerous methods available that involve collecting data from, or generating data with, research participants. In the most general terms, the methods that are available can be classified as either quantitative or qualitative. Quantitative and qualitative approaches to research are based on different philosophical assumptions about the nature of social life and human experience, what can be studied, and how the research process should proceed. Beyond classifying methods as quantitative or qualitative, we view the methods available for working directly with research participants on a continuum with respect to two factors: (1) the level of interaction

128

between the researcher and participant(s), and (2) the depth of the relationship between the researcher and participant(s). (See Figure 6.1.)

The methods reviewed in this chapter flow from those involving the lowest level of interaction between the researcher and participants in the maintenance of a distanced relationship, to those with increasing interaction, and finally to those with the highest level of interaction in which the researcher and participants are full collaborators.

Quantitative Methods

Today, quantitative research is grounded in postpositivist or empiricist philosophy. This tradition asserts reality exists independently of the research process and can be measured via the objective application of the scientific method. **Postpositivism** or **empiricism** is based on probability testing and building evidence to reject or support hypotheses, but not conclusively prove them (Crotty, 1998; Phillips & Burbules, 2000). Given the premium placed on objectivity, quantitative methods that involve working with research participants involve low levels of interaction between the researcher and participants and the maintenance of distanced relationships. Quantitative methods value a breadth of data and result in statistical descriptions of phenomena. So, these methods are well suited for exposing rates of phenomena. For example, quantitative methods can tell us the percentage of women who have suffered a sexual assault. These methods can further tell us how those rates are impacted by any number of factors such as race/ethnicity, religion, sexual orientation, gender identity, geographic location, and age. Further, these methods can be used to study the consequences of sexual trauma, such as how surviving sexual assault is statistically related to other issues, including depression, eating disorders, self-harm, suicide attempts, and so forth.

While the feminist critique of empiricism has been strong, as reviewed in Chapter 3, feminist researchers nonetheless capitalize on the unique potential of quantitative research to address feminist concerns, particularly survey research.

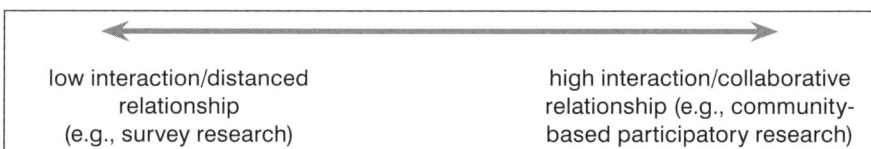

low interaction/distanced relationship (e.g., survey research)	high interaction/collaborative relationship (e.g., community-based participatory research)

FIGURE 6.1 Continuum of researcher participant level and depth of interaction.

Survey Research

In 2013 White women in the United States earned 77 cents for every dollar earned by White men. African American and Latina women earned even less.[1] This simple statistic that women earn 77%, 68%, or 60% of what men earn, which you have likely heard many times, illustrates the power of survey research to advance feminist issues.

Survey research is the most widely used quantitative method in the social sciences. Surveys typically rely on collecting data from large samples that is then analyzed and represented statistically. Surveys are well suited for learning about individuals' attitudes, beliefs, and opinions or their reporting of their experiences or behaviors (Leavy, 2017). While many feminist researchers have critiqued quantitative research for producing androcentric bias and favoring male ways of knowing, others contend there is great power in numbers. Accordingly, feminist researchers and activists have been employing surveys for over 100 years.

In the late 1800s and early 1900s feminist researchers at the University of Chicago created surveys to aid social reform efforts on causes including child labor, unemployment, and reducing poverty (Miner & Jayaratne, 2014; Miner-Rubino, Jayaratne, & Konik, 2007; Miner, Jayaratne, Pesonen, & Zurbrugg, 2011; Spalter-Roth & Hartmann, 1996). These researchers used their data to educate the public and influence public policy (Miner & Jayaratne, 2014; Miner-Rubino et al., 2007; Miner et al., 2011). As times have changed, the topics feminists have studied via survey research have also evolved. In the 1960s and 1970s feminist survey researchers studied issues including rape, divorce, discrimination, and women's health in order to advance public policy (Miner & Jayaratne, 2014; Miner-Rubino et al., 2007; Miner et al., 2011; Spalter-Roth & Hartmann, 1996). Today feminists employ surveys to study any number of topics, including violence, body image, eating disorders, biases in education and employment, sexually transmitted infections and diseases, sexuality, and a host of other topics.

Designing Feminist Survey Research

Survey research begins with transforming your topic into a research purpose statement and a hypothesis *or* a research purpose statement and research questions. Feminists contend two factors distinguish *feminist*

---

[1] In 2013 the per capita earnings of African American women were 68.1% of all men's earnings, and Latinas' per capita earnings were 60.4% of all men's earnings. (Source: U.S. Census Bureau, Current Population Survey, 2014, Annual Social and Economic Supplement, Series PINC-05.)

survey research: the research purpose/
questions investigated, and how data are
interpreted and used (Kelly, 1978; Miner
& Jayaratne, 2014). Feminist researchers ask questions that advance feminist
concerns. In quantitative research these
statements and questions are constructed

> **Girls and women:** Femi-
> nist research questions
> advance the concerns and
> circumstances of girls
> and/or women.

in terms of variables. A **variable** is a characteristic that can be different
from one element to another, or can change over time. For example, sex is a
variable that can differ from one person to another: male, female, intersex.
An **independent variable** is one that likely affects or influences another
variable. A **dependent variable** is a variable that is affected or influenced
by another variable. An **intervening variable** (also called a **moderator** or
mediator) is a variable that can mediate the effect of the former on the latter. Here is an example:

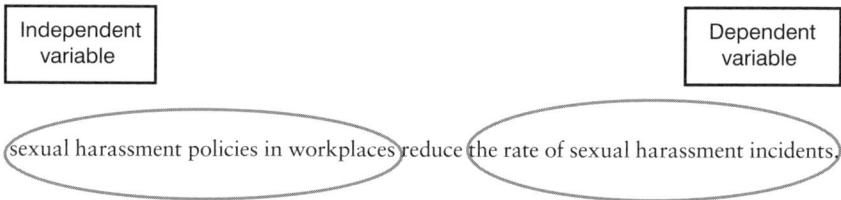

Independent variable		Dependent variable
sexual harassment policies in workplaces	reduce	the rate of sexual harassment incidents.

From a *statistical perspective* (which is important in terms of the tests
you can ultimately run on the data), variables can be classified in two ways:
categorical and continuous (Fallon, 2016). **Categorical variables** have
names and distinguish classes (e.g., male/female/nonbinary, insured/not
insured, religion, race, class year); **continuous variables** differences steadily
progress and "preserve the magnitude of difference between values" (e.g.,
age, income, precise time running a race) (Fallon, 2016, pp. 16–17).

A **research purpose statement** specifically states the purpose or objective of the research project and may note the variable relationship being
tested. A **hypothesis** is a statement predicting how variables relate to each
other that can be tested through research. There are three primary kinds
of hypotheses: A **null hypothesis** predicts there is no significant difference
between two groups with respect to the variable being tested. A **directional
hypothesis** relies on prior research to make a prediction that there is a
specific difference between two groups with respect to the variable being
tested. Finally, a **nondirectional hypothesis** predicts a difference between
two groups with respect to the variable being tested but does not predict
what that specific difference will be.

Weuve, Pitney, Martin, and Mazerolle (2014) conducted a cross-sectional online survey to study workplace bullying (WPB) among female and male athletic trainers (ATs) in college settings.

They state their first two hypotheses as follows (p. 697):

"H1: Female ATs experience more WPB than male ATs."
"H2: Male bullies will be more common than female bullies."

The preceding are examples of directional hypotheses.

As an alternative to a hypothesis you may pose a series of central questions. **Quantitative research questions** are generally deductive and focus on the variables under investigation and how they relate to each other, how they affect different groups, or how they might be defined.

With a working purpose statement and related hypotheses or research questions, you can move on to **sampling,** which determines who participates in your study. Sampling is the process by which you select a number of individual cases from a larger population. An **element** is the kind of person, group, or nonliving item that you are interested in (sometimes the word "unit" or "case" is used in lieu of element.) A **population** is a group of elements that you might later make claims about. So for example, if you are interested in exploring the qualities that draw some college students to feminist activism, the element in your study is individual college students involved in feminist activism. The population you might later like to make claims about is all college students who engage in feminist activism. The **study population** is the group of elements from which you actually draw your sample. If the population you are interested in is "all college students who engage in feminist activism," it will be impossible to draw a sample from that entire population. Therefore, you create a study population, such as all students at two identified local colleges who are engaged in a specific feminist club or program after school. A **sample** is the number of individual cases that you ultimately draw from the study population. These are the participants in your study.

Survey research uses **probability sampling,** which is any strategy in which samples are selected in such a way that every element in the population has a known and nonzero chance of being selected. This means the chance that each element in the population will be included in the sample can be statistically determined, and their chance of inclusion, no matter how small, will be a number above zero. Here are the main types of probability sampling strategies:

• **Simple random sampling (SRS):** Every element in the study population has an equal chance of being selected.

- **Systematic sampling:** The first element in the study population is selected randomly and then every *k*th element after the first element is selected. For example, if your study population is a feminist club membership list comprised of students at multiple colleges, you may randomly select student number 18 on the list and then if you decide *k* = 5, you would select every fifth student on the list after 18 (so 18, 23, 28, and so on until you reach the end of the list).

- **Cluster sampling:** In this multistage sampling strategy, first, preexisting clusters are randomly selected from a population. Next, elements in each cluster are sampled (in some cases all elements in each cluster are included in the sample). For example, if your population is all college students who participate in feminist activism clubs, you might get a list of all the universities in the Northeast with such clubs. Then you randomly select several of those schools—each serving as a cluster—and the students in activism clubs at those schools are your sample.

- **Stratified random sampling:** Elements in the study population are divided into two or more groups based on a shared characteristic (these groups are called strata). Then you conduct simple random, systematic, or cluster sampling on each strata. For example, if you want to compare student feminist activism across class year, divide your elements into four categories: freshman, sophomores, juniors, seniors.

Data Collection in Feminist Survey Research

Questionnaires (or **survey instruments**) are the primary data collection tool in survey research. There are many preexisting surveys available on a wide range of topics. Consult published research on your topic and available online databases to determine whether or not there are preexisting surveys that you can use or draw from to answer your research questions. Survey items (questions in the questionnaire) are designed to help you test your hypotheses or answer your research questions.

Question construction is at the heart of survey research, and there are many books devoted to the topic if you are designing your own instrument; however, we present some guidelines for creating effective survey questions. It's vital to use clear, understandable, and whenever possible highly specific language (Ruel, Wagner, & Gillespie, 2016). For example, avoid slang, abbreviations, contractions, and ambiguous phrases—all of which could be unclear to respondents (Ruel et al., 2016). Pay careful attention to how you word sensitive questions, as they are more likely to elicit nonresponses from respondents (Ruel et al., 2016; Tourangeau & Yan, 2007).

Feminist researchers are particularly attentive to using language that isn't biased (e.g., sexist, racist) (Miner & Jayaratne, 2014, citing Eichler, 1988). Likewise, cultural sensitivity and attention to cultural differences must also be accounted for during question construction (Miner & Jayaratne, 2014, citing Fowler, 1984). Questions should not be leading or biased, or contain built-in assumptions, all of which may pressure respondents toward particular responses (Ruel et al., 2016).

Forced-choice or **fixed-choice questions,** which is what most surveys use, provide respondents with a range of response options to select from. These responses are easily quantified. Different types of forced-choice questions include but are not limited to multiple choice, dichotomous, checklists, and scales (rating scale, Likert scale) (Ruel et al., 2016). Response choices must **be mutually exclusive** and **exhaustive.** Mutually exclusive means there is no overlap in response items, and exhaustive means that all of the possible responses a respondent might wish to select are available.

The organization of your survey instrument (questionnaire) is also important. The layout should be simple, clear, and uncluttered (Fowler, 2014). Consider font style and size as well as the spacing of items on the document. Begin with a short introduction to the survey, providing general instructions. Next carefully consider question order, beginning with engaging questions, locating highly sensitive questions in the middle, logically ordering questions and subsets of questions, and placing demographic questions last in order to reduce respondent fatigue for the substantive questions (Ruel et al., 2016, p. 42). Finally provide a brief conclusion in which you thank respondents for their participation and which may also include a space for open-ended comments regarding their experience (Ruel et al., 2016, p. 37). **Respondent burden** occurs to the degree that respondents experience their participation as too stressful and/or time consuming (Biemer & Lyberg, 2003; Ruel et al., 2016). High burden causes respondent fatigue, which leads to a higher nonresponse rate and lower-quality responses (Ruel et al., 2016). Consider these issues carefully as you determine how many questions are needed to ascertain the data you are after and how many more "burdensome" questions there will be, such as those on highly sensitive or personal topics, those that require respondents to recall past events (Ruel et al., 2016), and those with longer statements or vignettes for respondents to read.

Survey delivery is another important decision. Available delivery methods include, from those with the highest to lowest response rates, in person, online (there are e-mail or web-based software programs such as Survey Monkey), mail, and telephone. For feminist researchers survey delivery is about more than pragmatic concerns such as time and budget. It's important to consider what the topic is, who the respondents are, and what strategy will be least burdensome to them, in terms of their schedules as well as emotionally. For example, Harding and Peel (2007) note web-based surveys are more convenient for single mothers, for whom scheduling a survey time may be challenging. They also suggest participants who wish to maintain their privacy, such as those who identify as LGBTQ, may be more comfortable participating privately via the web rather than in person. A final issue to consider is creating a **respondent inventory** (or a **respondent audit**) in which you keep track of respondents and reduce the risk of multiple responses from one individual (Ruel et al., 2016). Each respondent can be assigned a number for anonymity.

> **Methodologies:** Feminist concerns guide all aspects of developing the research methodology, minimizing the burdens placed on participants.

Analysis and Interpretation of Quantitative Data

Data analysis procedures allow you to determine what the findings are. Has the hypothesis been supported or refuted? What are the answers to the research questions? The analysis process leads to a statistical rendering of the data generally represented in a set of tables or charts along with a discussion. Use a statistical methods book to assist you through this process.

First, **prepare the data** by entering it into a spreadsheet or statistical software program. Before getting into statistical data analyses, it's important to report on the members of the sample who did and did not complete the survey, and note **response bias** (the effect of nonresponses on the results) (Creswell, 2014; Fowler, 2009). There are numerous statistical tests you may run on your data set. It depends what you want to know from the data.

Descriptive statistics describe and summarize the data (Babbie, 2013; Fallon, 2016). There are three kinds of descriptive statistics (Fallon, 2016, pp. 16–18):

1. **Frequencies:** count the number of occurrences of a category. Frequencies are generally reported as percentages.
2. **Measures of central tendency:** use a single value to represent the sample.
   a. **Mean:** the average
   b. **Median:** the "middle" value
   c. **Mode:** the most frequent value in the sample

3. **Measures of dispersion:** illustrate how spread out the individual scores are and how they differ from each other.

    a. **The standard deviation:** the most commonly used measure of dispersion lets you see "how individual scores relate to all scores within the distribution" (p. 18).

Descriptive statistics can be represented visually in tables, graphs, and charts.

Inferential statistics test the research questions or hypotheses and make inferences about the population from which the sample was selected (Adler & Clark, 2011). One common approach to inferential statistics is **null hypothesis significance testing (NHST)** (Vogt et al., 2014). NHST or statistical significance tests are used to test the null hypothesis (which states there is no relationship between the variables). Even though you are actually interested in the alternative hypotheses (the relationships that do exist between variables, and in some cases, the direction of those relationships), you test the null hypotheses in order to avoid **Type I error** (Fallon, 2016). Type I error occurs when you infer a relationship exists that *does not* exist (Adler & Clark, 2011). Significance testing results in a p value (p refers to probability). You are looking for a p score of less than .05, which is expressed as follows:

$$p < .05$$

A p score of .05 means 5 in 100. If your p score is higher than .05 you should not infer a relationship between the variables. A **Type II error** occurs when you do *not* infer a relationship that *does* exist.

Typically, you conduct a significance test on the null hypotheses and any number of inferential statistical tests depending on your questions/hypotheses and the kind of variable relationship(s) you wish to test.

Feminist researchers place their findings in a context to aid interpretation. For example, you may use literature to highlight the implications of the findings. Feminist researchers may also use the results of a survey to seek change. For example, Toby Epstein Jayaratne, Nancy Thomas, and Marcella Trautmann (2003) conducted feminist survey research to evaluate a program intended to keep middle school girls involved in science. They sought to evaluate the effectiveness of different components of the program for nonminority and minority girls. They conducted

> **Girls and women:** Jayaratne, Thomas, and Trautmann's study is an example of using survey research to promote social justice on behalf of girls.

the study in order to generate information that could be used to develop programs that increase girls' participation in science across race.

Qualitative Research

Qualitative research is diverse both methodologically and theoretically. Today qualitative research is conducted from numerous paradigms or worldviews, including interpretive or constructivist, symbolic interactionism, phenomenology, ethnomethodology, dramaturgy, postmodern theory, poststructuralism, as well as feminist, critical race, indigenous, and queer theoretical perspectives

> **Intersectionality:** When using qualitative methods to study microaggressions in any setting, apply an intersectional approach that examines the interlocking nature of two or more status characteristics.

(Leavy, 2017). Regardless of the particular perspective employed, qualitative research values people's subjective experiences and how people attribute meaning to their own lives and within the broader culture. Given the focus on meaning-making processes and experiential knowledge, qualitative methods that involve working directly with participants involve high levels of interaction between the researcher and participants. Cultivating rapport and nurturing those relationships can be an important part of the research process. Therefore, qualitative methods value a depth of meaning. Qualitative methods are well suited for developing rich descriptions of social life and the exploration of phenomena. For example, qualitative methods can unpack the different contexts in which women of different races experience microaggressions in their workplace due to the intersection of their gender and race. These methods can be used to study how they feel when these instances occur, how they respond to these incidents and their reasons for responding that way, how it impacts their work life, and how it impacts them in other areas of life.

Interview Research: In-Depth Interviews, Focus Groups, and Oral History

Interviews of various kinds are commonly used across the disciplines and are a main staple in feminist research. Many feminist researchers have turned to methods of interview in order to document women's experiences and perspectives. Sue Armitage, a champion of women's oral history, says she turned to the method in 1974 when she was slated to teach women's history, searched for local stories about women, and discovered there weren't any (Armitage, 2011). Similarly, Sherna Berger Gluck wrote the following in a 1977 special issue of the feminist journal *Frontiers:*

> Refusing to be rendered historically voiceless any longer, women are creating a new history—using our own voices and experiences. We are challenging the traditional concepts of history, of what is "historically important," and we are affirming that everyday lives *are* history. Using an oral tradition, as old as human memory, we are reconstructing our own past. (p. 170)

Regardless of the particular method, interview formats highlight participants' words and value their subjective knowledge.

In a general sense, interview methods use conversation to elicit data from research participants. Methods of interview differ based on the level of structure imposed, how many interview sessions are conducted with each participant, and whether one or more participants are interviewed at a time. With respect to the level of structure, one-on-one interviews can range from highly structured to semistructured to unstructured. Highly structured interviews resemble survey research, which was discussed in the last section and will not be reviewed further. The three primary qualitative interview methods, all of which are routinely used by feminist researchers, are in-depth interviews, focus groups, and oral history.

Methods of interview are useful for gaining detailed data directly from participants about their experiences and attitudes. Interviews are generally organized around a topic or experience of interest. In-depth interviews and focus groups are typically topical, focusing on a particular issue or experience. For example, participants may all share a common experience (motherhood, adoption, divorce, sexual assault, eating disorders, caregiving for an aging parent or ill spouse, drug addiction, a certain profession) or they may all be responding to a topic or issue (body image, dating culture in college, a political campaign, gender identity). Oral history interviews may be topical and center on a particular experience (surviving a tragedy such as September 11 or the Pulse nightclub killings, surviving a particular genocide, living with chronic pain or a particular illness, immigrating, being a racial minority in a particular job) or they may cover a long period of time in a participant's life or even their whole life, providing a "life history." Here are overviews of the three primary kinds of qualitative interview:

- **In-depth interview:** Inductive or open-ended interviews conducted with one participant at a time. Questions do not have a finite set of acceptable responses, such as yes or no, but rather, participants can use their own language to respond. Responses may be lengthy and involve descriptions, stories, or examples. These interviews may be conducted face-to-face (optimal when possible) or via videoconferencing, Skype, telephone, or e-mail. Interview sessions generally last from 45 to 60 minutes but may be shorter or longer depending on the project. In-depth interviews are appropriate when you want to gather qualitative data from a moderately sized sample of individuals.

• **Focus groups:** A method for interviewing several participants at one time. These interviews are conducted in person. Focus groups produce a "happening" in which data are collected from individuals and the group as a whole. The group dynamic or "group effect" may be a part of the data you collect (Carey, 1994; Morgan, 1996; Morgan & Krueger, 1993). For example, in a mixed-race focus group you may be interested in the dynamic between Black, Hispanic, and White participants (whether/how some people dominate the discussion, cut other people off, agree with each other, whether/how "whitesplaining" occurs, etc.). Focus groups are appropriate when you are exploring a new or underresearched topic, working with a population that may feel disenfranchised (Kitzinger, 1994; Leavy, 2007), want to study the group dynamic as a part of the data, or want to compare groups (e.g., groups of women and men).

• **Oral history:** A type of inductive interview in which one participant is interviewed over several sessions or more, in person. This method is uniquely suited for accessing a significant portion of a person's life or their life history and uncovering processes, and requires very close collaboration between the researcher and participant. Oral history has a political agenda (Turnbull, 2000), as it is a method for bearing witness as it unearths, chronicles, and documents knowledge previously excluded from the historical record (Leavy, 2007, 2011b). Oral history is appropriate when you want to gather rich, qualitative data from one participant or a very small sample of participants. This is a very popular method for feminist researchers.

A brief selection of the many topics feminist researchers have investigated with these various forms of interview includes eating disorders (Hesse-Biber, 2006; Holmes, 2016; Leavy & Sardi, 2006); women's romantic and familial relationships (Leavy & Scotti, 2017); women's sexual experiences (Fahs, 2016); body image and sexual identity (Chmielewski & Yost, 2013; Leavy & Hastings, 2010); menstruation and birth experiences (Moloney, 2011); Jewish women in concentration camps (Saidel, 2004); lesbian physical education teachers (Sparkes, 1994); violence/abuse/intimate partner violence (Allen, 2011; DeShong, 2013); the socioeconomic contexts of women in Cape Town, South Africa (Slater, 2000); cultural identity (Ramji, 2008); the feminist movement (Stephens, 2010); men in court-ordered treatment for domestic violence against female partners (Anderson & Jack, 1991); and adolescent girls and sexual risks (Oliveira, 2011).

Designing Feminist Interview Research

Interview research begins with transforming your research topic into a research purpose statement and research questions and selecting the appropriate method of interview. A **qualitative research purpose statement** focuses on the primary focus or goals of the project. It includes a concise statement of the main topic, problem, or phenomenon, the participants and setting, the method, and the primary reason for conducting the research. It is also typical to include one to three central research questions (which may have subquestions). These questions are designed to focus the research and help you achieve your research purpose. **Qualitative research questions** are inductive and often begin with the words "what" or "how." For example:

- How do female college students describe the nighttime social environment on their campuses?
- How do female college students feel regarding personal safety at on-campus parties or social gatherings?
  - What do female college students think about how their college deals with issues of student safety and sexual assault on campus?

As the process of creating a research purpose statement and research questions is the same across qualitative methods, this description will not be repeated in the section on ethnography.

You also need to determine which method of interview to use. While for the sake of reader ease, we reviewed writing purpose statements and questions prior to selecting an interview method, in practice, you may be working all of these issues out at the same time. In fact, your purpose statement likely notes the kind of method selected. Here's an example:

> This focus group study will compare how female and male college students describe the nighttime social environment on their campuses, including their personal safety, and their perspectives about how their college deals with issues of student safety and sexual assault on campus.

Once you have the purpose and questions and know which method of interview you're employing, it's time to determine who the participants will be. First you have to figure out what kind of participant you're looking for and then you can proceed to sampling. In terms of the kinds of participants you're looking for, feminist researchers generally employ interview methods to learn about women's lives, to compare women's and men's experiences, or to work with groups that may be marginalized, disenfranchised, or feel unsafe (Kitzinger, 1994; Leavy, 2007). Individuals may fit into the latter group based on the intersection of any number of status characteristics or membership in a stigmatized or historically oppressed community. In this regard, feminist oral historians Kristin L. Anderson and Dana Jack (1991) write about oral history as a method for reclaiming "voice." As you think about what kinds of people to interview, consult the literature on your topic and consider whose perspectives, experiences, and voices have been left out. Have women's experiences been included in published research? What about women across racial and ethnic groups? What about women along the sexual orientation spectrum?

Once you know what kinds of participants you're looking for, you can select a sampling strategy. Qualitative research typically relies on **purposeful sampling,** which is based on the premise that seeking out the best cases for the study produces the best data (Patton, 2015). Therefore, it is important to be strategic when sampling in order to find "information-rich cases" that best address the research purpose and questions (Morse, 2010; Patton, 2015, p. 264). Patton (2015, pp. 265–272) identifies 40 kinds of purposeful samples. Here are a few purposeful sampling strategies commonly used by feminist researchers:

- **Snowball sampling:** a process whereby each participant leads to another (Adler & Clark, 2011; Patton, 2015). You may directly ask participants to suggest others who would make good interviewees (Babbie, 2013). For example, if a participant is a particularly good source of information and/or seems to be well connected with the larger group you are interested in, you may ask them to suggest additional participants.

- **Convenience sampling:** involves identifying participants based on their accessibility to you (Hesse-Biber & Leavy, 2011).[2] For example, if you are interested in studying how college students experience peer pressure and you work in a university setting, you may begin your sampling process on your own campus. You look for the best cases within the larger group that you have access to.

---

[2]Some don't consider convenience sampling a true purposeful sampling strategy because you're selecting the most convenient cases, not necessarily the best.

• **Quota sampling:** a strategy whereby you identify the relevant characteristics of the population you are interested in and their overall presence in the population. Then you select cases (participants) to represent each of the relevant characteristics in the same proportion as they are represented in the population.

In some projects you may be looking for a **single case**. For example, oral history may involve the selection of one robust case. There are numerous strategies for selecting a single case. For example, you may seek a single significant case that is an exemplar (Patton, 2015, p. 266).

There are additional considerations regarding selecting and grouping participants for focus groups. Will the groups be comprised of participants who are similar to each other (**homogeneous**) or dissimilar from each other (**heterogeneous**)? For example, in a study about dating on college campuses, do you want to have female, male, and nonbinary students in the same or different groups? Do you want to have students who identify as homosexual, bisexual, and heterosexual in the same or different groups? If you're interested in the group dynamic among male and female students, for example, you may decide to have mixed-sex groups. However, if you are interested in making comparisons across groups, for example comparing male and female students, you may separate groups by sex. The practice of separating groups based on one or more characteristics is called **segmentation**.

It's also important to select a **setting** for the research. Interview research usually occurs in an artificial setting, meaning one in which both the researcher and participant would not otherwise be at that time. Common settings include the researcher's office, a private room in a public library, or the participant's home.

Data Collection in Feminist Interview Research

In order to prepare for data collection researchers create **interview guides** that range from a list of general "lines of inquiry" (Weiss, 1994) to detailed lists of open-ended questions. While oral history interviews generally involve the lowest level of structure, in-depth interviews and focus groups can vary with respect to the structure imposed. If you intend to impose a high level of structure and ask all interviewees the same questions, you need a detailed guide. In focus group research there are two additional considerations. First, if you are employing segmentation and want to compare responses across groups, it's important to standardize the questions. The second consideration, related to standardization, is moderation. When conducting a focus group, the researcher embodies the role of **moderator** (Morgan, 1996). If you want to study the natural group dynamic, the level of moderation should be low; however, if you want to standardize the interviews so that every participant answers the same questions, the level of moderation will be high (Leavy, 2007).

During the interview, the most important aspect of data collection is active listening. Build rapport with participants by demonstrating an interest in what they're saying. Use eye contact, gestures, and probes to show you are listening. A probe can be as simple as "Can you tell me more about that" or "What do you mean by that" or "Do you have a story about that" or even a nonverbal gesture such as a nod (Leavy, 2017). You should also attempt to pick up on **markers**. Participants often drop markers when they are talking about something else (Weiss, 1994). In other words, while they are speaking to one topic, they say something about a different topic that you think may be worth returning to for exploration. While you do not want to interrupt the participant until they have completed their response, you can jot down markers when you hear them and when they have finished their current line of talking, you can return to the marker. For example, in an interview with women about their experiences during their first year of motherhood, you may ask a participant about breastfeeding. In the context of telling you about breastfeeding she describes how exhausted she is and says, "He woke up every few hours and sometimes because he often took so long to start eating, before you know it I was feeding him again, I was exhausted all the time. I felt like I was constantly breastfeeding. It was my main activity. My husband thought we should try bottle feeding but I think it was because he hoped I'd have more energy since we never had time for sex. Anyway . . . " While your participant is speaking you may pick up on the marker she dropped about her sex life with her husband, which you could note on a small notepad with the word "sex" or "husband." Once she has finished with her train of thought you could say, "Thank you for sharing that. When you were talking about breastfeeding you mentioned that you were too tired at that time for relations with your husband. Can you tell me about that?" While not all markers lead to information that is important for your project, often they do. In this example it is possible the participant could go on to describe relationship strain, body image issues postpregnancy, how time-consuming motherhood was during that time, conflicts about parenting, or many other things. In those instances, what is revealed might bear directly on the larger topic of how your participant experienced the first year of motherhood. In short, there may be vital data that would not come out otherwise simply because you wouldn't know to ask.

In addition to direct questioning, there are alternative techniques for ascertaining data in interview contexts. **Enabling techniques** are a way of modifying a question to make it easier for participants to express themselves, and these strategies can be quite useful in social research (Roller & Lavrakas, 2015, p. 140). Examples noted by Roller and Lavrakas include:

- Sentence completion/fill in the blank (e.g., During breastfeeding I felt _____.)
- Word association (e.g., What is the first word you think of when you hear "breastfeeding"?)
- Storytelling (e.g., Tell me a story about something that happened when you first began breastfeeding.)

The preceding approaches are appealing to feminist researchers because they open up storytelling possibilities and allow participants to guide the interview.

Feminist approaches to active listening extend beyond these standard interviewer techniques. Feminist researchers consider the context in which women and men—and women and men across other status characteristics—live their lives and have developed communication styles. There are cultural and institutional contexts for participants' stories (Collins, 1990). Feminist oral historians have added immeasurably to practices that address issues of **sociocommunication.**

Kristina Minister (1991) explains that to interview women we need to alter "the communication frame" because male speaking practices have been normalized and practices of interview have been developed in a "male sociocommunication system" (p. 31). We would add that it isn't simply male ways of speaking, but specifically White, Western male ways of speaking that devalue non-White, indigenous, nonbinary, and female ways of speaking. Minister eloquently states that "interviewers who validate women by using women's communication are the midwives for women's words" (p. 39). How do we enact this? As feminists, how do we validate the sociocommunication styles of our participants and account for the context in which those styles developed?

First, we need to listen to *how* stories are told—the form (Anderson & Jack, 1991). What form do participants use? Male forms of sociocommunication have been normalized and may influence participants' storytelling processes as well as the specific language and concepts they employ, so as feminist researchers, it's important to be aware of those ways of speaking and to remain open to women's communication processes, which may differ from those generally legitimated in the culture (Anderson & Jack, 1991; Minister, 1991). Gwendolyn Etter-Lewis (1991) studied Black women's life story interviews and asked, "How do their unique experiences influence the manner in which they tell their own life stories?" (p. 45). In her research she found three distinct narrative styles: unified, segmented, and conversational. She suggested there's "a connection between the narrator's verbal performance and her views of self and the world" (p. 45).

Second, we need to listen to *what* is said and *what* is omitted—the content. Anderson and Jack (1991) suggest there are three things to listen for: (1) moral language, (2) meta-statements, and (3) the logic of the narrative. **Moral language** refers to "self-evaluative statements" a participant makes (p. 20). Such statements may reveal a disjuncture between the participant's sense of self and cultural norms that dictate what is appropriate. For example, if a woman is talking about sexual partners and then says, "I guess it was sort of promiscuous . . . ," the statement may indicate that her self-concept is influenced by norms around female sexuality and the slut-shaming women often experience in society. **Meta-statements** are moments when a participant cycles back to reflect on something she said earlier. Such statements may reveal that a participant is monitoring her own thoughts and is concerned that something she has said conflicts with expectations of what she thinks should be said. For example, if a woman is talking about sexual partners, moves on to other topics, and then cycles back and says, "When I said I slept with those guys in college it may have sounded slutty but it was just a weird time and . . . " Finally, the **logic of the narrative** requires researchers to pay attention to "internal consistency or contradictions" in statements about themes that recur in the interview (p. 22). For example, if in some instances a participant describes her sexual activities during college in a positive way and then in other statements she reflects judgmentally on those experiences, there may be valuable data about how the participant's story is shaped by cultural forces.

DIY Oral History in the Digital Age

We would like to note one recent development in oral history research in the digital age that carries implications for feminist researchers: DIY (do-it-yourself) oral histories (Armitage, 2011). In a **DIY oral history** there is no trained researcher, rather people record their own stories, sometimes with the assistance of a loved

> **Feminist digital media:** DIY oral histories are an example of an emergent method that has developed in the context of feminist digital media.

one, and the interviews are archived online. Armitage (2011) notes two exemplars of this new trend: YourStory and StoryCorps.

YourStory is a project that emerged out of an interdisciplinary course, "The Life Story," taught by Professor Meg Brady in the English department at the University of Utah in 2003/2004. Students in the course have, since that beginning, collected biographical interviews with various communities in Utah as a means of documenting locals' lives. StoryCorps is an independently funded organization whose "mission is to preserve and share humanity's stories in order to build connections between people and create a more just and compassionate world" (*https://storycorps.org*). They further contend, "Everyone's story matters." On their website stories can be searched for by theme, for example LGBTQ issues, and they have a section devoted to stories told in Spanish.

The extent to which feminist researchers will ultimately take advantage of this new approach remains unclear. For example, feminist researchers could develop project sites in which participants upload their own interview audios around particular themes, or general life story interviews. Or, researchers may, with proper permission, analyze preexisting audios created in this manner, applying a feminist lens to analysis and interpretation. Eroding the power divide between the researcher and participant during data collection and honoring participants' voices as primary seems to be in alignment with core feminist principles. For that reason, feminist oral historian Kathryn Anderson thinks the practice may gain legs, while by contrast Armitage views this approach as "oral history lite" and fears the quality and depth of storytelling may diminish without a trained interviewer to guide the process (Armitage, 2011).

Ethnography

Field research (ethnography) is the oldest qualitative genre, with its roots in cultural anthropology. **Ethnography** refers to writing about culture or a written text about culture. Field research is research that occurs in natural settings, referred to as "the field." The result of field research is an ethnography. Sarah Pink defines ethnography as "a process of creating and representing knowledge (about society, culture and individuals) that is based on ethnographers' own experiences" (2007, p. 22). Traditionally, field research relies on direct observations of people in their natural settings in order to understand social life from the perspective of participants (Bailey, 2007). **Participatory observation** requires the researcher to engage in the activities of the participants, and to record systematic observations. **Nonparticipatory observation** involves direct participation without engaging in the activities of the participants. Ethnographers aim to describe the culture in which the research participants are enmeshed. These approaches to research result in "thick descriptions" of social life (Geertz, 1973). Researchers spent extended periods of time in the field with their participants, often visiting or even living within the community site for months or years.

While feminist ethnography truly emerged in the 1970s as a means of challenging the male-centered ways of thinking about and doing ethnography that dominated the field, women ethnographers have been conducting research on women's lives since the 1800s (Buch & Staller, 2014; Lewin, 2006). Shulamit Reinharz (1992) provides a historical sketch of key publications by women ethnographers, which we summarize. In 1921 Frances Wright, a British woman, published *View of Society and Manners in America, in a Series of Letters from That Country to a Friend in England, during the Years 1818, 1819, 1820.* This work critiqued gender norms and institutions of slavery. In 1837, sociologist Harriet Martineau published *Society in America,* which explored the role of women in American society. In the 1880s Alice Fletcher, an American anthropologist, studied the Sioux people, including camping with them for weeks. Fletcher made an enormous contribution to the field through her contention that "ethnography could be an observational science" (Reinharz, p. 50, quoting Mark, 1988, p. 39). *Middletown: A Study of Modern American Culture,* published in 1929 with a follow-up book in 1937, is one of the most well-known ethnographies. Originally Robert Lynd was using it as his dissertation, and he had a staff of four people on the research team assisting him. His wife, Helen Merell Lynd, one of the staffers, contributed significantly to the book and became its coauthor. However, it was another team member, Faith Williams, who suggested interviewing people in addition to direct observations. Today, interviewing people as a part of ethnographic fieldwork is a norm.

Elana D. Buch and Karen M. Staller (2014) note that while there is a history of American and European ethnographers traveling to study people and places they deemed "exotic," there are now multiple forms of ethnography feminists engage with, which they identify as follows:

- **Native ethnography:** research that is conducted in familiar settings
- **Urban ethnography:** research conducted in cities, also considers "global flows of people, money, and goods" (p. 112)
- **Global ethnography:** research that looks at interconnections between people located in disparate places

- **Critical and applied ethnography:** research that involves collaboration with a community for a real-world intervention (e.g., to study a social policy and lobby for its revision)
- **Visual ethnography:** research that focuses on visual aspects of culture (e.g., photographs, films, social media)
- **Digital ethnography:** research conducted in virtual spaces/cyberspace. With respect to this rapidly growing area, Hsu (2014) distinguishes "media ethnography," which aims to study the role of digital media in society, and "virtual ethnography," which is research that describes life in digital social environments.

To the preceding list created by Buch and Staller, we add the following two practices:

- **Sensory ethnography:** Sarah Pink, a leader in the field, advocates "sensory ethnography," which she describes as "a way of thinking about and doing ethnography that takes as its starting point the multisensoriality of experience, perception, knowing and practice . . . a process of doing ethnography that accounts for how this multisensoriality is integral in both the lives of people who participate in our research and how we ethnographers practise our craft" (2009, p. 1). Pink defines this as a "critical methodology."
- **Autoethnography:** the researcher engages in a rigorous writing practice using his/her/their personal experience as the starting point for inquiry, as a method for connecting the personal to a larger cultural context or phenomenon (Adams, Holman Jones, & Ellis, 2015).

Designing Feminist Ethnographic Research

As with interview research, ethnographic research begins with moving from your topic to a research purpose statement and research questions (already reviewed in the interview section). Participants are generally selected in conjunction with selecting a setting (the field site). In other words, answering the question of *where* the research will occur leads to determining *who* will participate, and vice versa. If you are interested in studying a particular community, that itself likely determines the site and pool of potential participants.

Field research is dependent on the researcher's ability to gain access to the setting and build relationships in the field. This is highly relational work involving deep levels of interaction between the researcher and participants. The first issue to consider is gaining entrance. There can be both **formal and informal gatekeepers** preventing you from accessing the site. Beginning with formal gatekeepers, these can be present in both private and public spaces. For instance, if you wish to conduct research in a members-only environment, such as a private club or rehab group, it is unlikely you will be able to gain entrance unless you are already a member or know a member who can assist you. If you wish to conduct research in a day care, hospital, school, prison, or work environment (e.g., office, construction site), you will need formal permission from a host of gatekeepers before you are able to gain entrance. However, every setting has informal gatekeepers. Each person in the setting in which you are conducting your research can decide whether or not they will participate, and in that sense they are, at a minimum, a gatekeeper to their own knowledge. If multiple participants in a setting do not want you there, then even if they can't keep you out of the space, they can still deny you the kind of access you need in order to conduct your research.

In some settings, feminist researchers may find they have to negotiate conflicting identities and "play the game" in order to make it past gatekeepers. An excellent example comes from Venus Evans-Winters's (2011) 3-year ethnographic project about Black girls' educational experiences. The participants were recruited from two majority-Black low-income schools, but not before Evans-Winters went through a host of formal gatekeepers. When seeking approval from the director of research, Mr. White, it became clear that he thought it would be worthwhile to learn why these students "fail" whereas the research purpose was to learn how they succeed in spite of adversity (p. 65). He also didn't understand why the study would focus only on girls. Evans-Winters made a strategic decision to explain it in a way that he could grasp by responding to his questioning as follows: "Actually, African American girls have one of the highest high school dropout rates, only second to Latinos." He approved the study, barring permission from the school principals. She explains why she shifted to this wording to gain access as follows: "I realized that the general public was accustomed to the language of failure . . . I survived the white man in a suit by using language that most educators and policymakers are accustomed to hearing, and by embracing patience with the system" (p. 66).

Evans-Winters's process of gaining access from formal gatekeepers continued as she met with school principals. She was quite nervous for these meetings and, as is often the case when meeting with school officials, the principal at one school was late for their meeting. She describes how she negotiated her nerves and hid her annoyance from the principal's secretary during this process, and the strategy behind doing so.

I know establishing rapport with the school secretary is the key to getting important information and avoiding excessive red tape. An initial
bad impression with a secretary could cut off access to important student
files, demographic information, easy access to the principal, and other
data. . . . Therefore, strategically I played down my irritation with the
late appointment, along with my anxiety over meeting the principal. I
took a seat next to a group of students, who were also pretending to be
patiently awaiting the principal. (p. 66)

From this example we see how feminist researchers often have to think
on their feet and strategically negotiate issues of access. Further, while the
research director and principal may be conceived of as the formal gatekeepers, Evans-Winters demonstrates that the principal's secretary also held significant gatekeeping power.

Data Collection in Feminist Ethnographic Research

Ethnographic research is dependent on building relationships in the field.
In order to collect data it is necessary to develop **rapport** with the participants in your setting. This is how you develop trust and build a working
relationship with participants. Some participants may become key infor-
mants who not only share their own experiences but also introduce you to
other possible participants and/or provide an overview picture of people
and activities in the setting. Feminist researchers have been at the forefront
of explicating and theorizing two key issues: insider/outsider statuses and
reciprocity. Attention to these issues is often a distinguishing factor of feminist ethnography. In practice, these two issues are often related.

Traditionally, ethnographers were warned that if they were too similar to research participants, it would discredit their research (Buch &
Staller, 2014; Pillow & Mayo, 2007). This is why the history of ethnographic research is rife with Western researchers traveling to other cultures
deemed "exotic" and producing colonizing research on "the other." Feminist researchers challenged the assumption that being similar to research
participants was problematic (Pillow & Mayo, 2007). As you attempt to
gain entrance into the field and cultivate relationships once you are there,
insider–outsider or outsider/within statuses come to bear. You may share
some status characteristics in common with the participants, such as gender, race, and/or age, but you may be an outsider as well, based on different characteristics such as education, job, and so forth. It is important to
be aware of these similarities and differences as you build relationships.
Insider statuses may assist you as you build rapport; however, it is equally
important to be sensitive to differences.

The statuses we bring to bear on ethnographic research, and how they impact our field relationships, are also tied to the key issue of **reciprocity**. Feminist ethnography, sometimes referred to as feminist critical ethnography, aims to problematize unequal relationships between researchers and participants (Junqueira, 2009). Rosalie Hankey Wax (1952) first raised the idea of reciprocity in field research. Influenced by the theories of George Herbert Mead and Sigmund Freud, Wax assumed that humans are capable of understanding what others are thinking and applied this principle to field research relationships. Wax suggested people know when they are being taken advantage of and participants will "resent a manipulative and patronizing attitude" on the part of a researcher who "takes pride in getting something for nothing" (p. 36). Wax urged researchers to consider why someone in the group you're interested in should take time out of their lives for your research. She explained fieldwork is an "exchange" in which the researcher and participants "are consciously or unconsciously giving each other something they both desire or need" (pp. 34–35). For Wax, reciprocity could be as simple as creating a space to listen to someone who doesn't normally have a chance to share their perspectives, experiences, or grievances. It could also involve demonstrating that you respect and value what another is sharing with you. In her own field research, Wax built rapport with working-class women with whom she shared gender identity but not social class by listening to their strategies for dealing with predatory men. Here we see how reciprocity and insider–outsider statues are connected in actual research practice.

> **Feminist epistemologies:** Theorizing reciprocity exemplifies how feminist epistemologies develop over time as researchers continue to engage in questions about power and the nature of participation in research studies.

Since the issue of reciprocity has first been raised, feminist researchers have been committed to putting it into practice, while simultaneously realizing it is a goal that perhaps can never be fully realized. We offer a few examples.

Anthropologist Perry Golde conducted research about decorative ceramics in a small rural village in Mexico in 1959, which was later published in 1970 (Junqueira, 2009). As an attempt at reciprocity, she gave food to her participants. Golde wrote: "How can I repay these people who give so much?" (1970, p. 10). She urged ethnographers to consider what "makes up for the trouble" ethnographers cause by intruding into the lives of those they study (1970, p. 10).

Another commonly cited example is Sofia Villenas's (1996) research on Latina immigrant mothers and their experiences with, and perspectives on, education (Junqueira, 2009; Pillow & Mayo, 2007). Villenas was a Chicana PhD student raised in the United States, and struggled with her insider–outsider statuses. As a means of reciprocity she wanted to become involved in the women's community as a bilingual tutor or teacher. Based on her experiences she advocates for an "ethnography of empowerment" that improves the lives of those in the community being researched. She cautions that feminist ethnography that does not seek to do so is implicated in imperialist agendas. The idea of empowerment promoted by Villenas is echoed by other feminist ethnographers. Eisenhart states ethnography should "empower participants to take greater charge of their own lives" (2001, p. 219).

Our final example comes from Judith Stacey, who has famously questioned whether or not there can be a "feminist ethnography." Stacey specifically turned to ethnography instead of interviews because she thought the method aligned more closely with the feminist principle of dismantling hierarchies in the researcher–researched relationships. In the course of her fieldwork she found herself subject to secrets, betrayals, and forced inauthenticity as she covered up secrets shared by some participants from others. She writes:

> I find myself wondering whether the appearance of greater respect for and equality with research subjects in the ethnographic approach masks a deeper more dangerous form of exploitation . . . fieldwork represents an intrusion and intervention into a system of relationships . . . the researcher is far freer than the researched to leave. The inequality and potential treacherousness of this relationship is inescapable. (1991, p. 113)

Stacey ultimately concluded that there is an unavoidable paradox in feminist ethnography. Because of the relationships developed in the field and the "apparent mutuality," there is far greater danger that participants will be exploited than there is in quantitative research in which no such relationships are formed (1991, p. 114).

Feminist ethnographers or critical feminist ethnographers are not able to reconcile these issues, per se; however, many advocate some form of "good enough" reciprocity or exchange as the answer (Junqueira, 2009). Luttrell (2000) wonders if we can ever really know if our efforts are *good enough,* as research participants may feel pressure to appear grateful (Junqueira, 2009). With this said, most feminist ethnographers make attempts at advocacy or making the concerns of their participants visible and heard as a means of reciprocity. Some refer to this as being a "mouthpiece" for participants and against the injustices they experience (1994, p. 81), or more commonly, an ally.

As you build relationships and follow the protocols of informed consent, it is also important to set expectations about your role in the setting, including how long you intend to be there, whether or not you intend to maintain relationships once you have left the setting, and if so, in what capacity. Setting expectations with participants with whom you are developing relationships is important so that when it is time to leave the field the participants are properly prepared for your departure.

Data collection itself entails a process of systematic note-taking—called **field notes**. Field notes are the written or recorded notes of your observations in the field—they are the data. It is important to date and time field notes to maintain a chronological record. It is also good practice to note the location, and if the field note refers to an interaction with a particular participant or group of participants, note that as well. Field notes should be written systematically. Typically ethnographers set aside a certain time or times in the day for extensive note-taking.

Keep a small notepad or telephone with a voice recording feature in order to "jot down" words or phrases that you want to remember. Those jottings are referred to as on-the-fly notes. There are numerous types of field notes you might collect including those labeled thick descriptions, summary notes, reflexivity notes, conversation and interview notes, and interpretation notes (Bailey, 1996, 2007; Hesse-Biber & Leavy, 2011). Table 6.1, reprinted from Leavy (2017), summarizes the different kinds of field notes (this is not an exhaustive list).

TABLE 6.1. Types of Field Notes

On-the-fly notes	Words or phrases you want to remember
Thick descriptions	Highly detailed descriptions of the setting, participants, and activities observed. When describing the setting use your senses to paint the scene, and when describing participants and activities use their exact language and other specifics when possible.
Summary notes	Daily or weekly summaries of what you learned in the field and things you intend to look for or follow up on
Reflexivity notes	An ongoing accounting, or regular gut check, of your role as researcher in the process. Comment on your feelings, ethical dilemmas or issues, and relationships in the field.
Conversation and interview notes	Notes about each informal or formal topic, details of what was said (using exact words when possible). Include follow-up questions or names of others you want to speak with.
Interpretation notes	Notes about your sense-making process (including what you think something means).

Try to capture as many details as you can, including the exact words of participants whenever possible. Given the breadth of data you will be collecting, it is vital to have a good organizational system and catalog your field notes regularly.

Memoing is also a vital part of data production in ethnographic research. **Memo notes** help you develop your ideas about your data (field notes), synthesize your data, integrate your ideas, and see relationships within the data (Hesse-Biber & Leavy, 2005, 2011).

In addition to observations (field notes) and your analysis and impressions (memo notes), you may also informally and/or formally interview participants. Field research typically produces an abundance of data in the form of field notes, memos, and interview notes or transcripts. As this kind of research occurs over a lengthy period of time, you'll know it is time to exit the field and cease data collection when you have reached the **saturation point**. This means that you are not learning new information and may be losing clarity. If you are engaging in a recursive process of collecting and analyzing data, sometimes referred to as data analysis cycles (Tenni, Smith, & Boucher, 2003), it can help you realize you've reached data saturation (Coffey, 1999).

Digital Ethnography

Feminist digital media: Digital ethnography has been one of the main areas in which feminist digital media has emerged.

We would like to elaborate on digital ethnography, which was briefly mentioned earlier, because this is a growing area with innumerable possibilities for feminist researchers. Digital ethnography has been rapidly developing over the past two decades. Although not the first publication on the topic, Christine Hine's 2000 book *Virtual Ethnography* was a pivotal work, and her 2013 book *The Internet* continues to push the field forward. Sarah Pink and colleagues define digital ethnography as:

> In digital ethnography, we are often in mediated contact with participants rather in direct presence . . . we might be in conversation with people throughout their everyday lives. We might be watching what people do by digitally tracking them, or asking them to invite us into their social media practices. Listening may involve reading, or it might involve sensing and communicating in other ways. (2015, p. 3)

Beyond studying people in mediated environments, many leaders in the field suggest that digital technology is "redefining" how ethnographic research is practiced across the board (Hsu, 2014; Pink et al., 2015). Wendy F. Hsu observes that most ethnographers already use digital media and technology:

> We use email and social media to identify and communicate with our research associates. We use cloud-based mapping systems like Google maps to locate sites during field work. We use Internet media hubs like YouTube and Facebook to find, post, and share documentation of culture in action . . . we use digital audio recordings, taking field notes on Twitter and Storify. (2014)

Webscraping is a software tool with innumerable possibilities. In essence, webscraping is able to "extract targeted information from web pages (Hsu, 2014)." This tool can be used to gather data from digital communities and websites and place findings from traditional ethnographic research into a context, and for many other purposes (Hsu, 2014). For feminist researchers this is an opportunity to contextualize field notes or interview data.

While the term "digital ethnography" has typically referred to a subject of inquiry or a set of tools used to assist inquiry, Hsu suggests, and we concur, it is also becoming a research method and "an emerging platform for collecting, exploring, and expressing ethnographic materials." Pink and colleagues note these practices may even replace traditional ethnographic writing with video, photography, and blogging (2015, p. 3). We pick up on this discussion in Chapter 9 as representing research in these ways contributes to public scholarship, a goal of much feminist research.

Analysis and Interpretation of Qualitative Data

The process of data analysis and interpretation helps us to answer the question: What does it all mean? This process allows us to create "intelligible accounts" of our data (Wolcott, 1994, p. 1). It is important to remember that "the data do not speak for themselves. We have to speak for them" (Vogt et al., 2014, p. 2). Allen Trent and Jeasik Cho define analysis as "summarizing and organizing data" and interpretation as "finding or making meaning" (2014, p. 652). These phases may blur as analysis and interpretation are often a **recursive process**.

The first decision feminist qualitative researchers need to make is the extent to which the analysis and/or interpretation process will be collaborative. To what extent, if at all, will participants help make sense of the findings? Will participants be directly involved in data analysis and/or interpretation, or have opportunities to offer input? This can occur in many ways. For instance, will interviewees have an opportunity to see their transcribed interviews and make amendments? Will field research participants be asked to collaborate on memo writing? It's also vital to consider how you will deal with interpretive conflict, should it arise.

Before analysis you need to **prepare the data** (e.g., transcribe interview recordings) and **organize the data in a repository**. As qualitative research produces a wealth of data, you will also need to **sort** the data for analysis as a part of the organizational process. Johnny Saldaña (2014) recommends a separate file for each "chunk" of data. For instance, one day's worth of field notes, one interview, and so forth. After preparation, analysis begins.

It's also important to **immerse yourself in the data** to get a sense of the data as a whole before beginning a systematic analysis process. Read, look at, and think about the data (Hesse-Biber & Leavy, 2005, 2011). Take the time to stew in it and let your ideas develop. Immersion helps you to "feel" the pulse of the data (Saldaña, 2014) and develop your initial ideas (Creswell, 2014). During this review of the data take brief notes about your thoughts, ideas, and things you want to remind yourself of (Hesse-Biber & Leavy, 2005, 2011; Saldaña, 2014). Initial exploration may also help you begin data reduction (Hesse-Biber & Leavy, 2005, 2011). You may begin to "prioritize" the data for analysis by noting what data will best help you address the research purpose and answer the research questions (Saldaña, 2014, pp. 583–584).

The **coding** process allows us to reduce and classify the data generated. Coding is the process of assigning a word or phrase to segments of data. The code selected should summarize or capture the essence of that segment of data (Saldaña, 2009). Coding may be done by hand or using computer-assisted software (CAQDAS). There are many programs available including NVivo, MAXQDA, ATLAS.ti, Dedoose, HyperRESEARCH, and NUD*IST. Regardless if you are coding by hand or with a computer software program, there are numerous approaches to coding qualitative data, a few of which follow:

- **In vivo coding:** relies on using participants' exact language to generate codes (Strauss, 1987).

- **Descriptive coding:** mainly uses nouns to summarize segments of data (Saldaña, 2014).

- **Values coding:** focuses on conflicts, struggles, and power issues (Saldaña, 2014).

Once you have coded your data, it is important to look for patterns and the relationships between codes. **Categorizing** is the process of grouping similar or seemingly related codes together (Saldaña, 2014). As you work with your coded data, you may also engage in a process of **theming** the data. As you study your codes and categories, what themes emerge? Differing from short codes, a theme may be an extended phrase or sentence that signals the larger meaning behind a code or group of codes (Saldaña, 2014).

During the process of coding, categorizing, and theming, which are likely occurring cyclically, you may engage in **memo writing**. Memo writing involves thinking and systematically writing about data you have coded and categorized. Memos are a link between your coding and interpretation, and they document your impressions, ideas, and emerging understandings (they also assist you later in your write-up) (Hesse-Biber & Leavy, 2011). Each memo further articulates your understanding of that particular topic/concept/data and thus allows you greater insight into the data (Saldaña, 2014). You may write different types of memos, including but not limited to detailed descriptions or summaries, key quotes from the data, analytic memos about different codes, interpretive ideas about how codes and categories are related and what you think something means, and interpretive ideas about how a theory or piece of literature relates to a segment of coded data (Hesse-Biber & Leavy, 2011, p. 314).

Interpretation addresses the question "So what?" (Mills, 2007). How do you make sense of what you have learned? What does it all mean? For feminists, the question also becomes: How do these findings relate to the larger project of feminism or advance feminist concerns?

In order to develop meaning out of your coded data, use your memo notes, look for patterns across your data, make note of anomalous data, and look for links between different categories, concepts, and/or themes. You can also turn to strategies of triangulation in order to build confidence in the summary findings you are developing. **Data triangulation** refers to using multiple sources of data to examine an assertion (Hesse-Biber & Leavy, 2011, p. 51). Explicitly use feminist literature and/or theory to coax meaning out of your data and to put it in a framework for understanding. **Theoretical triangulation** refers to looking at the data through more than one theoretical lens in order to allow different interpretations to emerge (Hesse-Biber & Leavy, 2011, p. 51). For example, examine the analyzed data using some of the different feminist theories reviewed in Chapters 3 and 4.

Community-Based Participatory Research (or Participatory Action Research)

Community-based participatory research (CBPR) or participatory action research (PAR)[3] involves forming research partnerships with nonacademic stakeholders to develop and execute a research project based on a particular community-identified problem or issue. CBPR values collaboration, power sharing, and different knowledges (scientific, lay, experiential). CBPR develops projects from the ground up with those whose lives are most impacted by the problem at hand in an effort to create needed change. Methodologically, these are problem-centered or problem-driven approaches to research that require flexibility. These approaches are generally used when the aim is to promote community change or action. CBPR is necessarily **social justice driven**. Researchers engage in CBPR and related approaches to research in order to address inequality, include marginalized people and perspectives in all phases of the research, empower disenfranchised or historically oppressed groups, and democratize knowledge production and dissemination. Feminist principles have been embedded in CBPR from its inception.

Feminist sociologist and activist Jane Addams (1860–1953) engaged in what would now be considered community-based research with immigrant women in Chicago (Boyd, 2014). In 1899 Addams made an impassioned call for applying knowledge in real-world settings, a cornerstone of what later became CBPR. She wrote:

> Just as we do not know fact until we can play with it, so we do not possess knowledge until we have an impulse to bring it into use; not the didactic impulse, not the propagandist impulse, but that which would throw into the stream of common human experience one bit of important or historic knowledge, however small, which before belonged to a few. The phrase "applied knowledge" or science has so long been used in connection with polytechnic schools and it may be well to explain that I am using it in a broader sense. (p. 39)

---

[3] Closely related practices include community-based research (CBR), community-based participatory action research (CBPAR), action research (AR), social action research (SAR), and others.

Education reformers John Dewey (1859–1952) and Paulo Freire (1921–1997) also directly influenced the philosophy of CBPR. Freire founded critical pedagogy, which posits that education must be used to liberate the poor from oppression, as they become active leaders in their own liberation (Boyd, 2014). In the 1940s Kurt Lewin challenged the borders between research, theory, and action in psychology and is widely credited with beginning "action research" in the United States (Fine et al., 2003). The social justice movements of the 1960s and 1970s also influenced the advancement of CBPR philosophical principles. More recently, indigenous theories have impacted the practice of CBPR. Critical approaches to indigenous inquiry emerged in the 1990s prompted by the theoretical approaches born from the justice movements coupled with the effects of globalization. These perspectives place indigenous knowledges, peoples, and circumstances at the center of research practices (Tuhiwai Smith, 2012). These approaches aim to access the subjugated knowledges of indigenous people for social justice purposes, determined, at least partly, by research participants (and non-Western researchers).

Today, the **transformative paradigm** serves as the philosophical basis for CBPR. Donna Mertens (2005, 2009) has pioneered the development of the transformative paradigm (which she formerly called the emancipatory paradigm). This is a human rights and social justice approach to research in which those historically forced to the margins of the research process are actively included in the entire process (Mertens, 2009). Inclusion extends far beyond participants serving as the "subjects" of research—rather, they are *partners* within the research endeavor. Mertens writes, "The transformative paradigm provides a metaphysical umbrella with which to explore similarities in the basic beliefs that underlie research and evaluation approaches that have been labeled critical theory, feminist theory, critical race theory, participatory, inclusive, human-rights based, democratic, and culturally responsive" (2009, p. 13). Under this perspective, research partners should include those who face discrimination and oppression on any basis (Mertens, 2005, 2009). For example, women, people of color, the poor, people with disabilities, indigenous people, and others confronting structural inequalities and exclusion are sought out for research partnerships, their concerns and perspectives brought to the forefront. By forming research partnerships with those marginalized persons or groups, for whom the research matters on practical levels, research is understood to be **participatory and action-oriented**. Further, this is a power-reflexive or power-sensitive approach to research (Haraway, 1991; Pfohl, 1992). This philosophy posits that research should be empowering, emancipatory, and transformative (in whatever ways are possible). Figure 6.2, reprinted from Leavy (2017), illustrates the major tenets of the transformative paradigm.

Design, Data Generation, Analysis, and Interpretation in Feminist Community-Based Participatory Research

In CBPR, design, data generation, and analysis usually occur as a responsive, recursive, or iterative process, so we are reviewing them together. This kind of process involves the research team cycling back and repeating steps, checking data, and adapting to new insights (Pohl & Hadorn, 2007). This approach builds recurring communication and evaluation into the process (Krimsky, 2000), which is vital in team research.

CBPR begins with determining a community-identified problem or issue to investigate. Determining the problem or issue involves a process of initially coming to a general topic, identifying key stakeholders and community partners, collaboratively identifying the problem or issue, conducting a literature review, and then collaboratively crafting a problem or issue statement.

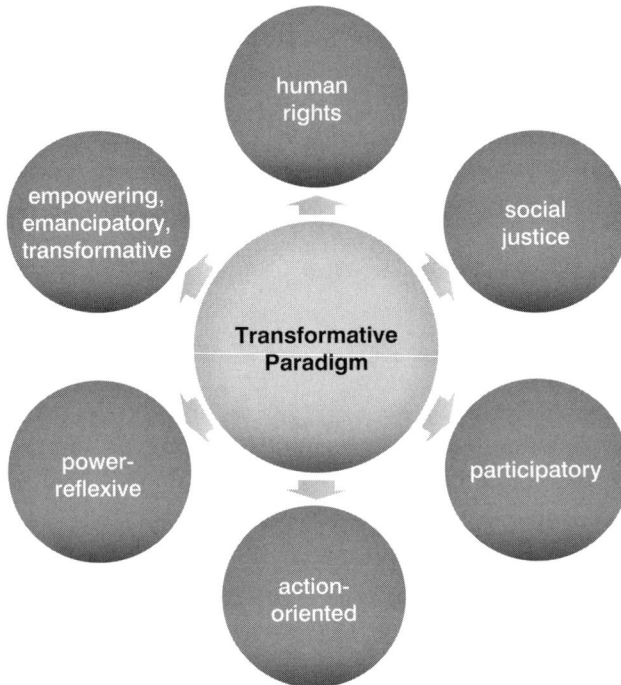

FIGURE 6.2 The transformative paradigm.

Identifying relevant stakeholders and community partners is a vital part of moving from a general idea to a researchable problem. Stakeholders are those parties who have a vested interest in your topic. For example, if the topic you're interested in is domestic violence, relevant stakeholders may include some combination of the following:

- Domestic violence victims/survivors
- Domestic violence perpetrators
- Nurses
- Doctors
- Psychologists/counselors
- Social workers
- Staff at domestic violence shelters
- Police
- Lawmakers
- Gender studies researchers

In addition to identifying stakeholders, finding **collaborators/coinvestigators/community partners** is essential. Depending on the topic, there may be an established **community-based organization (CBO)** or CBOs with whom you can try to forge a partnership. For example, in a study about domestic violence you may partner with a local shelter or related not-for-profit.

Regardless of how many people are on the formal research team, you may also establish a **community advisory board (CAB)** in order to incorporate community perspectives into the project (Israel, Eng, Schultz, & Parker, 2005; Letiecq & Schmalzbauer, 2012). Soliciting formal input from differently positioned members of the community can be essential as you seek to formulate the problem and develop a **culturally competent** approach to investigating it. Members of advisory boards may "serve as cultural guides, bridges to the most marginalized community members, research consultants, and sources of critical feedback" (Letiecq & Schmalzbauer, 2012, p. 248).

Multiplicity is also an active part of problem identification. Everyone comes to the project with different perspectives, experiences, and skills, all of which must be valued. It's often useful to take an inventory of where each person is coming from, including their stake in the topic and personal hopes and expectations with respect to what will come from the research. This process helps hone in on how to conceptualize the problem or issue so that the project is beneficial for all participants and takes proper advantage of the different skills sets and knowledge people bring to bear.

Terms used to build the conceptual framework and any data collection instruments must be relevant to the communities the research serves—to **community understandings** of relevant concepts. This is even more challenging in transcultural or transnational research in which various cultural perspectives are also brought to bear.

An excellent example comes from a 10-year cross-cultural project in eight developing countries called "The Household, Gender, and Age Project." A primary challenge during the first year was developing a definition of "the household" that worked across disciplines and in the eight different cultural contexts. The researchers worked together and came to view the term

> from an economic point of view in terms of income; from a sociological point of view in terms of numbers of members of the household; from a psychological perspective in terms of interrelations within the family; from a historical point of view in terms of changes in the household; and from an anthropological point of view in terms of co-residence. (Masini, 2000, p. 122)

With respect to how cultural understandings of "the household" differ across contexts, the team considered the conventional Western notion of the household (coresidence) and other cultural understandings of the household such as kinship and obligations of nonresident "household" members toward resident members (e.g., financial or childcare obligations) (Masini, 1991).

The research team collectively moves from the general topic to the specific problem or issue and ultimately to the research purpose and "community-generated research questions" (Stoeker, 2008, p. 50). CBPR research questions are generally inductive, change oriented, and inclusive (Leavy, 2017). They may employ words and phrases such as "co-create," "collaborate," "participatory," "empower," "emancipate," "promote," "foster," "describe," and "seek to understand from the perspective of various stakeholders" (Leavy, 2017).

As with ethnography, research may occur in formal or informal community settings and there may be formal and informal gatekeepers. With respect to selecting research participants, given the nature of CBPR, snowball sampling (reviewed earlier) is a popular strategy.

Methodologically, CBPR is **"an orientation"** to research, not a particular set of methods (Boyd, 2014; Langhout, Fernandez, Wyldebore, &

Savala, 2016; Reason & Bradbury, 2008). Any of the methods reviewed in this text may be used in a CBPR project. However, there are core principles of CBPR that are used in conjunction with particular methods in order to build the methodology.

Collaboration is at the heart of CBPR. Collaboratively delineate a clear division of labor that serves each stakeholder's interests and abilities. Participation in the research should be mutually beneficial for all parties. Community needs must be identified collaboratively to avoid the power imbalances that often occur when academic research-

> **Power sharing:** A core principle of CBPR that emphasizes collaboration during all phases of the research endeavor.

ers go into communities in order to conduct research. In this regard, many practitioners regard **power sharing** as a core principle (Boyd, 2014). Different stakeholders should be given leadership roles in the various stages of the research process to avoid research that occurs within communities, but not *with* communities (Minkler, 2004; Montoya & Kent, 2014). For example, with respect to data collection instruments, cultural understandings shape the kinds of questions asked in a survey or interview (content and language). The goal is to be *effective* in addressing the problem at hand, thereby maximizing the benefits to the community. Intervention strategies must also be culturally competent (Montoya & Kent, 2014). Multiplicity and different forms of knowledge—experiential, scientific, and lay—are valued.

Recruitment and retention often prove challenging in CBPR (getting appropriate participants to participate for the duration of the project). It is important to build trust and rapport with community members, research partners, and participants. CBPR is a highly "relational" approach to research (Boyd, 2014). One challenge is that the idea of "research" may be poorly received by members of some communities, particularly disenfranchised, marginalized, or historically oppressed populations (Meade, Menard, Luque, Martinez-Tyson, & Gwede, 2009). Insider–outsider statuses come to bear. As with ethnography, negotiating insider–outsider statuses requires building genuine and reciprocal relationships.

It's important to bear in mind that the principles outlined can be applied to the use of any particular methods and are central to building your methodology. These principles carry through to analysis and interpretation. The research findings should be credible to all research partners.

Let's look at an example of feminist participatory action research. Gouin, Cocq, and McGavin (2011) conducted a study about Inter Pares, a

Canadian social justice organization founded in 1975. *Inter Pares* supports organizations in the global south that work on behalf of issues such as violence against women, women's health and reproductive rights, and civil liberties. Over time, the organization developed an egalitarian organizational structure informed by feminism. Gouin and colleagues conducted a study, working with the staff, to evaluate how this structure worked on a day-to-day basis. They employed an entirely iterative process, with cycles of data collection, analysis, and writing. The staff was broken into clusters, and all decisions about the project were made by consensus at the cluster level and then presented to the entire team of clusters for final decision making. This egalitarian and participatory approach worked very effectively. Based on their experience, the authors suggest feminist participatory action researchers place four things at the forefront of their projects: a commitment to process, consensus, building relationships out of a common cause, and working collaboratively to achieve common objectives.

Photovoice

> **Feminist digital media:** Feminist approaches to photovoice represent an emergent form of feminist digital media that can be viewed as a qualitative or arts-based approach to research.

While CBPR can draw on any methods, **photovoice** is on the rise. Photovoice is a practice that merges photography with participatory methods. Some refer to this as a method for conducting **arts-based action research** (Chilton & Leavy, 2014). Research participants are given cameras and a particular prompt, based on which they take photographs of their environment and circumstances (these days participants may use the cameras on their smartphones). Research goals and instructions to participants vary greatly, but generally, participants are documenting their circumstances as they relate to a larger goal, such as improving their community, affecting public policy, or increasing self- and social awareness around a particular topic. When people are invited to tell their own stories, a "decolonial space" is opened that aligns with feminist principles (Langhout et al., 2016).

Photovoice developed as a feminist methodology (Langhout et al., 2016; Wang & Burris, 1994). Gunilla Holm (2008) suggests that the practice of this method can be grounded in critical consciousness-raising theories. We suggest this is a part of feminist practice. The method was first used in a CBPR project about Yunnan Chinese women's health and related work experiences (Wang, Burris, & Ping, 1996). The method continues to be used in projects about women's and girls' lives. For example, the Witnesses to Hunger project involves having low-income mothers in Philadelphia take photos and record their stories in order to influence social welfare policy (Chilton, Rabinowich, Council, & Breaux, 2009; see *https:// witnessestohunger.blog*). Janet Newbury and Marie Hoskins (2010) used photovoice to study the experiences of adolescent girls who used methamphetamines. They conceived of the girls as coresearchers, which allowed the adult researchers and girls to interact in ways that might not otherwise have been possible (Chilton & Leavy, 2014). The photography led to conversations with the adult researchers that would not otherwise have happened, which in turn prompted a deeper level of understanding.

In terms of research design, consider the following general guidelines:

> Conceptualizing the problem; defining broader goals and objectives; recruiting policymakers as the audience for photovoice findings; training the trainers; conducting photovoice training; devising the initial theme/s for taking pictures; taking pictures; facilitating group discussion; critical reflection and dialogue; selecting photographs for discussion; contextualizing and storytelling; codifying issues, themes, and theories; documenting the stories; conducting the formative evaluation; reaching policymakers, donors, media, researchers, and others who may be mobilized to create change. (Wang, 2005, as quoted in Holm, 2008, p. 330)

It will be interesting to see how changes in the technological landscape continue to influence these practices.

CONCLUSION

Feminist researchers employ many methods and research designs when working with participants. Each has a different utility and therefore methods should be selected in accord with research goals. As we move throughout this chapter from survey research to community-based participatory research, the level and depth of interaction and collaboration between researchers and participants grows exponentially. However, as some of those cited in this chapter caution, issues of hierarchy, relationships, and potential exploitation do not disappear simply because we develop close relationships with participants. Each method brings its own set of challenges for feminist researchers working with human participants. Whether conducting surveys, interviews, ethnography, or CBPR, feminist researchers aim to create reciprocal relationships with participants by, at a minimum, serving as an ally and advocate on their behalf.

DISCUSSION QUESTIONS

1. What are the primary differences between survey and interview research? What are the advantages of each for feminist researchers?

2. What are the main issues feminist ethnographers have to deal with during data collection?

3. Discuss reciprocity and why it is such a complicated issue for feminists.

ACTIVITIES

1. Visit an online oral history repository and select one transcript from a feminist research project. Read the transcript and write a one-page response answering the following: What did you learn? Do you think that data could have been ascertained with a different method? (Explain your answer.)

2. Analyze the oral history transcript using the inductive coding process reviewed in this chapter (you can do it by hand or use a CAQDAS program if you have one available). What codes emerge? What themes emerge?

3. Find a photovoice project online that focuses on the experiences of girls or women. Explore the website and write a one-page response stating what you learned about the substantive topic and your assessment of the effectiveness of the method in the project (explain your answer).

SUGGESTED RESOURCES
. . . .

📖 Article

Narayan, K. (1993). How native is a "native" anthropologist? *American Anthropologist, 95*(3), 671–686.

📚 Books

Davis, D., & Craven, C. (2016). *Feminist ethnography: Thinking through methodologies, challenges, and possibilities.* Lanham, MD: Rowman & Littlefield.

An excellent book on feminist ethnography that covers topics from the historical context to how to do feminist ethnography. The book includes multiple perspectives, partly in the form of excerpts from published works by leading feminist ethnographers as well as original interview material.

Smith, L. T. (2012). *Decolonizing methodologies: Research and indigenous peoples* (2nd ed.). London: Zed Books.

An important book that explores the intersections of imperialism and research. The author makes a powerful argument that the decolonization of research methods will help to reclaim control over indigenous ways of knowing and being.

Visweswaran, K. (1994). *Fictions of feminist ethnography*. Minneapolis: University of Minnesota Press.

A classic collection of essays in which the author draws on her work with women in India to explore what feminist ethnography is and how it might be practiced and represented.

Digital Resources

Feminist Oral History Online

VOAHA II: Virtual Oral/Aural History Archive at CSULB (California State University, Long Beach)

www.csulb.edu/voaha

Audio recordings of oral histories that have been deposited in Special Collections of the University Library, ranging from women's social history, labor, and ethnic studies to Long Beach area history and musical development in Southern California. Major topics include the following: American Indian Studies, Asian American History, Labor History, Long Beach Area History, Mexican American/Chicano Musical Developments in Southern California, Southeast Asian Communities, The Sixties: Los Angeles Area Social Movements/Activists, Women's History

The Women's History section (*www.csulb.edu/voaha*. Please visit the Women's History section on the main page.) hosts topics including Asian American Women's Movement Activists, Chicana Feminists, Feminist Health Movement, Los Angeles Feminists, Professionals and Entrepreneurs, Reformers and Radicals, Suffragists, Welfare Mothers, Welfare Rights, Women's Lives, Women's Work 1900–1960.

YourStory Project at the University of Utah

www.yourstory.utah.edu

Record and Remember (the full name of the project) is a program that initially grew out of a course taught by Professor Meg Brady of the Department of English at the University of Utah. As the 2003–2004 University Professor, Brady developed a new interdisciplinary course in "The Life Story" to train students in interviewing strategies and the narrative genres of memoir and life history; this course was at the core of the YourStory endeavor. It provided students with the necessary skills and understandings to carry out the important work of life story preservation, and at the same time created a vital link between the students' university experiences and their service to the larger community.

StoryCorps
https://storycorps.org

An independently funded organization, StoryCorps has a mission to preserve and share humanity's stories in order to build connections between people and create a more just and compassionate world. They do this to remind one another of our shared humanity, to strengthen and build the connections between people, to teach the value of listening, and to weave into the fabric of our culture the understanding that everyone's story matters. You can sort the audio stories by theme, and as examples, they offer those on LGBTQ issues and in Spanish: *https://storycorps. org/listen*. Choose Collections under the drop down menu and filter stories by different categories.).

Schlesinger Library at Radcliffe Institute, Harvard
www.radcliffe.harvard.edu/schlesinger-library/collections

Highlights from the Schlesinger Library's digital collections can be found on their home page.

Black Women Oral History Project Interviews, 1976–1981
www.radcliffe.harvard.edu/schlesinger-library/collection/black-women-oral-history-project

Smith College Voices of Feminism Oral History Project

The Voices of Feminism Oral History Project documents the persistence and diversity of organizing for women in the United States in the latter half of the 20th century. Narrators include labor, peace, and antiracism activists; artists and writers; lesbian rights advocates; grassroots antiviolence and antipoverty organizers; and reproductive justice leaders who were women of color.

www.smith.edu/libraries/special-collections/research-collections/resources-lists/oral-histories/voices-of-feminism

Oral Histories on Women's History Matters

Here you can find audio clips from an oral history of a farm woman who grew up on a homestead near Cut Bank; bibliographies of women's oral histories held at the Montana Historical Society; information on how to conduct your own oral history project; and information on ongoing statewide oral history projects focused on women's experiences.

http://montanawomenshistory.org/oral-history/

Chinese Historical Society of New England's Chinese-American Women Oral History Project

This project documents the lives and activities of Chinese American women living in New England. This glimpse into the Chinese experience in America focuses on women from a broad range of life experiences.

www.chsne.org/programs/chinese-american-women-oral-history-project/

Cambodian Women's Oral History Project: Life Stories of Survival under the Khmer Rouge Regime

This project collects testimonials from women who survived the genocidal Khmer Rouge regime that ruled Cambodia between 1975 and 1979. Unique in its life story approach, the project aims to increase understanding of the ways in which women were uniquely impacted by the atrocity, including as victims of widespread sexual violence and gender-based abuse.

http://cambodianwomensoralhistory.com/about/

The Civil Rights History Project: Survey of Collections and Repositories

Subjects covered in this collection include the NAACP, the National Council of Negro Women, the Urban League, the YWCA, the Tuskegee Syphilis Study, Actresses, Women and education, Women and employment, civil rights, Greek letter societies, race relations, women artisans, women artists, women authors, women clergy, women clerks, women educators, women in community development, women in medicine, women in politics, and women in trade unions.

www.loc.gov/folklife/civilrights/

The Women in Military Service for America Oral History Program

Oral history is a vital tool in recording and preserving the diverse experiences of U.S. servicewomen in their own voices. The Women's Memorial Foundation Oral History Program promotes research and understanding of all aspects of the history and culture of the women who have served in defense of our nation.

www.womensmemorial.org/oral-history

GSU Gender and Sexuality Oral History Project

The Gender and Sexuality Oral History Project was established in 2011 and forms part of the Archives for Research on Women and Gender. It aims to document LGBTQ history in Atlanta, Georgia, and the South through interviews with activists and leaders in grassroots movements as well as established organizations and public offices.

http://research.library.gsu.edu/gender_sexuality

CHAPTER 7

Feminist Methods for Studying Nonliving Data, Organizations, and Programs

The way to right wrongs is to
turn the light of truth upon them.
—IDA B. WELLS-BARNETT

LEARNING OBJECTIVES

- To introduce you to feminist content analysis, why these approaches are popular, and how feminists have employed content analysis to study print texts (with or without images), film and television, and the Internet or blogosphere

- To learn how to design and carry out a research project using content analysis

- To introduce you to feminist evaluation research, including the main principles

- To learn how to design and carry out a project using feminist evaluation methods

- To provide a discussion of the impact of geospatial technologies in evaluation

- To provide a discussion of the roles of advocacy and public policy in feminist evaluation

The previous chapter focused on methods whereby data is collected from individuals. In this chapter we review methods for studying nonliving and noninteractive data, as well as methods for studying organizations and/or programs. In other words, this chapter centers on methods for investigating "things" created by human beings that in turn shape us.

170

Content Analysis (or Unobtrusive Methods)

Content analysis is a method for studying **cultural materials,** sometimes referred to as *cultural artifacts* or *cultural content.* Those materials are wide-ranging and may include written texts/documents, visual images, audiovisual texts, digital platforms and media, music, and objects (e.g., toys, technology). These cultural materials, which become the data in content analysis, share three distinctions. First, they have been *created by human beings.* As Shulamit Reinharz and Rachel Kulick note, "cultural artifacts are the products of individual activity, social organization, technology, and cultural patterns" (2007, p. 258). Second, they *exist independent of the research* and are thus naturalistic (Reinharz, 1992). Third, because the data are nonliving they are *noninteractive* (Reinharz, 1992). As a result, content analysis is often referred to as unobtrusive.

Differing from most research methods, which are either quantitative or qualitative, content analysis can be employed in quantitative or qualitative ways. Quantitative content analysis is useful for identifying rates and patterns. For example, quantitative content analysis can tell us how frequently female athletes are represented by sports media as compare to male athletes. Qualitative content analysis is useful for identifying and fleshing out themes, providing context, and in some instances generating theory. For example, it can tell us the nature of representations of female athletes as compared to male athletes, including the context of the stories and images.

Content analysis, often in the form of media analysis, is one of the most popular methods employed by feminist researchers. Questions about the **politics of representation** lie at the center of this work. How are cultural norms about gender created and maintained? For example, how do we create, re-create, and resist a gender binary? How do we get our ideas about what it means to be female or feminine, male or masculine? How are cisgender norms

> **Representation:** The ability to represent individuals and groups is always imbued with power.

constructed? How do our ideas about gender connect with ideas about sexuality? How is gender inequality constructed? What systems are in place to maintain injustices? How is power at play? Specifically, how is dominant ideology that serves patriarchal power and White supremacy created and reified through representations?

Historically and culturally specific ideas about gender are constructed and reconstructed through representations. In other words, meanings associated with being female (e.g., ideas about femininity) and meanings associated with being male (e.g., ideas about masculinity) are created through

> **Socially constructed (gender) categories:** Feminist content analysis focuses on the social construction of gender via media and other texts.

representations, and are reinforced by their circulation within the culture. Furthermore, culturally specific ideas about sexuality, race, class, age, and ableness, which intersect with dominant narratives about gender, are constructed through representations.

For example, there are print advertisements that sell beverages using a conventional image of female beauty that is at once gendered, sexualized, racialized, aged, and able-bodied. Further, the particular messages about sexuality are highly objectified, perhaps most clearly in instances in which the female body literally becomes part of the product in the image. The mainstream Western female beauty ideal propagated by the commercial media is at once highly gendered portraying stereotypical views on cisgender identity and femininity, and also White, heterosexual, and able-bodied. These are overarching and inter-

> **Cisgender:** Feminist analysis of media exposes the widespread construction of cisgender norms, which become taken for granted within the culture.

locking sets of ideas and assumptions about "female beauty." The images of "female beauty" repeated throughout the culture, even when female beauty is not the topic per se, communicate this set of meanings. So to simplify, for example, the media create associations between "beauty" and "ableness" that become taken for granted within the culture. Many feminist researchers thus understand "representation as a prevailing locus of female and gender subordination and liberation" (Reinharz & Kulick, 2007, p. 260).

Feminist researchers concerned with *the politics of representation* often turn to media analysis to examine how gendered power operates through representations in multiple ways, including around issues such as voice, agency, spectacle, and stereotypes. (McIntosh & Cuklanz, 2014). In this regard, feminist researchers investigate how media representations "support traditional power structures" and how we might create new representations that promote social justice (McIntosh & Cuklanz, 2014, p. 267).

In addition to analyzing existing cultural content, feminist researchers also identify and investigate exclusions and erasures (Karon, 1992; Reinharz & Kulick, 2007). George Gerbner coined the term **symbolic annihilation** in 1976 to refer to the underrepresentation or total absence of representation of a group based on shared status characteristic (e.g., gender, sexuality, race). Symbolic annihilation is understood as a strategy of dominance that promotes inequality. It is important to understand that contemporary

feminists can apply this concept with an intersectional approach. For
example, let's take representations of female protagonists on prime-time
television in the United States and consider the intersections of gender and
race. A content analysis might find that there is a slight underrepresentation
of White women relative to men, significant underrepresentation of Black
women, and the total absence of representation of Asian and Native American women. This is merely an example. It becomes more complex when
we consider multiple dimensions of symbolic annihilation. What groups,
ideas, and values are *not* visible in cultural texts? Whose stories and perspectives are *not* shown? In "Introduction: The Symbolic Annihilation of
Women by the Mass Media," the groundbreaking opening chapter of the
coedited volume *Hearth and Home: Images of Women in the Mass Media,*
Gaye Tuchman (1978) related "the reflection hypothesis" and "symbolic
annihilation." The **reflection hypothesis** states that the mass media reflect
dominant cultural values (Tuchman, 1978, p. 7).[1] Images and narratives
that correspond with these values, such as the nuclear family ideal, become
taken for granted, reinforced, validated, and elevated. Working in concert
to reinforce *those* values is the exclusion of other values or ideas. So at
once some ideas are reinforced and take on an air of status, while others
are rendered invisible or delegitimated. Tuchman broke down the concept
of symbolic annihilation into three categories: absence, trivialization, and
condemnation. Many feminist researchers adopt her conceptualization as a
framework for their content analysis.

   Another way that feminist researchers tackle the study of erasures is by
examining the cultural and economic processes that obstruct certain texts
from being produced (Reinharz & Kulick, 2007, p. 259). In this respect,
"feminist researchers seek to understand the ways certain topics came to be
missing and the implication of these gaps. Thus, feminist content analysis
is a study both of texts that exists and of texts that do not" (Reinharz &
Kulick, 2007, p. 259).

   While feminist content analysis took off over the last 50 years, feminists have been shaping the field for far longer.

   In 1838 British sociologist Harriet Martineau published her renowned
book *How to Observe Morals and Manners* based on her observations in
the United States.[2] In this volume she paved the way for the development
of content analysis in the social sciences, and arguably the importance of

---

[1]Contemporary feminists note the media also create these cultural values, and that individuals do not all consume and internalize media messages in a unifom way.

[2]It is widely suggested in feminist literature that Martineau was the first female sociologist
or even the first sociologist.

studying "things" for generations of feminist researchers to come. Flipping the script from learning directly from individuals, she famously wrote, "The grand secret of wise inquiry into Morals and Manners is to begin with the study of THINGS, using the DISCOURSE OF PERSONS as a commentary upon them." Martineau argued that "the action of the nation is embodied" in its records, and is both "more comprehensive and more faithful than that of any a variety of individual voices" (1838/1998, pp. 73–74).

Another significant force in the development of feminist content analysis, Ida B. Wells-Barnett investigated the lynchings of Black people in the South. It was commonly said that Black men were lynched for raping White women. In 1891 Wells-Barnett researched the circumstances around 728 lynchings. She conducted multimethod research, studying newspaper reports of the lynchings, visiting crime scenes, and interviewing witnesses (Giddings, 1984). Her findings contradicted the often promulgated rape narrative (e.g., women and children were lynched, alleged crimes included "arguing with Whites" and "making threats") (Giddings, 1984). During the course of her research she also discovered and bravely wrote about interracial relationships, many initiated by White women (Giddings, 1984). What is perhaps most revolutionary about her research is her strategic use of content analysis, specifically her systematic use of newspaper reports written by Whites to legitimate her findings. Wells-Barnett's research is one of the earliest examples of using content analysis in social justice work.

Betty Friedan's 1963 book *The Feminine Mystique* also made lasting contributions to the practice of feminist content analysis. In this celebrated text, Friedan explored the lives of suburban homemakers, looking at the underbelly of the culturally idealized version of femininity. As a part of her investigation she analyzed media and advertisements, particularly women's magazines. Her research pointed to the frivolity that White middle- and upper-class women were socialized into via these texts. Although this book has been rightly critiqued for its overemphasis on the experiences of White middle- and upper-class women, it represents a pivotal moment in the development of feminist content analysis.

Genres

As feminist content analysis is conducted across mediums and disciplines, researchers categorize types of content in numerous ways. For example, the literature is often categorized *topically* (e.g., pornography across media, sports media research). Heather McIntosh and Lisa Cuklanz (2014) categorize content by *format*: print, TV, film, Internet, and advertisements. Shulamit Reinharz and Rachel Kulick (2007) created the following four *categories:* written records, narratives and visual texts, material culture, and behavioral residues. Based on the primary areas of study we have identified in the literature, we use the following categories:

1. **Print texts with or without images** (e.g., newspapers, books, diaries, magazines, pamphlets, comics)
2. **Film and television** (e.g., romance films, action adventure films, sitcoms, dramas, cop shows, cable programs, broadcast news, broadcast sports media)
3. **Internet or the blogosphere** (e.g., sports blogs, pornography, online feminist communities).

Print Texts with or without Images

Feminist researchers have content-analyzed numerous forms of print texts. For example, feminist researchers have studied texts produced within academia or for educational purposes, including but not limited to the extent of published feminist content analysis in peer-reviewed psychology journals (Angelique & Culley, 2000), marriage and family textbooks from 1950 to 1987 to examine depictions of abortion and adoption (Hall & Shepherd Stolley, 1997), representations of women in world history books (Commeyras & Alvermann, 1996), representations of feminist and antiracist scholarship in American introductory social work textbooks (Wachholz & Mullaly, 2000), and representations of masculinity in elementary school textbooks (Evans & Davies, 2000).

Another popular area of study is gender and sport print media. For example, feminist researchers have found that less than 10% of print sports media coverage is devoted to female athletes (Bruce, 2013). In the most comprehensive study to date, including 80 newspapers in 22 countries, researchers found that female athletes are the focus of only 9% of articles (Toft, 2011), and only 9.7% of *Sports Illustrated* feature articles are about female athletes or women's sports (Lumpkin, 2009). Feminist researchers have shown that gender differences can be found at every level of sport too. A visual content analysis of newspaper photographic coverage of female and male high school athletes that consisted of 827 photographs from 602 randomly selected newspapers found rampant gender inequities (Pederson, 2002). They coded for features such as still or action shots.

A lot of research in this area attempts to counter arguments or assumptions that representations of female athletes have improved over time. Kent Kaiser and Erik Skoglund (2006) analyzed the column inches and feature photos "above the fold" on the front page of the sports section in two U.S. newspapers from 1942 to 2005. They found coverage of female athletes *decreased* over time and never exceeded 10%. They argued Title IX has not produced significant change in sports media coverage. Jonetta D. Weber and Robert M. Carini (2013) analyzed the covers of *Sports Illustrated* magazine from 2000 to 2011. They found female athletes appeared on only 4.9% of covers, excluding the swimsuit issue. That statistic is similar to those from the 1980s and 1990s. It is actually lower than 1954–1965, when female athletes appeared on 12.6% of covers. In addition to this quantitative data they studied the representations qualitatively. They found female athletes were typically sexually objectified, appeared along with a man, and were featured in ways that did not highlight athleticism. Through these examples we can see Tuchman's expanded framework of symbolic annihilation in action, particularly in the forms of absence and trivialization.

Women's magazines are a staple of feminist content analysis because they represent cultural ideas about gender roles, beauty and body image, consumerism, and romantic relationships, which are common spaces of gender inequality. For example, feminist researchers have studied teen magazines (e.g., *Seventeen*) (Carpenter, 1998; Levin & Kilbourne, 2009; Kilbourne, 1999, 2000; McRobbie, 2000; Peirce, 2011; Schlenker, Caron, & Halteman, 1998). While these magazines are often subject to harsh criticism, some feminists see them as a female-centered space that brings girls and young women enjoyment (Currie, 1999). Suzanna Danuta Walters (1995) asserts that we cannot assume all girls and women are similarly impacted by the messages that circulate in magazines. She suggests inviting research participants into the interpretive process.

Less common print texts can also be studied. For example, Melvin L. Williams and Tia C. M. Tyree (2015) performed a feminist content analysis of the *Fame* comic book 2013 Nicki Minaj issue. The *Fame* series launched in 2010 as a biographical comic series that explores celebrity culture. It has only featured two Black women (Beyoncé and Nicki Minaj) and only two rappers (50 Cent and Nicki Minaj). Minaj is the only Black female rapper to be featured in the comic. Williams and Tyree analyzed the plot, setting, clothing, and physical and behavioral characteristics presented in the issue. They used two frameworks for their analysis. First, they drew on Dionne P. Stephens and Layli D. Phillips's (2003) sexual scripts: Diva, Gold Digger, Freak, Dyke, Earth Mother, Baby Mama, Gangsta Bitch, Sister Savior. Second, they applied Anna Sainai's framework of three Black superheroines: Quiet Queen, Dominant Diva, Scandalous Sojourner. They found that the representations of Minaj in the issue fit into many of Stevens and Phillips's categories but were not "deeply rooted" in any (2015, p. 60). For example, they found links to the Diva category through her physical image, which fit Eurocentric beauty ideals and found that she had attained success on her own. They also found references to the Freak category based on the sexual script presented, which included hypersexuality and objectification (e.g., an image of her sitting on a rocket). With respect to Sainai's framework, they concluded that Minaj's portrayal fit into the Scandalous Sojourner category because ultimately she was represented as a self-empowered heroine (2015, p. 61).

Film and Television

Film and television are frequent domains for feminist research. Audiovisual data is considered a "multiple field" because it contains several components: visual, audio, and text (discourse) (Rose, 2000). British feminist film theorist Laura Mulvey's (1975) essay "Visual Pleasure and Narrative Cinema" has been pivotal to the field. Mulvey posited that women in film are generally depicted in passive roles and are sexually objectified. Viewers are positioned as voyeurs. Feminist research on film and television often explores "patterns of objectification" and stereotypes (McIntosh & Cuklanz, 2014, p. 275).

Feminist researchers have content-analyzed a wide range of films. Some projects focus on a specific film, such as *Fifty Shades of Grey* (Boyd, 2015), *The Sisterhood of the Traveling Pants* (Projansky, 2011), *13 Going on 30* (Radner, 2011), and *Underworld* (David Magill, 2015). Other projects consider genres of film or themes across films, including but not limited to violent women in film (Neroni, 2005), women in martial arts films (Chen, 2012), and gender in vampire films and pop culture (Anyiwo, 2016).

Research on television is quite common. Some studies focus on a particular television show or character. For example, feminists have investigated *The Mary Tyler Moore Show* (Dow, 1990), *Law and Order: Special Victims Unit* (Cuklanz & Moorti, 2006), *Ally McBeal* (Leavy, 2000, 2006), *Ugly Betty* (Esposito, 2009), *Will & Grace* (Battles & Hilton-Morrow, 2002), *Buffy the Vampire Slayer* (Boyle, 2008), *Sex and the City* (Arthurs, 2008), and *The Vampire Diaries* (Nicol, 2016). Recently, April Kalogeropoulos Householder (2015) conducted a feminist content analysis of the television series *Girls*. She explored various dimensions of the show's feminism, including casting and production decisions (e.g., hiring unknown female actresses), the title, and topics and themes including women's solidarity and intersectionality, sex, and body image. Feminist research on television is increasingly applying an intersectional perspective. For example, Rachel Alicia Griffin (2015) content-analyzed *Scandal*

> **Intersectionality:** Feminist researchers applying intersectional approaches to media analysis consider how gender intersects with at least one other status characteristic.

and the character Olivia Pope, applying Black feminist thought that considers the intersection of gender and race. Lauren J. Decarvalho and Nicole B. Cox (2015) studied *Orange Is the New Black* applying a queer theory perspective that emphasized the intersection of gender, sex, and sexual orientation.

Some studies focus on genres of television. For example, there are feminist analyses of talk shows (Gamson, 1999), reality television (Pozner, 2010), and cop shows (Buist & Sutherland, 2015). Some projects apply intersectional approaches. For example, Joshua Gamson's study of talk shows is grounded in queer theory. There are also longitudinal studies aimed at identifying and evaluating change over time. For example, Nancy Signorielli and Aaron Bacue (1999) analyzed lead characters on prime-time television from 1967 to 1998. Their results contradicted the public's perception that there had been great change toward gender equity.

Feminist media analysis also, at times, investigates overall patterns across mediums. For example, Casey Cipriani (2015) reported on an annual study by the Center for the Study of Women in Television and Film that investigated the kinds of roles male and female characters had in both television *and* film in 2014. The findings indicate:

- Male characters were more likely than females to be identified only by a work-related role, such as doctor or business executive (61% of males vs. 34% of females).

- Female characters were more likely than males to be identified only by a personal-life-related role such as wife or mother (58% of females vs. 31% of males).

- Male characters were more likely than females to have an identifiable goal (60% vs. 49%).

- Male characters were more likely than female characters to have work-related goals (48% vs. 34%) or crime-related goals (7% vs. 2%).

- Female characters were more likely than males to have goals related to their personal lives (14% vs. 5%).

This kind of combined study illustrates that media culture overwhelmingly presents women as relational, with personal relationships taking primacy in their lives, much more so than for men.

Feminist researchers also study television news. Feminist research tells us, for example, that men were on camera in evening broadcast news 68% of the time in 2014, with women on camera only 32% of the time (Women's Media Center, 2015). This includes appearances by anchors as well as correspondents. To return to the genre of sports media, fewer than 5% of all sports media broadcasts feature female athletes (Bruce, 2013).

Internet or the Blogosphere

As noted throughout this text, feminist researchers are embracing digital media. One area in which we see that occurring is Internet-based content analysis. Feminist researchers have used content analysis in numerous subject areas. For example, digital sports media research is an emergent area. Galen Clavio and Andrea N. Eagleman (2011) studied portrayals of female athletes in the 10 most popular sports blogs. They found that female athletes, teams, and leagues are rarely featured. When there are photos of females, they are sexualized and predominantly nonathletes (e.g., dancers, models).

Internet pornography has been an area that has received considerable attention from feminist researchers. For example, feminist content analysis of online pornography has shown that Internet-based pornography is more violent than print-based pornography (Barron & Kimmel, 2000). Internet research has also shown 40.8% of the stories published in Internet group sex sites feature a nonconsent element (e.g., rape, child molestation, forced slavery) (Harmon & Boeringer, 2004). Jennifer Gossett and Sarah Byrne (2002) conducted a content analysis of Internet "rape sites." Their research centered on websites that feature female victims. They analyzed the content of 31 free sites, which include links to pay-per-view sites. Among their findings they found an overrepresentation of Indian women featured on the sites. They posit that narratives about race are the subtext of rape on the Internet.

> **Feminist digital media:** The Internet is an increasingly popular source of data for content analysis. In some cases feminists may focus specifically on sites that are male or female dominated.

The preceding examples of sports media research and online pornography represent male-dominated Internet spaces. Feminist researchers also study female-dominated spaces, including feminist sites themselves (see for example, Choi, Steiner, & Kim, 2005; Nip, 2004). This work represents feminists investigating **cyberfeminism** (Reinharz & Kulick, 2007).

Designing Feminist Content Analysis

Content analysis begins with transforming your topic into a research purpose statement and developing a set of research questions, or questions and hypotheses. Please consult the last chapter to review this process. Once you have a research purpose statement and research questions, it's time to determine what the data will be as well as your sampling strategy. While these issues were discussed in the last chapter, as we are now dealing with nonliving data we briefly review this process. You may employ probability or purposeful sampling strategies (both reviewed in the last chapter). Let's say you're analyzing advertisements in women's magazines. First you will need to determine which magazine or magazines, and during what time frame. Let's say you select all issues of *Cosmopolitan* magazine from 2016 to 2017. You may employ a probability sampling strategy in which you randomly select the first page of the first issue, and then you select every fifth page (omitting those pages which do not include ads). Or, you may employ a purposeful strategy in which you go through the magazine and select those images that relate to your larger research purpose and research questions. These are merely examples.

Data Collection, Analysis, and Interpretation

The majority of feminist content analysis projects are either qualitative or combine qualitative and quantitative approaches, so we focus primarily on how to conduct qualitative content analysis, and then note how to add a quantitative component to a study. Feminist content analysis generally involves **initial immersion** into the content to get a sense of the "big picture," determining the units of analysis, coding, analysis, and interpretation (there are typically multiple rounds of coding and analysis). During initial immersion, or what Margaret R. Roller and Paul J. Lavrakas (2015) call "absorbing the content," take notes on your overall impressions and ideas for how you might approach coding based on what you are seeing. Next determine the units of analysis you will study and begin coding.

   Units of analysis can be thought of as **chunks of data** (Leavy, 2017). For example, in a written text such as a newspaper, you may define the units of analysis as individual stories, each column of text, each paragraph of text, or each sentence of text. Or, instead of predetermining the unit of analysis based on the "amount" of text, you may do it thematically. So, every time theme *x* (something in your study) is mentioned, that is considered a unit of analysis. For instance, if you are conducting a content analysis to understand how female politicians are portrayed by the television media with respect to marriage, motherhood, and gender presentation (e.g., body, clothing, femininity), you may decide that each time one of those topics is mentioned in a chunk of reporting, it constitutes a "unit of analysis." As you determine your units of analysis consider the type of data you are working with. If it is a *multiple field*, will all the fields be coded? For example, if you're studying television (audiovisual data), will you code the visual aspects, the sound, and the dialogue? Or, will you code only one or two forms of data?

The process of coding data can begin once the units of analysis are determined. Some qualitative feminist researchers use computer-assisted qualitative data analysis software programs (CAQDAS), lauded for their efficiency, reliability, and ability to handle large quantities of data. CAQDAS can be used to code, group codes, memo, and collapse codes, as well as other functions (Roller & Lavrakas, 2015; Silver, 2010). There are numerous programs suitable for conducting content analysis, including ATLAS.ti, MAXQDA, NVivo, HyperRESEARCH, Ethnograph, Qualrus, NUD*IST, and Dedoose. Other researchers choose to code manually, without a software program. CAQDAS may miss important nuances or latent meanings, and further, each program's utility differs (Roller & Lavrakas, 2015). Roller and Lavrakas remind us that even when using CAQDAS, it is merely a "tool" and researchers remain "instrumental" to the research outcomes and their quality by the questions they ask, how they code, and how they explore latent or underlying meanings (p. 252).

Whether doing so by CAQDAS or manually, during initial immersion into the data it is customary to generate a **code** for each unit of analysis. So if you are using sentences as your unit of analysis, for each sentence you would assign a word or phrase that captures the essence of that sentence. Typically this process starts with literal codes (exact words, concrete ideas). As you continue to analyze or reanalyze the data, you may refine your codes, or collapse several literal codes into a larger category or more abstract code. Eventually you identify themes. Memo writing can assist you during this process. As noted in the last chapter, **memo writing** involves thinking and systematically writing about data you have coded and categorized. Memos are a link between your coding and interpretation, and they document your impressions, ideas, and emerging understandings (they also assist you later in your write-up) (Hesse-Biber & Leavy, 2005, 2011).

Qualitative content analysis is **inductive,** with codes and themes developing out of a recursive process of data collection and analysis (Hesse-Biber & Leavy, 2005, 2011). One inductive approach to employ is **grounded theory.** Developed by Barney Glaser and Anselm Strauss in 1967, grounded theory refers to an approach by which one collects and analyzes data, develops new insights, and then uses those insights to inform the next round of data collection and analysis. These steps are repeated until the saturation point is reached. Codes, concepts, and insights develop directly out of the data, and hence are *grounded* in the data. Qualitative researchers use grounded theory to develop concepts and ideas that directly emerge from data. Grounded theory approaches to content analysis involve an inductive coding process in which data are analyzed, typically line by line, and code categories emerge directly out of the data (see Charmaz, 2008). Using this approach, you sample a small portion of data (content), analyze the data-generating codes, and based on what you learn, you collect and analyze more data, refining your codes and creating memo notes, continuing on until you reach data saturation (the point at which new data does not produce new insights). This approach is often favored by feminists as a way of building credibility into their findings.

Quantitative content analysis is **deductive,** beginning with preconceived codes. If you are building a quantitative component into your project, develop a list of codes and then account for their presence within the data. If employing a true **mixed methods approach** to the study, the qualitative and quantitative components of the project should be **integrated**. You may use the code categories that emerged through the inductive qualitative phase that you have explored thematically, and now count for the presence or absence of these codes within segments of data. Conversely, you may begin with a predetermined set of codes and conduct a quantitative analysis to determine rates in patterns, and then build a qualitative component to the research in which you thematically investigate those codes.

The data analysis strategies for quantitative and qualitative research discussed in the last chapter also apply to content analysis. While interpretation—or answering what Mills (2007) called the question of "So what?"—was also reviewed in the last chapter, given the prominence of feminist content analysis we would like to briefly expand on how to relate findings to the larger project of feminism. Feminist researchers conducting content analysis, typically in the form of media analysis, are contributing to a vast repository of previous research. As a whole, this research paints a picture about the media context in which we live, and how girls and women across various differences are represented and may be impacted. Therefore, during the interpretation of findings it is important to make explicit connections to previous research and/or theories.

Evaluation Research

Evaluation research centers on studying a program, intervention, or what is referred to as an "evaluand" in order to make judgments about the program moving forward. This is a systematic and applied approach to research in which evidence is collected about a particular program or "evaluand." Michael Quinn Patton, a leader in the field, defines program evaluation as "the systematic collection of information about the activities, characteristics, and results of programs to make judgments about the program, improve or further develop the program effectiveness, inform decisions about future programming, and/or increase understanding" (2015, p. 178). Evaluation research is typically **problem centered** and seeks to determine the **dynamics** of the program in its current state (how it is designed and how it functions for various stakeholders) and the **outcomes** of that program (the extent to which it is effective in its stated purpose) in order to make future recommendations (Brisolara, 2014; Brisolara & Seigart, 2012). We follow the comprehensive definition of evaluation put forth by feminist evaluators Donna M. Mertens and Nichole Stewart:

> *Evaluation* is an implied inquiry process for collecting and synthesizing evidence that culminates in conclusions about the state of affairs, value, merit, worth, significance, or quality of the program, product, person, policy, proposal, or plan. Conclusions made in evaluation encompass both an empirical aspect (that something is that the case) and a normative aspect (judgment about the value of something). (2014, p. 330)

Evaluation research differs from the other methods reviewed in this text in two distinct ways: (1) the value-based, judgment aspect is an *essential* part of evaluation, and (2) evaluation is not only a method, but a discipline in its own right.

Beginning with the former, when using the other approaches to research, researchers may or may not make evaluative judgments and recommendations. However, such judgments are a constituent part of *all* evaluation research. Feminist evaluator Sandra Mathison (2014) explains "*evaluation* as the process and product of making judgments about the value, merit, or worth of an evaluand" (p. 42). Patton defines **merit** as the value of the program for those it is intended to help and **worth** as the value of the program for those outside of the program (e.g., the community or society) (2008, p. 113). For example, consider a researcher studying the success of a welfare program that gets recipients jobs. The *merit* would be the extent to which the program is successful in getting jobs for program participants and the *worth* would be the value of the program societally (e.g., reducing welfare) (Patton, 2008). Mertens and Stewart (2014) note that explicit values guide the determination of merit and worth in a particular project. Those values "should reflect real-world considerations" (Mertens & Stewart, 2014, p. 332). In other words, they must be realistic and useful. Evaluators need to **synthesize facts and values** in order to determine merit and worth (Mathison, 2014; Scriven, 1997).

In addition to the explicit judgment aspect of evaluation research, this approach to inquiry also differs from the others reviewed in this text because evaluation was established as a discipline in the 1960s. Evaluation is now considered an integral part of decision making for numerous types of government, public, and private organizations as they develop or assess the success of programming (Mertens & Stewart, 2014).

There are numerous models that guide evaluation research. Each model provides "an explicit or implicit perspective on the relationship of the evaluator to stakeholders, the evaluator's role in the project . . . and use of evaluation findings" (Brisolara, 2014, p. 21). Feminism is one such model. Feminist evaluation did not develop in a vacuum. It's important to understand the context in which feminist evaluation has recently emerged, as well as key moments in its development. Over the past several decades evaluation research has become increasingly focused on "action research models and participatory forms" (Brisolara & Seigart, 2007, p. 279). Numerous models have emerged that place a premium on stakeholder participation and a democratic approach to knowledge building (including the transformative paradigm discussed in the last chapter in the section on community-based participatory research). In the 1990s, several models that combine social action and collaborative, participatory approaches developed, one of which was feminist evaluation (Brisolara & Seigart, 2007).

In 1995 the American Evaluation Association created a feminist TIG (topical interest group). In the mid-1990s feminist evaluators, including Elizabeth Whitmore, Donna Mertens, and others, developed a proposal for an edited volume on feminist evaluation (Brisolara, 2014). They faced many challenges. Reviewers asked for extensive revisions, and the researchers ultimately felt that mainstream journals were not ready to support feminist evaluation (Brisolara, 2014). According to Sharon Brisolara, the researchers were not surprised by the debate surrounding feminist evaluation. In addition to raising methodological questions, a feminist approach to evaluation "raised questions about the meaning of utility, the role and responsibilities of the evaluator, and what relationship can or should exist between evaluation and social justice objectives" (Brisolara, 2014, p. 21). Brisolara and Seigart (2007, p. 280) note that a feminist evaluation perspective necessarily raises questions about

- Objectivity
- Our role(s) and positionality
- Obligations to clients
- Voice (who is heard)
- Assumptions we bring to bear
- Ethical praxis

It is not surprising this model has been met with resistance from the larger evaluation community. Years after the derailed attempt to create an edited volume, Denise Seigart and Sharon Brisolara took up the task. They built on the original proposal, which ultimately resulted in the breakthrough 2002 publication *New Directions for Evaluation.*

What exactly is feminist evaluation? How is it different from other evaluation models? Drawing on the work of Seigart, Mathison (2014) writes: "Like all evaluation approaches, feminist evaluation is fundamentally about ascertaining the value, merit, or worth of an evaluand, but with particular attention to gender issues, the needs of women, and the promotion of change" (Seigart, 2005, p. 155; 2014, p. 54). Some suggest that women and their material realities are placed at the center of the research process (e.g., Ward, 2002) while others focus on gender inequities, which is more inclusive (Brisolara & Seigart, 2007). Applying an intersectional approach, we take the latter position and suggest, in accord with others in the field, that feminist evaluation focuses on gender inequalities that lead to social injustice (Brisolara & Seigart, 2007; Mertens, 2010). In this regard, gender is a *starting point* for research, but a feminist evaluation model also examines **multiple identities** (such as sexuality and race) and advocates for social action (Podems, 2014). Feminist evaluation is thus political, activist, and action oriented.

> **Intersectionality:** Most contemporary feminist evaluators suggest that *gender inequities,* and not women per se, are central to their projects. Although gender is a starting point for inquiry, evaluators ultimately consider the complexity of multiple identities and how they intersect.

Feminist evaluators bring a critical and gender-focused lens to the evaluation process (Podems, 2010; Seigart, 2005). Feminist evaluation is not about studying programs intended for women, but rather bringing this critical and gender-focused lens to the study of *any* program (Mathison 2014; Seigart, 2005). A feminist lens influences everything from topic selection to the dissemination of research findings (Podems, 2010). Building on her earlier work with Seigart, Brisolara (2014, pp. 23–30) proposes eight key feminist evaluation principles:

1. Knowledge is culturally, socially, and temporally contingent.
2. Knowledge is a powerful resource that serves an explicit or implicit purpose.
3. Evaluation is a political activity; evaluators' personal experiences, perspectives, and characteristics come from and lead to a particular political stance.

4. Research methods, institutions, and practices are social constructs.

5. There are multiple ways of knowing.

6. Gender inequities are one manifestation of social injustice. Discrimination cuts across race, class, and culture and is inextricably linked to all three.

7. Discrimination based on gender is systemic and structural.

8. Action and advocacy are considered to be morally and ethically appropriate responses of an engaged feminist evaluator.

In the following three tables, reprinted with permission, Brisolara elaborates on each key concept.

TABLE 7.1. Feminist Evaluation Positions on Feminist Concepts Related to the Nature of Knowledge and Associated Questions		
Concepts	Positions	Questions
Knowledge is culturally, socially, and temporally contingent.	• Feminist evaluation contextualizes programs and findings in their social, cultural, economic, and historical contexts and asks questions that reflect these understandings. • Feminist principles encourage evaluators to make their own identities and interests in the program clear and known. • Involvement and participation by a range of stakeholders in the evaluation, including program participants, is important to widening understanding of program realities.	• What are the prevalent social issues and cultural values of various stakeholders? • How do current understandings differ from understandings from the recent past? • Considering various stakeholders, what is needed in order to recognize and elicit meaningful and credible results in this context? • What forms of communicating findings would participants find most credible or appropriate?
Knowledge is a powerful resource that serves an explicit or implicit purpose.	Feminist evaluators make initial intended purposes and possible uses that emerge through inquiry known to all who might be affected by the evaluation and engage with participants to discover and articulate the other important uses of findings.	• Who/what gatekeepers to sources of knowledge exist? • In what ways are the types of knowledge of interest already utilized by stakeholders? • What are the consequences of sharing/not sharing what is learned? • For whom are we producing "knowledge" and for what purposes?

Source: From Brisolara (2014).

TABLE 7.2. Feminist Evaluation Positions on Feminist Concepts Related to the Nature of Inquiry and Associated Questions

Concept	Positions	Questions
Evaluation is a political activity; evaluators' personal experiences, perspectives, and characteristics come from and lead to a particular political stance.	Feminist evaluation approaches a project seeking to understand the political nature of the context from the very beginning of the project through reflexive processes, engagement with stakeholders, open-ended inquiry, and establishing trust among research participants.	• Whose voices are ostracized or limited in this context? • What power issues exist among stakeholders? • To what extent do power differences need to be addressed in order to allow for fuller participation? • To what extent can power imbalances safely and ethically be acknowledged? • To what extent is a feminist evaluation possible? • What personal political stances might interfere with an ability to see or represent project politics and what steps can be taken to mitigate this effect?
Research methods, institutions, and practices are social constructs.	• Methods are not value-neutral. • Through mixing methods, thinking critically about how to give space to silences, and using inclusive approaches, evaluators can work to counteract the influence of limiting ideologies.	• What procedures and stances do we introduce to ensure that we are making the best effort to understand program context and dynamics? • Who is asking the questions and from what position? • Whose voices or what perspectives are potentially excluded or diminished using the methods proposed?
There are multiple ways of knowing.	Feminist evaluation honors and searches for multiple ways of knowing, in part through deep and real engagement of a range of stakeholders.	• What ways of knowing are valued in this (cultural, social) context (e.g., stories, emotions, artistic representations)? • Do these ways of knowing vary by stakeholder/participant group? • Which forms of knowledge have the highest credibility (and does this depend on the source of information)?

Source: From Brisolara (2014).

TABLE 7.3. Feminist Evaluation Positions on Feminist Concepts Related to Social Justice and Associated Questions

Concept	Position	Questions
Gender inequities are one manifestation of social injustice. Discrimination cuts across race, class, and culture and is inextricably linked to all three.	Feminist evaluation begins its investigation by examining sex and sexual identity and expands its inquiry to understand how gender interacts with, shapes, and is shaped by other critical identities.	• In what ways are women (men, bisexual, transgendered people, etc.) treated differently within the program and how do their experiences and outcomes differ? • How does viewing participants/stakeholders from the perspective of class illuminate program dynamics? • In what ways do class, race, and gender combine to expand or contract possibilities for participants?
Discrimination based on gender is systemic and structural.	Efforts must be made to uncover policies and practices that lead to discrimination if programs and outcomes are to be more accurately understood. Care must be taken, however, to investigate what the possible repercussions of bringing these dynamics to light might be.	• What structural and gender inequities exist within this context? • What are the personal, social, and political consequences of these inequities? • What are the consequences of bringing systemic and structural inequities to light?
The purpose of knowledge is action.	Advocacy with or for people central to the evaluation, such as facilitating action on evaluation findings, is one of the most important intended outcomes of the evaluation. In order for advocacy to be ethical, the evaluator must discuss possible actions with participants most likely to be affected by advocacy and respect their experiences and concerns.	• What is the appropriate role of the evaluator given the circumstances and potential consequences of advocacy? • What are evaluation participants' most pressing needs for action, according to them? • What is gained and lost by acting? By not acting?

Source: From Brisolara (2014).

Feminist evaluators have conducted projects on numerous topics, including mental health and substance abuse treatment programs (Bowen, 2011); women's substance abuse programs (Beardsley & Miller, 2002); programs for sex workers (Magar, 2012; Podems, 2010); HIV/AIDS outreach centers and programs (Ross, 2003); welfare-to-work programs for women (Gilbert & Masucci, 2006; Warren, 2004); school-based health care (Seigart, 1999, 2014); programs of the UN and governments in Latin America (Faundez & Abarca, 2011); a development program in Angola (Nichols, 2014); an interactive multimedia instructional program for social work students (Thurston, Cauble, & Dinkel, 1998); an in-service training program for teachers (Thurston, 1989); tutoring procedures (Thurston & Dasta, 1990); and numerous other topics.

Because evaluation is itself a discipline and an overarching approach to research, evaluators may use any of the methods reviewed in this text, which is why we are reviewing it last. Evaluators typically use **multimethod research** or even more commonly, **mixed-methods research (MMR)**. Multimethod research involves using two or more methods from one paradigm (e.g., two qualitative methods such as in-depth interviews and ethnography). Mixed-methods research involves collecting and integrating quantitative and qualitative data in a single project (Leavy, 2017). For example, in her evaluation of the program for an HIV/AIDS outreach center that intended to teach women to use the female condom, Wilson employed both surveys and interviews. In Magar's (2012) evaluation of programs for sex workers in India, she used focus groups and in-depth interviews.

In addition to relying on mixed-methods research, feminist evaluators often use strategies similar to those discussed in the section on community-based participatory research. These are often highly participatory and collaborative designs. Mathison (2004) notes that feminist evaluators place a premium on stakeholder input throughout the evaluation process. Participant input beyond data collection is integral to feminist evaluation whether or not the project follows a participatory design (Brisolara & Seigart, 2007). Other feminist evaluators advocate for the use of the transformative paradigm in conjunction with the feminist lens (Mertens, 2009; Mertens & Stewart, 2014).

Let's take an in-depth look at a research example. In her evaluation of school-based health care, Seigart (2014) conducted case studies in the United States, Australia, and Canada from 2008 to 2009. Her mixed-methods approach included 73 in-depth interviews with various stakeholders (e.g., health care providers, teachers, administrators, parents, and community leaders involved with school-based health care) in multiple locations in each of the three countries. The interviews were generally conducted face-to-face and lasted approximately 1 hour. Seigart employed a method of "active listening" and "extensive conversations" (2014, p. 271). In addition to the interviews she included on-site observations and a review of institutional reports and other relevant literature. She aimed to build "thick descriptions" in order to be able to transfer the research findings from one context to another. In an effort to build credibility into the findings, she both sought triangulation of the data sources *and* shared her analysis with stakeholders and other researchers involved in order to ascertain their comments, which contributed to the final analysis (2014, p. 272). In these ways she developed a mixed-methods design and used a participatory approach (one that is inclusive of various stakeholders) that is in line with feminist principles.

Feminist evaluators may also conduct multiphase research. Let's take the example of Bowen's (2011) evaluation of a rural mental health and substance abuse treatment program in Appalachia. The study did not initially have an explicit feminist lens. Rather, it began with a quasi-experimental one-group design. Data were collected at three points: baseline, discharge, and 6 months after completing the program. The evaluation also included interviews and observations, but it was in year two that a feminist lens was applied. At this point a variety of methods, including life histories, were used in order to learn about the women comprehensively. For example, the challenges and strengths they brought with them into the treatment program and thus how they were or were not positioned for success within the program and after treatment.

Designing Feminist Evaluation Research

Each evaluation design will look different according to the specific topic, goals, and methods employed. Any research method or combination of methods may be used in evaluation research.[3] Quantitative, qualitative, and CBPR designs have already been reviewed, and you can refer to those sections of the last chapter as appropriate to your project. Because evaluators often rely on mixed-methods designs, which have not been reviewed, we briefly describe that process.

MMR begins by moving from your topic to a research purpose statement that outlines the **primary purposes or objectives** of the study. Include

---

[3]While evaluators typically use a combination of quantitative and qualitative methods— those reviewed in this text and others—there have been some methods created specifically for evaluation. Mathison (2014) notes Davies and Dart (2005) created the "most significant change methods" and Brinkerhoff (2005) created the "success case method," which borrows from existing methods and disciplines but "packages" them in distinct ways.

the research topic (phenomenon), the participants and setting, the methodology (quantitative and qualitative data collection methods, the selected mixed-methods design, and the theoretical framework guiding the study as applicable), and the primary rationale for conducting the evaluation (Leavy, 2017).

It is then customary to create research questions. MMR necessarily involves at least one quantitative research question or hypothesis, at least one qualitative research question, and generally at least one mixed-methods question (although sometimes it is omitted). It is necessary to have **integrated research questions** (Brannen & O'Connell, 2015; Yin, 2006). Integration can take various forms. For example, the qualitative question may be formulated to explain or contextualize the answer to the preceding quantitative question. Or, the quantitative question may be formulated in response to what was learned by addressing the qualitative question. Quantitative and qualitative research questions were addressed in the last chapter. The MMR question directly addresses the mixed-methods nature of the project by asking something about what is learned by combining the quantitative and qualitative data, or it may ask something about how the mixed-methods design aided the project. These questions may employ **relational language,** aimed at addressing the relationship between the quantitative and qualitative phases of research, including words and phrases such as "synergistic," "integration," "connection," "comprehensive," "fuller understanding," and "better understanding" (Leavy, 2017).

There are three issues feminist evaluators carefully consider as they develop a research purpose statement and a set of research questions. First, feminist evaluation is typically highly **participatory,** and therefore it is important to collaborate with various stakeholders during the research design process. Second, as evaluators create research questions, it is important to consider the **reasons** the evaluation is being undertaken. Mathison notes the evaluation may be occurring for any number of reasons including,

> to determine if goals are met; to determine outcomes, both anticipated and unanticipated and intended and unintended; to improve the evaluand; to make decisions about an evaluand (including decisions about adopting, funding, or dismantling the evaluand); to inform public discourse and policy about an evaluand; and to demonstrate accountability. (2014, p. 49).

Finally, feminist evaluators must ask questions that **focus on gender inequities,** if that is what they want to learn about, or else those issues may be rendered invisible (Mertens & Stewart, 2014).

Regardless of the particular method or combination of methods employed, any other evaluation models or values guiding a feminist evaluation will also influence the methodology. For example, if you are combining feminist and transformative models, the research design will likely involve various stakeholders at every phase of the evaluation, employ a responsive design, and use multi- or mixed methods (Mertens & Stewart, 2014). With respect to the multi- or mixed-methods approach, Mertens and Stewart advocate using qualitative research first and then determining if further qualitative or quantitative research is appropriate (2014, p. 337).

Data Collection, Analysis, and Interpretation

The procedures used for data collection, analysis, and interpretation depend on the method or methods employed in the evaluation (consult the last chapter as appropriate). However, it is customary in feminist evaluation to include stakeholders in these processes, at least to some extent. In their review of feminist evaluation in Latin America, Silvia Salinas Mulder and Fabiola Amariles (2014) note that participation often refers only to the evaluators and program managers. Further, they contend the attitudes of evaluators often end up limiting the participation of women and other excluded groups. This is because evaluators often focus on their own questions and interests. This is referred to as a "fact-seeking drive" (Salinas Mulder, Rance, Serrate Suarez, & Castro Condori, 2000, as quoted in Salinas Mulder & Amariles, 2014, p. 229). This is akin to the "drive-by scholarship" we discussed in the ethics chapter. Enacting reflexivity and soliciting stakeholder feedback at various points of the project are both good measures toward attaining true participation. Salinas Mulder and Amariles also offer an extensive list of tips, some of which we paraphrase here (2014, pp. 231–243):

- Consider interviews as dialogues.
- Employ context-relevant approaches to diminish unequal power relations.
- Give all relevant stakeholders a genuine opportunity to choose whether or not to participate.
- Organize a group of diverse staff members. ("The group will be the voice of staff in matters related to evaluation design and development" p. 233).
- Map stakeholders' roles, interests, and relationships, including our own as evaluators in order to better understand the data.

- Discuss the client and/or donors' expectations regarding the evaluation.
- Enact active listening and develop theory directly out of the data.
- Foster buy-in with the participants through a careful explanation of the purpose and process of the evaluation (which is a necessary part of ethical practice).
- Employ methods creatively and with flexibility.

Geospatial Technologies

The use of geographic information systems (GIS) and other geospatial technologies in feminist evaluation is on the rise. Geospatial technologies including GIS have existed for over 40 years but became readily available to nonspecialists in the mid-1990s (Steinberg & Lakshmi Steinberg, 2011). These technologies can be used to help bring stakeholders, including those who are typically marginalized,

> **Feminist digital media:** Feminist evaluators are increasingly using geospatial technologies to spatially represent gender inequities in communities of interest and find better ways to be of service to stakeholders.

into the evaluation process (Mertens, 2008, 2010; Mertens & Stewart, 2014). These technologies can be used to help identify and make visible the gender inequities that lead to injustice (Mertens & Stewart, 2014). Feminist geographer Mei-Po Kwan has been at the forefront of this trend. Drawing on Kwan (2002) and McLafferty (2002), Mertens and Stewart suggest:

> The utilization of GIS for feminist visualization seeks to represent gendered experiences and spaces of women by using geographic data to link trajectories of women's everyday lives with geographical contexts, and to challenge traditional power relations to strengthen and empower women's activism. (2014, p. 350)

Feminist evaluators have used these technologies in numerous types of projects.

For example, Warren (2004) wanted to map child care facilities for women entering welfare-to-work programs. Data on licensed programs were readily available, but many poor women were using unlicensed providers. Warren had to gather that information directly from the community in order to properly map the facilities. In another example, Melissa Gilbert and Michelle Masucci (2006) wanted to teach women going from welfare to work how to use GIS in order to assist them in job searching. However, the women didn't have time to learn how to use the technology and instead wanted their children to learn. The researchers adapted and collaborated with community organizations to develop an after-school program to teach the kids.

As evident by these examples, communities are often actively involved in generating mapping data. Feminist evaluators also need to be able to adapt based on the realities of the stakeholders and the communities in which they are enmeshed.

Dissemination, Advocacy, and Public Policy

The role of action and advocacy is highly contested in the field of evaluation. Notwithstanding the debate, most in the field agree that findings should be useful in a real-world context and evaluators may have a role in that process (Brisolara & Seigart, 2007). There are multiple models, including feminism, that strongly advocate for both social action and advocacy. Jennifer Greene (1995) has been a vocal proponent for advocacy as an integral part of evaluation. Greene suggests it is our responsibility to advocate for program participants. While there is debate even among feminist evaluators, there is consensus that findings should be put to use to combat gender inequities (Brisolara & Seigart, 2007).

What does it mean to be an advocate? What does this look like in practice? Kristin Ward (2002) proposes two strategies: (1) collaborating with activists and disseminating the findings, and (2) advocating for, and along with, participants. This harkens back to discussions earlier in this book about what it means to be an ally. The issue is not necessarily how you think the findings would best be put to use, but what your participants think is in their own best interest. An excellent example of this difference comes from Salinas Mulder and Amarile's (2014) review of the Latin American feminist movement that challenged the common practice of calling the target population of a program "beneficiaries." That framing is biased, assuming that women are so poor or disempowered "that they will benefit from any external action. It may also ignore women's self-determination and critical capacities" (p. 229). The Latin American feminist movement rejects the word "beneficiary" promoted by the "women in development (WID)" perspective, which mainly gives "assistance" to women

> **Ally:** In the context of feminist evaluation, being an ally may mean being an advocate along with participants—prioritizing their agenda for change and using the evaluation findings to assist them.

without challenging gender inequality. They instead favor a "gender and development (GAD)" perspective which seeks to remedy gender inequality (Salinas Mulder & Amariles, 2014, p. 229).

Salinas Mulder and Amarile also suggest that feminist evaluators plan their research dissemination and advocacy *strategically,* advocating that they

> sensitize politicians, decision-makers, and society about prevailing human rights and gender injustices and their negative impact on poverty reduction and development. Provide decision-makers with evidence, arguments, and concrete ideas for gender responsiveness in culturally sensitive policy design and implementation. (2004, pp. 245–246)

Finally, and significantly, they suggest feminist evaluators consider what happens after advocacy. They suggest building capacity "for the construction of an ex-post advocacy strategy by the program staff and feminist groups—tools, information, results, and also for building a theory of change for the program or project" (p. 239). While any of the research methods reviewed in this text may include attempts at social action, advocacy, and influencing public policy, feminist evaluation *necessarily* includes these in some measure. Further, it is good practice on both practical and ethical levels to consider what you leave stakeholders with even after that formal phase of the process.

CONCLUSION

Content analysis, particularly in the form of media analysis, has long been a staple for feminist researchers. By studying those texts that both appear and do not appear in a particular culture at a particular time, as well as the context of production, feminists are able to create knowledge about pervasive sexism, how sexism relates to other "isms," and how girls, women, and others may be impacted by these representations. How is gender socially constructed? What is included in those constructions? What is left out? In addition to studying "things," feminist researchers are increasingly committed to studying programs and organizations in order to understand how they function with respect to gender issues. What programs do business, private agencies, or governments create? What are the gender dynamics within those programs? How is gender linked up to other status characteristics? What outcomes are produced by new or emerging policies? How might they be improved in order to create more gender equity?

DISCUSSION QUESTIONS

1. Why are feminist researchers so drawn to content analysis?
2. How does evaluation differ from the other research approaches reviewed in this book?
3. What distinguishes feminist evaluation from other evaluation models?

ACTIVITIES

1. Conduct a small "mock" feminist content analysis. Take a research topic in which you are interested and select a small sample of sources from which to extract your data (e.g., three to four magazines, newspapers).
   a. Determine the unit of analysis.
   b. Code your data, refining your codes as you go.
   c. Write memo notes about your impressions and ideas.
2. After completing the "mock" feminist content analysis, describe how your feminist perspective influenced the project (consider topic selection, your coding process, how you developed memo notes: up to one page).
3. Find a peer-reviewed journal article or book chapter that details a feminist evaluation project. Respond to the following (one to two pages):
   a. What was the purpose of the evaluation?
   b. What methodology was employed?
   c. How, specifically, did the feminist perspective shape the project?
   d. Describe the social action or advocacy component. What worked well? What could be improved?

SUGGESTED RESOURCES

Books

Brisolara, S., Seigart, D., & SenGupta, S. (Eds.). (2014). *Feminist evaluation and research: Theory and practice.* New York: Guilford Press.

An excellent edited volume on feminist evaluation that provides historical context, design guidelines, and rich interdisciplinary and international exemplars from leading evaluators.

Kilbourne, J. (2012). *Can't buy me love: How advertising changes the way we think and feel.* New York: Free Press.

A powerful book about how contemporary advertising affects people, with a special emphasis on young girls.

Mertens, D. M. (2008). *Transformative research and evaluation*. New York: Guilford Press.

The author offers an in-depth and persuasive case for using the transformative paradigm in evaluation research, which she defines as a human rights approach. This perspective allows one to design projects around the concerns and perspectives of those who have been pushed to the margins based on gender, sexuality, race, ableness, social class, and other social identities.

☐ Digital Resources

www.mediaed.org
The Media Education Foundation

http://idabwellsmuseum.org
Ida B. Wells-Barnett Museum

▬ *Films*

Miss Representation (2011)
Killing Us Softly: Advertising's Image of Women (1979) (Note: Several updated versions are available.)
Slim Hopes: Advertising and the Obsession with Thinness (1995)

PART III

Being a Feminist Researcher

GETTING THE WORK OUT

CHAPTER 8

Writing and Publishing Feminist Research

Research is formalized curiosity. It is
poking and prying with a purpose.
—ZORA NEALE HURSTON

LEARNING OBJECTIVES

- To introduce issues related to the ethics of representation
- To explain how and why the personal is political in feminist writing
- To offer guidance on the craft of writing with specific instruction for traditional academic forms, arts-based and literary forms, and public forms such as op-eds, blogs, and vlogs
- To provide a discussion about what it means to publish work as a feminist and become a public intellectual (to varying degrees)
- To offer advice about navigating the publishing world

You have conducted a project—gathered, analyzed, and interpreted data. Now what? Research needs to be represented and distributed so that others have access to the findings. It is the representation, publication, and dissemination of research findings that makes what we have learned available to others, thereby contributing to feminism. The ethics surrounding representation, issues of audience, and writing as critique are all issues taken seriously by feminists.

> **Ethics** permeates the representation stage of research.

Feminist researchers have a complicated relationship to representation. There is an **ethics of representation** that is vital to feminist research because women and other minority groups have been egregiously misrepresented (Preissle, 2007). Women's lives, for example, have been distorted, marginalized, and excluded in research findings (Preissle, 2007; Richardson, 1997). In this regard, for feminists there is an acknowledgment of, and a wrestling with, the inescapable issue of power that permeates representation. What does it mean to speak for another? What does it mean to represent another's story? Feminist participatory action researcher Michelle Fine (1994) has long been writing about the struggle representing others. For her, collaborative writing with participants provides a solution; however, even that isn't a magic potion. Every feminist researcher has to develop an ethical writing practice in accord with their belief systems.

> **Power sharing:** Collaborative writing is one way to enact power sharing.

Another issue that is paramount for feminist researchers is **audience,** those groups we are trying to reach. The target audiences for research, within and/or beyond the academy, must be identified and appropriate choices made for how to reach them. This influences the formats feminists use, as well as the venues in which they distribute their findings. For example, if one writes an essay, will it be published in an anthology or an online blog? If online, which blog, and how will it be distributed/promoted in order to maximize its audience?

What distinguishes a feminist write-up from a nonfeminist write-up? Because of the diversity in feminist research, there is no one way to answer that question; however, it is clear that feminist writing, in one way or another, is a form of **critique.** Feminist research is value laden and seeks to uncover, disrupt, and challenge prevailing systems of inequality and the knowledge that supports them. Critique can thus be understood as a form of intervention. Judith Roof proposes, "feminist research in general believes in the power of critique and inquiry to change materially the structures of culture and the lives of individuals" (2007, p. 426).

In an effort to reach and persuade audiences, feminist researchers often merge the personal and political, pay careful attention to the craft of writing, engage multiple formats, and publish strategically, including taking advantage of opportunities afforded by the Internet.

The Personal Is Political

Although historically researchers were mandated to render distanced and "objective" research reports, feminist researchers have persuasively demonstrated how false claims of neutrality mask and perpetuate the construction of gendered, racialized, sexed, and classed knowledge (see Halpin, 1989; Smith, 1987). There is a continuum of subjectivity and objectivity, with innumerable points that blur both ways of knowing (Charmaz, 2007, 2012). Feminist researchers have a long history of challenging the objective/subjective dichotomy, including by writing from a place that is both personal and political. By imbuing our work with personal experiences, stories, and emotions, feminist research aims to personalize political and social issues and engage the consumers of research on deep levels. Even more so, the use of the personal is a way of positioning oneself as an authority—an expert with unique insights (Roof, 2007, 2012). We are each an authority on our own experiences.

Virginia Woolf perhaps paved the way for incorporating the personal into feminist writing with the 1929 publication of *A Room of One's Own*. In this famed essay written in the first person, Woolf described a woman's struggle to be an artist at a time when only men were afforded material support, time, and space. Woolf challenged prevailing ideologies through the use of women's personal experiences. Roof writes, "Woolf's essay deploys the personal as a most influential mode of persuasion. Woolf's use of the personal model has become a persuasive trope for feminist writers and researchers" (2007, p. 439). Indeed, this strategy is a mainstay of contemporary feminist writing. For example, bell hooks's significant body of work consists primarily of collections of personal essays that blur the subjective and objective. The 2014 *New York Times* best-seller *Bad Feminist: Essays* by Roxane Gay is likewise a collection of personal essays aimed at cultural critique.

Over the past three decades, use of autobiographical data has been on the rise across the academy, perhaps most clearly evidenced by the emergence of autoethnography (mentioned in Chapter 6). Carolyn Ellis (2004), the founding mother of the method, conceptualizes autoethnography as a way of using personal experience to write critically about culture. Another leader in the field, Stacy Holman Jones (2005) has specifically written about autoethnography as a way of making the personal political. Many autoethnographies takes the form of essays. Today, blogs are a very popular format feminists use to merge the personal and political (discussed later in this chapter).

The Craft of Writing

In order to persuade and engage audiences, it's vital to write well. You've done all of the work studying your topic and reaching your findings, but unless you are able to communicate what you have learned effectively, it's of little consequence. Writing is a skill that can be learned and improved with practice and commitment. All writing takes **discipline**. As you have set aside certain time to collect data, for example, so too you should set aside time for writing. Marianne Fallon (2016) suggests setting "concrete, actionable goals" (p. 34) to help develop a discipline around writing. You may have times when you're feeling inspired and others when writing feels like a chore, but waiting for inspiration to strike is a fool's errand. Some feminist scholars suggest making writing collaborative so that you are accountable to your writing buddy (Charmaz, 2007, 2012; Faulkner & Squillante, 2016; Leavy, 2013). Writing also follows stages: outlining, drafting, revising, soliciting feedback, and additional rounds of revising as needed. As you go through these stages, you come to a deeper understanding of the research findings and how to best represent them. There are some core features of good writing that you can read about in virtually any instructional book on writing. Here we review those that are particularly salient in feminist research.

Show, don't tell is standard writing advice. Showing is important in feminist research for two interconnected reasons. First, showing is a strategy for engaging readers—drawing them in. Second, by showing instead of telling, we create some degree of a buffer against critique. This is not to say we can ever fully protect our work from critique, or even that such insulation would be desirable; however, by using data to show readers about the people, places, or circumstances we've researched, we are better able to convince others our conclusions are legitimate. Engaging readers with details and descriptions and using data to illustrate our assertions are tools of **persuasion**. An excellent example comes from feminist sociologist Jessica Smartt Gullion.

Language is the tool with which writers sculpt. Good writing requires rigorous attention to language. Specificity makes writing compelling. Use language clearly, crisply, and effectively. Words carry meaning(s), histories, emotion, tenor, and lyrical qualities. Feminist writers are hyperattentive to the ways that words shape our perceptions of socially constructed realities. Words can be used to expose, challenge, or disrupt dominant ideologies and stereotypes. Sometimes this means something as simple as challenging a binary like he/she and instead *flipping* the binary with she/he or *challenging* the binary with she/he/they.

Metaphors and similes "are figures of speech that compare an abstract concept with something concrete—an object we can see, hear, feel, taste, or smell" (Caulley, 2008, p. 440). The use of metaphors and similes makes for richness of writing. Feminist researchers may create **original metaphors** or uncover, expose, and challenge **taken-for-granted metaphors** (Charmaz, 2007, 2012). With respect to creating your own, metaphors and similes may be used to establish micro–macro connections, challenge, disrupt,

An Example of Showing, Not Telling

In telling, it is easier for your critics to pelt you with accusations of bias, particularly when your colourful adjectives read like your personal opinion rather than based in your research. For example, I can write, "The conditions at the county jail are deplorable." That sounds like my opinion, like I personally believe the conditions at the jail are deplorable, but that an objective observer might not draw the same conclusion. And while it may in fact be my opinion, my argument becomes much stronger when I *show* you the deplorable conditions at the county jail, when I give you enough information to enable you to reach my conclusion on your own:

Joan wakes with a start—someone is pulling her hair. She reaches through the darkness to find a warm furry mass. She leaps from her bunk, squealing, disgusted. It's the third night in a row she's woken to rats chewing on her hair. Her bunkmates scream at her: "Shut the fuck up, bitch!" She lays back down on the concrete platform, puts her arm under her head as a pillow, and cries.

The details of Joan's story are gathered from interview transcripts and observations conducted at the jail. I put them into a narrative form to tell the story of the deplorable conditions at the jail. Readers do not have to rely on me to tell them that the conditions are deplorable—they can see that for themselves. Rats chewing your hair? Concrete bunks with no pillow? People cursing at you? Yeah, that sounds pretty deplorable to me. There are additional details that the writer could include to further round out the story. The room smells like sewage because the toilet backs up nearly every day. A glob of rotten milk goes in Joan's mouth when she takes a sip from her carton. Show the reader this slice of the social world. Lead them through your theoretical argument with your words. Give them pieces of information to help draw them to the conclusions you found.

Gullion (2016, p. 75). Reprinted with permission.

or subvert taken-for-granted assumptions, or create subtext. They "allow writers both to interpret and construct meanings" (Watson, 2016, p. 12). In terms of challenging preexisting metaphors, renowned feminist scholar Emily Martin (1999) suggests there are "sleeping metaphors in science" that favor males that feminists must "awaken." Charmaz explains the importance of sleeping metaphors as follows: "They shape the text and, moreover, our conceptions of the realities it addresses. Such metaphors shape *what* we see and *how* we see it and contain hidden reasons that explain, justify, and perpetuate *why* we see it in that way" (2007, p. 450).

Rhetorical devices beyond metaphors and similes, such as foreshadowing, understatements, or posing questions to readers can be employed to engage readers (Charmaz, 2007, 2012). Feminist researchers may use these devices to cultivate reflection and critical thinking.

Finding your voice as an author is an essential part of developing your style or personal signature, which in turn helps you build an audience for

your work. Do you incorporate humor into your writing? Do you use rhetorical devices? How do you approach sentence structure? How do you
end pieces? These are just examples of the kinds of decisions that help create your unique fingerprint. Feminist authors Sandra Faulkner and Sheila
Squillante explain that different writers sound different on the page. They
note the elements that create that *sound* include "diction and word choice,
sentence or line structure, punctuation, tone, use of dialogue, figurative
language (or lack of), and even subject matter" (2016, p. 45). They go on
to astutely observe that while we often talk about finding our voice, in
fact, we each have many voices and need to consciously decide which to
use in each piece of writing. This becomes clearer in the next section on
different formats. For example, if you have conducted a study about gender
inequality in education, it is possible you will represent that research in a
traditional research article for an academic journal as well as an op-ed for
a local newspaper. Surely you will write each in a different *voice*, but both
will represent you as an author.

   While we have provided an overview of good writing practices, there
are specifics to consider depending on the format used.

Formats

> **Representation:** Feminists
> strategically engage with
> multiple formats in order to
> represent research findings.

Feminist researchers have numerous
formats available for the representation of research findings, including
those traditionally used for scholarly
research, emergent practices involving
the arts, and popular forms intended
for public audiences. Because feminists are often trying to reach audiences
both inside and outside of the academy, they may engage with multiple
formats in one project in order to best communicate their findings to each
identified audience for their work. Roof (2007, 2012) suggests that the
mixed media feminist researchers turn to mirrors the mixing of disciplinary knowledge required by feminism. In the following section we review
these three representational genres, offering guidance about the building
blocks of each form.

Traditional Academic Forms

Traditional academic forms developed in a Eurocentric, male-centered academy and include peer-reviewed journal articles, conference presentations,

monographs, and essays. Feminist approaches draw "attention to the inherent phallocentrism" within these forms (Roof, 2007, p. 426). Wanda S. Pillow and Cris Mayo (2007) report that "a review of ethnographies" showed "feminist researchers are paying attention to *how* they write as well as what they write" (p. 165). Long gone are the days when academic writing has to be dry. Storytelling can be a highly effective form of writing because it engages readers.

As peer-reviewed journal articles have long been considered the gold standard in academic writing, we would like to expand on them briefly. Notwithstanding the limitations of academic journal articles (e.g., their highly limited audience within the academy) it's important for feminists to contribute to scholarly research in this form in order to diversify the knowledge that the academy deems "legitimate." The organization of a journal article depends on the methodology. The best thing to do is to read many articles in your subject area that use your research method (e.g., if you have conducted qualitative interview research, read other articles that have used that method, including those in your subject area). This will teach you the basics of the format. The box below includes the components of most research articles, but again, this is only a template and will differ based on the methodology.

The Components of Research Articles

- Title
- Abstract
- Key words
- An introduction to the project: the topic investigated (including the significance of studying this topic)
- Research purpose statement and research questions or hypotheses
- Literature review
- Theoretical or philosophical perspective guiding the project
- The methodology (what research method or methods were used and how)
- Participants (including the sampling strategy used to find them)
- Data analysis and interpretation procedures
- Discussion of the findings (including how the findings move feminist concerns forward)
- Conclusion (may include strengths and weaknesses of the study and ideas for future research)
- References (follow the style guidelines of the journal)

Marianne Fallon (2016) offers a host of "rules" for strong academic writing. Here are a few of her top tips:

- "Write to learn, then write to teach" (p. 41).
- "Report, support, do not distort" (p. 42).
- "Collect and connect the dots" (p. 45).
- "Seek ye the 3 C's—clear, concise, coherent" (p. 48).

While academic texts are important, many feminists also represent their work in alternative forms. Research projects are likely to have more than one outcome.

Arts-Based and Literary Forms

Arts-based research (ABR) has emerged as a distinct paradigm over the last three decades (although feminists have been drawing on the arts for far longer). ABR involves researchers in any discipline adapting the tenets of the creative arts in order to address research questions (Leavy, 2009, 2015). ABR can be used during any or all phases of social research, and is commonly used to represent research findings. Arts-based research practices have been influenced by the creative arts therapies, neuroscientific research about how people consume art (including literary neuroscience), the rise in autobiographical data across the academy, and moves toward public scholarship. For feminist researchers, who have long used the personal in their work and have always given special consideration to the audiences they reach, including those outside of the academy, ABR offers a useful set of approaches. By harnessing the unique capabilities of the arts to tap into issues in new ways, jar people into seeing and thinking differently, promote self and social reflection, and open a multiplicity of meanings, these practices are highly effective for research centered on sensitive or controversial subject matter, and aimed at social justice. Feminist researchers can draw on any of the literary, performative, or visual arts in order to represent and share their work. As with any research practice, it is necessary to learn the craft you are working with. While space does not permit us to review each arts-based practice, as they are as extensive as arts practices themselves, we review ethnographic fiction and "social fiction" as they are increasingly being used by feminist researchers looking for alternatives to traditional academic written formats.

Ethnographic Fiction and Social Fiction

Fiction has long been used by feminist researchers as a means of interrogation and representation. Two of the best-known authors to explicitly blur anthropological ethnography and fiction are Zora Neale Hurston and Alice Walker. Their work can be termed **ethnographic fiction** or **anthropological fiction.**

Zora Neale Hurston never completed her PhD in anthropology and endured repeated criticism at Columbia University for failing to conform to standards of "rigor" (Harrison, 1995; Visweseran, 1994). Nevertheless, Hurston is widely considered an anthropological novelist. She went beyond the confines of traditional anthropology and decided to use literary tools to write "against the grain" of both the academy and the larger dominant culture (Behar, 1995; Harrison, 1995). Hurston's turn to ethnographic fiction allowed her to use an intersectional approach to writing that challenged dominant understandings of race, class, and, gender as she simultaneously challenged an academy that excluded her work. Alice Walker's fiction also blurs anthropology and fiction. In composing her work, she

> **Intersectionality:** Both Zora Neale Hurston and Alice Walker applied intersectional approaches to their ethnographic fiction.

drew on historical and anthropological sources as well as literary devices (Harrison, 1995). Also writing through an intersectional lens, her fiction seeks to tell complex stories about the social construction of gender, class, and race, the multiplicity of identity, and identity as a source of cultural and political struggles. Harrison (1995) termed Walker's short stories and novels "ethnographic and ethnohistorical" (p. 235). She writes, "Walker's novel [*The Temple of My Familiar*] is a world cultural history from a pluralistic Third World feminist perspective. As feminist 'her-story,' the novel should be seen as an integral part of the broader literature on the politics of representing gender, race, and culture history" (1995, p. 237).

More recently, **social fiction, fiction-based research (FBR)**, or **fiction as a research practice**[1] was popularized by the work of Patricia Leavy as a research practice whereby researchers in any discipline adapt the tenets of fiction to represent their research. Leavy has used social fiction as a means of analyzing and representing her feminist interview research with women about their relationships, gender identities, and body image issues (Leavy, 2011a, 2013, 2015, 2016, 2017). Social fiction is also being used to present contemporary intersectional feminist narratives. For example, A.

---

[1] These terms were coined by Patricia Leavy in 2010 and 2013, respectively.

Breeze Harper's (2014) novel *Scars: A Black Lesbian Experience in Rural White New England* follows protagonist Savannah Penelope Sales, a Black girl, from a White, working-class, rural New England town, struggling to accept her lesbian identity. Harper describes the novel "as a work of social fiction born out of years of critical race, Black feminist, and critical whiteness studies scholarship." She notes, "*Scars* engages the reader to think about USA culture through the lenses of race, whiteness, working-class sensibilities, sexual orientation, and how rural geography influences identity" (preface).

For another recent example, J. Sumerau's sociological novel *Cigarettes & Wine,* written in the first person and based partly on personal experience, explores bisexual and transgender experience. The novel investigates "relationships and intersections," including the complex ways different status characteristics and social norms shape our identities and experiences (Sumerau, 2017). Social fiction is increasingly being used by feminist researchers for reasons including being accessible to nonacademic audiences, opening up multiple meanings instead of presenting an authoritative view, and, as Elizabeth de Freitas (2003) notes, being uniquely able to promote "empathetic engagement."

As we realize academics are more likely to have some training with respect to writing in the traditional academic forms reviewed in the previous section, we offer some additional instruction for writing in a literary form. See the box on pages 211–212 for the main components of a literary story, which also bears similarities to the components of a play script or ethnodrama (originally developed in Leavy, 2013).

Public Forms

Public scholarship that is accessible and relevant outside of the academy is on the rise, broadly speaking. Research institutions are increasingly concerned with the **impact** of research. How does research reach and affect relevant stakeholders outside of the academy? What is the real-world usefulness? While the rise in public scholarship is relatively recent, for feminists, using public forms has always been important for several reasons. First, just as many feminists reject hierarchies within researcher–researched relationships, so too they reject an elitist system that makes knowledge available only to those in academic institutions. Feminist research is for the many, not the few. Second, as feminists seek to conduct research in order to, in some way, make the world a more just and equitable place, research is intended to matter beyond the academy. Finally, in efforts to create social change, it's important to demonstrate what the key issues are and how individuals and

The Components of Literary Stories

. . . .

Structural design elements: these features give the writing its form.

Master plot or master narrative: Stories that are told repeatedly in the culture in different ways and draw on deeply held values, hopes, and fears (Abbott, 2008). These are powerful literary tools because they resonate deeply with people and therefore carry "enormous emotional capital" (Abbott, 2008, p. 46).

Plot and story line: A plot refers to the overall structure of the narrative. The process of plotting involves ordering the major events or scenes of the story and sketching a general outline of the beginning, middle, and end of the narrative. Delineate major "plot points" during this process. The story line refers to the progression or sequence of events within the plot (Saldaña, 2003).

Scenes and narrative: Scenes are a dramatic way of writing—by showing what is happening as if the action were unfolding before the reader's eyes. When done well, scenes offer a high sense of realism and appear like slices of reality (Caulley, 2008, drawing on Gutkind, 1997). Scenic writing often uses active verbs (Caulley, 2008). Narrative writing is a means of summarizing or offering information beyond what is transpiring. Narrative is helpful for communicating information that happened outside of the scenes and/or providing commentary on characters and/or situations, including background information from the narrator's point of view. Narrative writing often uses passive verbs.

Endings/closure and expectations: Readers develop expectations based on (1) signs the writer has created, and (2) their previous experiences consuming stories (novels, films, etc.). Expectations do not necessarily need to be fulfilled, as in some circumstances it is beneficial to violate readers' expectations (Abbott, 2008). Closure refers to "resolution of the story's central conflict" (Abbott, p. 57).

Literary design elements: these features give the writing its feeling or gestalt.

Genre: A genre is a "recurrent literary form" (Abbott, 2008, p. 49). The novel, novella, or short story are all broad genres. Within each of those literary forms are thematically driven genres such as romance stories, "chick lit," mysteries, adventure stories, and so forth. Each genre comes with its own set of conventions.

Themes and motifs: A theme is a central idea and a motif is a recurrent idea, subject, or symbol.

Style and tone: Style refers to the author's personal fingerprint and may include attention to the dramatic effects of language (such as the use of short statements and emotionally charged language); emphasis on the lyrical nature of language; use of humor or sarcasm; and the particular balance between scenic and narrative writing, or between the different voices (e.g., the narrator, interior monologue, and dialogue or interaction between characters). The tone communicates the "mood" of the story (e.g., humorous, hopeful, tragic).

Characterization: the creation of those who people your story.

Types and character profiles: Recurring kinds of characters referred to as "types." Character types are often linked to master plots and can carry emotional

(continued)

and symbolic weight for readers. It's important to develop robust character profiles that result in sensitively portrayed, multidimensional characters. Character profiles can be created with descriptions of the following: physical appear-
ance, activities the character engages in, personality, core motivation, flaws and
strengths, and the character's name.

Dialogue and interaction: Dialogue can be thought of as "captured conversations" that enhance characterization and show the way people communicate
daily (Caulley, 2008, p. 435). Dialogue illuminates who individual characters are
and how characters relate to one another. It's important to consider the way a
character uses language, relationships between characters (e.g., dialogue may
denote familiarity between characters and many other aspects of their relationships), the tenor and pace of conversations, and the context in which the dialogue
is unfolding. Please note that if you are writing a play script or ethnodrama,
which favors action over description, "dialogue itself becomes the action as we
watch characters do battle with words and silences" (Harris & Holman Jones,
2016, p. 19).

Internal dialogue/interiority: The ability to represent a character's interiority
is one of the greatest benefits and distinctions of fiction. Representing interiority allows writers to make conceivable what is otherwise hidden (Caulley, 2008).
Internal dialogue can be used for purposes such as exploring sociopsychologi-
cal processes (readers have access to what a person thinks and feels in regard to
him, her, or themselves, in response to interactions with others, and in response
to particular events, situations, or circumstances), creating empathetic engagement, and establishing micro–macro connections (illustrating how larger social,
political, economic, cultural, or other forces are interpreted and internalized by
individuals).

Literary tools: these features help make fiction compelling.

Description and detail: Rich and multisensory descriptions of places, people, and situations engage readers and help create verisimilitude.

Language and specificity: Elizabeth de Freitas explains that "nothing is
sloppy in fiction" and we must work rigorously to achieve "exactness" in our writing, rewriting and crafting sentences over and over again (2003, pp. 269–70).

Metaphors and similes (discussed earlier in the section "The Craft of Writing").

groups are impacted, and then to persuade people that feminist knowledge
holds some answers. The research has to reach the public domain in order
to achieve any of these objectives.

Accessibility is central to public scholarship. The work needs to be
accessible in two ways (Leavy, 2011a, 2015). First, it has to be written
accessibly, that is to say, in clear, simple, widely understandable, and jargon-
free language. Second, it needs to circulate in venues relevant stakeholders
have access to. Blogs, vlogs, and op-eds are the most common public forms
feminists use. While there are formal gatekeepers with op-eds, anyone with

access to a computer can start a blog. While turning to established blogs, which require formal submission, is more likely to garner higher circulation (impact), if your work isn't accepted, you can always start your own blog and promote it on social media, a tactic many feminists use. Blogs have become a mainstay in feminist writing.

Blogs often begin from, or are centered around, a personal place or experience. The personal is used as a vehicle to raise social, cultural, and political issues. Blogs are thus a contemporary form in which feminists make the personal political. Feminist scholar and respected blogger Robin M. Boylorn writes autoethnographic blogs as a means of cultural critique. She notes:

> **Feminist digital media:** Blogs have become a popular form of feminist digital media.

> Blog entries are intentionally brief, informative, and pointed with a (political) purpose. The journalistic quality of blogs . . . makes them a combination of objectivity and subjectivity . . . blogs gain credibility by incorporating cultural, social and political components into subjective personal reflections . . . auto/ethnographic blogs resonate with readers due to their realness, subjectivity, emotionality, vulnerability, reflexivity, and bravery. (2013, p. 77)

Like most who engage with blogging, Boylorn had initial concerns. She called the prospect of blogging and receiving immediate feedback "uniquely risky" (2013, p. 75). However, during Women's History Month in 2010 Boylorn and colleagues launched Crunk Feminist Collective (CFC), now a wildly popular blog collective focusing on hip-hop generation feminists of color. At the time of this writing, they have over 39,000 followers on Facebook. Boylorn's first piece was titled "You are Pretty for a Dark-Skinned Girl." Boylorn quickly developed a loyal following. She describes the experience of blogging along with others in the collective as a way of building community and integrating activism into her writing, something she feels is often missing from her academic work, sentiments that are echoed by many feminist bloggers.

If you're interested in blogs, vlogs, or op-eds, the best thing to do is to read/view many examples. What titles draw you in? What kinds of writing styles do you respond to? How do authors use first-, second-, or third-person narration, sometimes alternating between them in order to share personal experience and then ask readers to envision their own situations?[2]

---

[2]For an example, read Boylorn's (2014) blog titled "Working While Black: 10 Microaggressions Experienced in the Workplace." The majority of the piece is written in the first person; however, the final list of 10 is presented in the second person so readers can imagine their own experiences.

How are the pieces organized? What do you find compelling? Which ones linger and inform your thinking? While there is great range in the word count and organization of blogs, op-eds are more rigid, so we provide a few tips in the box below.

As noted earlier, feminists often engage with multiple representational forms in a single research project. Let's take the example of a feminist interview study about women's romantic relationships to examine possible configurations of primary and secondary outcomes (see Tables 8.1–8.4).

Representational Formats, Visibility, and Feminists as Public Intellectuals

Now that we've reviewed the different formats feminists use, it's important to highlight the issue of **visibility**—the extent to which your work is consumed *and* you as an author and/or advocate become known. The representational forms available exist on a continuum of potential visibility, as illustrated in Figure 8.1.

Tips for Writing Op-Eds

Consult the guidelines for the newspaper you are submitting to. It's vital to follow the submission guidelines to a tee. There are typically instructions for subject lines, bios, and whether to cut and paste the op-ed into the body of the e-mail or provide an attachment. Strictly adhere to word counts. Most newspapers require between 600 and 900 words (some are capped at 600, some at 700, and so forth). Make sure you understand their policy on simultaneous submissions (which most newspapers do *not* allow). Use a hook or clever turn of phrase for a title.

Often a five-paragraph model is followed—the opening paragraph sets up the topic, the next three paragraphs present your argument and evidence, and the final paragraph summarizes, leaving readers with a final thought.

Busy op-ed editors often read the title and the first and last paragraphs in their initial review, and nothing in between. Those parts need to grab their attention for them to read the entire piece. Insert something relevant to your topic that is witty, funny, or clever into the opening and closing paragraphs. Strong opening and closing lines are essential to break through the clutter of an editor's in-box.

TABLE 8.1. Traditional Academic and Public Forms

Outcome	Form	Content
Primary	Traditional academic	Peer-reviewed article that details the study (research purpose and questions, participants, method and methodology, findings)
Secondary	Public	Blog or op-ed that outlines the five features of women's romantic relationships and asks readers to reflect on their own relationships. (Tip: a piece of this nature could be released during women's history month or in conjunction with a holiday such as Valentine's Day.)

TABLE 8.2. Arts-Based/Literary and Traditional Academic Forms

Outcome	Form	Content
Primary	Arts-based/ literary	Social fiction novel that draws on the interview research to create composite characters that exemplify key themes, issues, and patterns
Secondary	Traditional academic	Peer-reviewed article that details the methodology used in the study (contributing primarily to the research methods literature)

TABLE 8.3. Public and Traditional Academic Forms

Outcome	Form	Content
Primary	Public	Series of blogs or vlogs, each one centered on a theme from the interview research
Secondary	Traditional academic	Conference presentation providing an overview of the study and findings

TABLE 8.4. Arts-Based/Literary, Traditional Academic, and Public Forms

Outcome	Form	Content
Primary	Arts-based/ literary	Social fiction novel that draws on the interview research to create composite characters that exemplify key themes, issues, and patterns
Secondary 1	Traditional academic	Peer-reviewed article that details the methodology used in the study (contributing primarily to the research methods literature)
Secondary 2	Public	Blog or magazine article that offers relationship advice based on the interview data

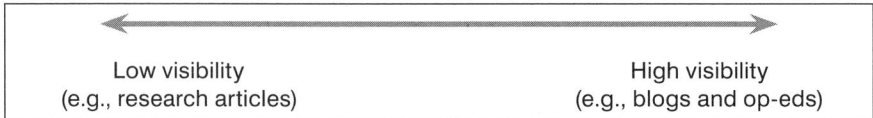

FIGURE 8.1 The continuum of visibility.

Traditional academic forms, such as peer-reviewed academic journal articles, have very small audiences, within the academy, consisting of other academics with similar research agendas. Accordingly, journal articles generally expose their authors to low levels of visibility. Further, there is a long lead time toward publication and feedback. It's common for it to take months or even over a year for an article to be published once it is submitted, and far longer to garner any feedback, if there is any at all. You may publish a journal article and never hear anything about it (although Google Scholar and other services are available to give you citation information so you know how many times the work has been cited). Likewise, monographs (scholarly books) typically have a small audience and also have a long lead time, and if there are published book reviews, this too can take months or years. In short, there is *relative* safety with publishing in these formats, meaning a buffer between the author and audience (itself likely quite small and homogenous). Arts-based forms have the potential to reach wider audiences, including nonacademic audiences. Feedback may also be immediate, visceral, and personal. For example, audience members at a play react as the art is unfolding, through their laughter, tears, applause, or lack thereof. While these are all strengths of these forms, they are not without consequence to the feminist researcher who places him/her/themselves out for immediate scrutiny. Furthermore, the art we create, even that which is intended as research, is likely to be quite personal, and critique can be especially difficult to take. As feminists, there is the additional dimension of safety, and the nature of reactions we provoke, as we expose our political and social positions and act on behalf of issues we care about. Finally, public forms are at the furthest end of the continuum as they necessarily reach public audiences and make the researcher highly visible. Blogs, vlogs, and op-eds are likely to reach broader audiences and to elicit immediate feedback. In the digital age, much of this occurs in the form of "comments" on social media, websites, and so forth. Some authors do not read the comments on pieces likely to inspire negative feedback, which is just about anything that is labeled feminist or that deals with social justice issues. This may be an important measure of self-care that you should consider if you take on this kind of public writing. We also must caution that many prominent feminist bloggers have written about the harassment and, at times, threats of violence they have endured. For example, high-profile feminist blogger Jessica Valenti recently took a break from social media when she and her young child received death and rape threats. By the same token, there can be immediate, positive feedback as well. Either way, engaging with popular forms requires vulnerability. Boylorn expresses the rewards well.

> I underestimated the impact that digital social justice work would have on me—expanding my audience from academe to the public sphere, and thrusting me into being recognized in the blogosphere. Until I became a blogger, few outside of the "ivory tower" knew my name . . . I realized through conversations about the growing popularity of the CFC that people rarely listen to phantom voices—I had to be visible to be heard. (2013, p. 80)

By acknowledging the range of responses public forms invoke, we in no way wish to discourage anyone from engaging in them. However, as a feminist researcher, one must consider and come to terms with issues of vulnerability and visibility. With that said, Melissa W. Wright (2008) suggests that any self-identified feminist within the academy is necessarily a "public" scholar, because the scholarship and teaching of feminist researchers is always being scrutinized and debated. While this bears merit, there are also different *levels* to which one may go "public" with one's research. No matter what form or forms your research takes, just labeling your work feminist is an important political act, and while there can be a host of personal consequences, this act also situates you in community with others.

Publication and Dissemination

Digital media has significantly aided the publication and distribution of feminist research. While we certainly don't suggest the Internet provides a panacea, there's no doubt that more of us are able to get our work out. Further, self-publishing, e-publishing, and print-on-demand publishing options all expand the possibilities for feminist researchers, who have historically been marginalized in the publishing world. The world of academic publishing has shifted too. Today there are feminist presses devoted solely to publishing feminist work. While gatekeepers abound in publishing, many academic and trade publishers actively publish feminist work. (Note that if you want to work with a trade publisher you need a literary agent.)

However you publish your work, it's important to promote it. Reaching relevant audiences inside or outside of the academy requires a commitment to talking about your publications, sending complimentary copies of books to journals for possible review, and sharing information on list serves and/ or social media. Help your work find an audience.

One issue feminists are likely to encounter in the publishing industry is **microaggressions** in publishing. These are most likely to occur when you submit your work to a traditional academic journal or monograph publisher. One example of a microaggression feminists often experience is that copyeditors change designations that you find important. For example, if you capitalize racial categories such as Black, Brown, and White, you may receive a copyedited version of your manuscript in which those words have been changed to lowercase. Another example might be using pronouns that challenge the he/she binary (e.g., she/he, he/she/they, she/he/they). You may protest only to be told that is their "style," putting you in the position of accepting a change that reflects politically and socially on you as an author, or continuing to argue with the publisher. If you know there are issues like this in your work, try to flag them in advance for copyeditors and ask them not to make changes; however, you also need to be prepared to do battle. Publishers typically give in, but the process can be difficult. In the case of books, no author wants to be on bad terms with their editor, who can ultimately showcase or bench their book so we recommend being pragmatic—be firm and clear while making it clear you want to work with them toward a solution.

Publishing Theses or Dissertations

If you're trying to publish your thesis or dissertation as a book, you'll find many publishers flat out don't publish dissertations, or do so rarely. This is because nobody wants to read a book that's written like a dissertation, with the lengthy citations and block quotes one usually includes to satisfy one's committee. After putting it in a drawer for at least a few months, look at it more objectively with fresh eyes and do some serious rewriting so it reads like a book and not a school assignment (Leavy, 2016). As a feminist scholar you already have publishing challenges, so do what you can to create a viable manuscript.

Archival

In oral history research archiving interview audios and/or transcripts is considered a part of ethical practice. This is especially important in feminist research as a goal is to document the lives of women for the historical record. There are a large number of library and online repositories for archiving your research. We note a small selection of those appropriate for feminist research in the suggested resources at this end of this book.

CONCLUSION

At the end of the day, whatever form our feminist writing takes, we need to publish and distribute it in order to make a difference. Publishing may be as simple as uploading something to our own blog or social media, or it can involve book proposals, rejections, and negotiations. No matter how we publish our work, tenacity counts. Don't be discouraged by the inevitable stumbling blocks (rejections, low readership). Keep going. Get the work out there. Build your audience over time. Try different formats. It's also important to make peace with your writing. Solicit feedback during the drafting and revising process, but once you let it go, really let it go. Have your own relationship with your work that isn't dependent on external praise or critique, because as a feminist writer, you are likely to inspire both.

DISCUSSION QUESTIONS

1. Why do some feminist researchers use autobiographical data?
2. What are the advantages of representing your research findings in more than one form?
3. What are the pros and cons of public forms?

ACTIVITIES

1. Select a peer-reviewed journal article written by feminist researchers in your subject area. Read the article and then write a critique of the writing. Was the article well organized? Explain. What worked well? What could be improved on? As a reader, did you find the writing engaging? Why or why not? (Up to one page.)
2. If you have conducted research with participants, such as interviews or field research, develop a character profile, based on one of your participants, which could be used in an FBR or ethnodrama (if you don't have your own data, go online to an oral history database and select an interview transcript to use for this exercise). Think about how you would describe the character in terms of his/her/their major values or motivations, challenges, and

relationships with others (e.g., family and friends) (one to two pages). Go a step further and write a sample monologue for the character, in which we learn what motivates him/her/them (at least one paragraph).

3. Practice writing a blog or op-ed. The goal of this exercise is to get you in the habit of writing accessibly, not to publish your piece. If you have conducted research, using any research method, write a piece intended for popular audiences about your research. If you have not conducted research, select a current event of interest. The topic doesn't matter. This exercise is about writing accessibly. Op-eds are ideally 600–800 words. Use a four-paragraph format: The opening paragraph introduces the topic with a hook or something catchy, the second and third paragraphs present the information or arguments, and the fourth paragraph recaps the piece with a final, strong statement with which to leave the reader. Don't forget to give your piece a catchy title.

SUGGESTED RESOURCES

Books

Boylorn, R. M. (2012). *Sweetwater: Black women and narratives of resilience.* New York: Peter Lang.

A stunningly written example of Black feminist narrative inquiry.

Faulkner, S. L., & Squillante, S. (2015). *Writing the personal: Getting your stories onto the page.* Leiden, The Netherlands: Brill-Sense.

An excellent, succinct guide to various forms of personal writing in which the authors draw on their own experiences and provide practical activities.

Harper, A. B. (2014). *Scars: A Black lesbian experience in rural White New England.* Leiden, The Netherlands: Brill-Sense.

A novel based on the principles of intersectional feminism.

Harris, A., & Holman Jones, S. (2016). *Writing for performance.* Leiden, The Netherlands: Brill-Sense.

An excellent, succinct guide to all aspects of writing for performance.

Leavy, P. (2013). *Fiction as research practice: Short stories, novellas, and novels.* New York: Routledge.

A detailed guide to writing research as fiction, from the development of the field to the nuts and bolts of designing a project—includes examples by leading scholars.

Sumerau, J. (2017). *Cigarettes and wine.* Leiden, The Netherlands: Brill-Sense.

   A novel about gender fluidity based on sociological research and autoethnographic experiences.

📖 Articles and Chapters

de Freitas, E. (2003). Contested positions: How fiction informs empathetic research. *International Journal of Education and the Arts, 4*(7).

   Harris, M. Y. (2005). Black Women writing autobiography: Autobiography in multicultural education. In J. Phillion, M. Fang He, & F. M. Connelly (Eds.), *Narrative and experience in multicultural education* (pp. 36–52). Thousand Oaks, CA: SAGE.

🖥 Digital Resources

The Crunk Feminist Collective
www.crunkfeministcollective.com

Zora Neale Hurston Official Website
www.zoranealehurston.com
Includes a book list.

Alice Walker Official Website
http://alicewalkersgarden.com
Includes a book list.

CHAPTER 9

Public Scholarship
and Critical Perspectives

#NeverthelessShePersisted
—VIRAL TWITTER HASHTAG (2017)

Truth does triumph over deception.
—NADEZHDA TOLOKONNIKOVA (2012), Pussy Riot member
who received a 2-year jail sentence for "hooliganism"
associated with her antichurch, feminist activism

LEARNING OBJECTIVES

- To explain what is meant by public feminist scholarship, and what different social role it plays from more traditional research engagements

- To offer a discussion concerning some contentious or debated areas of feminist scholarship, including postfeminism, pornography, and "moral panics" surrounding girlhood and popular expressions of feminist subjectivities

- To provide insights into how digital media (and social media in particular) have changed the way feminist research is "done"

Pussy Hats and Nasty Women

What is **public scholarship** in an era when almost everything is public, and scholarship can be constituted by nontraditional outputs such as performances, artworks, flash mobs, and intimate GoPro video footage of home increasingly networked into/within our lives and endeavors, via a proliferating range of self-tracking devices? One of the most exciting aspects of working in feminist scholarship today is the speed with which the field is expanding, proliferating, and branching out into new areas. The emergence of digital and online technologies has added a new landscape where issues of gender performance and inequities remind us of the promises of new kinds of gendering and sociality, but also the repetitions of old patterns of bias and exclusion. It is a rich and exciting landscape in which to wander, work, and network with other feminist researchers.

This chapter will discuss feminism in the mainstream and what it means to be a feminist researcher, which necessarily has public, activist components or implications. Ideas for activism beyond the classroom will also be offered. Global research, transnational research, arts-based research (including photo blogs), hybrid approaches (combining traditional and emergent methods), evolving feminisms and social media, and other emergent forms are covered in this chapter, which recognizes that a new generation of young scholars and activists is approaching feminist research from new directions.

Where Does 21st-Century Feminist Research Praxis Happen?

On January 21, 2017, the day after the U.S. presidential inauguration, over 5 million people around the globe mobilized themselves into Women's Marches—over 600 marches in the United States alone, but also protests from one side of the globe to another; from Iceland to Antarctica—to protest the misogyny and racism of the 24 months of the Trump presidential campaign. A Twitter message calling Hillary Clinton a "nasty woman" became a worldwide feminist rallying cry, bolstered by a global flood of pink knitted "pussy hats," which have come to represent womanpower and solidarity (they were also worn by men and nonbinary marchers at the gatherings).

The issues are not new, but seemingly overnight we went from the performative creative protests of Russia's Pussy Riot collective to neon-pink pussy hats, and through the immediacy of social media, a global wave of feminist direct action has taken hold, including the popular appeal of feminist activism.

The ubiquitous role of technology and social media has meant that heads of state and other high-ranking officials and public figures are more frequently nabbed saying offensive things, frequently concerning race and gender. That those perpetrators still manage to be elected, retain their jobs, and keep their public profile was suddenly, in early 2017, enough to drive many to the streets, to their phones, and to online groups and funding campaigns.

In a series of unprecedented (and, some believe, undemocratic) actions, including the firing of acting attorney general Sally Yates for refusing to defend a ban on travelers from seven mostly Muslim countries entering the United States, the current American president has enacted or validated a series of overt racist and misogynist behaviors. His anti-abortion "global gag rule," which defunds American support of international abortion-related services was brought in through executive orders. Unprecedented misogyny has been emboldened in the Republican-controlled House of Representatives and Senate, exemplified by the silencing of Senator Elizabeth Warren. For many, the accumulation of these and other unabashedly misogynist acts worldwide, such as the shooting of 15-year-old Malala Yousafzai by the Taliban in 2012, has prompted a passionate return to popular feminism.

But a positive part of this global pattern that should not be disregarded is this: the voices of women in these events have not been silenced; they have gone viral in greater numbers, including the final speeches of Pussy Riot while on trial and Senator Warren's resilience on the floor of the Senate. Women are asserting the power and right of their own (and other women's) stories, and they are being heard. As Maria Alyokhina argued in the closing statement of her 2012 Pussy Riot trial:

> But nobody can take away my inner freedom. It lives in the word, it will go on living thanks to openness [glasnost], when this will be read and heard by thousands of people. This freedom goes on living with every person who is not indifferent, who hears us in this country. With everyone who found shards of the trial in themselves, like in previous times they found them in Franz Kafka and Guy Debord. I believe that I have honesty and openness, I thirst for the truth; and these things will make all of us just a little bit more free. We will see this yet.

Journalists and feminist scholars following the Women's Marches in January 2017 noted that so many people may be taking to the streets because of the wide and diverse range of threats to women, but also the cumulative frustration from those threats over such a long time. But today's so-called alt-right (alternative far right) is threatening not only the rights of women, but also those of undocumented immigrants, as well as affordable health care, the natural environment, lesbian, gay, bisexual, trans*, and other sexual and gender rights, racial equality, freedom of religion, and workers' rights, to name a few—thus demonstrating in the public sphere the pervasiveness of intersectionality, and the ways in which patterns of oppression almost always occur simultaneously. In fact, it's almost possible to imagine the need for, and relevance of, a new Combahee River Collective Statement today, as if it were 1977 all over again.

Today's feminism and feminist research are inextricably intertwined with politics and digital media (where almost everything, including politics, gets played out in the 21st century). Digital media has radically changed (and is continuing to change) the ways that feminist research is done, received, and understood. It offers a revised and expanded set of analytic lenses as well as methodological tools for feminist researchers. Instagram, Twitter, Snapchat, Facebook, and others are all asking us to consider **representation,** gender, sexuality and sociality in different ways (Handyside & Ringrose, 2017), and their impacts on concepts of time, space, and community.

Digital media, many believed, was going to change the ways social codes and relationships were created and enacted, but as the 21st century progresses, it becomes clearer that the feminist research goal of social change and transformation might be even more difficult with the evolutions of gendered space and practices in the digital and **hybrid** (online/off-line) worlds (see Figure 9.1). Following in the footsteps of Rosi Braidotti (1996), several scholars (Senft, 2008; Senft, 2014; Hunsinger & Senft, 2013; Boler, Macdonald, Nitsou, & Harris, 2014; Boler & Nitsou, 2014; Ringrose, 2011; Retallack, Ringrose, & Lawrence, 2016) have looked at forms of **cyberfeminism** and social media, in which the principles of second- and third-wave feminism have reemerged as patterns of production and reproduction of gender inequities online (see Figure 9.1). The remainder of this chapter looks at some of the major categories of public scholarship and the ways in which those critical perspectives are enacted online and off.

A recent raft of **feminist manifestos** (also known as **femifestas** or **womanifestos**) is amassing new calls to early-21st-century feminist action, in a range of textual and online forms (see, e.g., Ahmed, 2017; Bennett, 2016; Sandberg, 2013; Harris, 2017; Hickey-Moody, 2016) in which women are called to unite against patriarchy, but often through a lens of work (Sandberg and Bennett) rather than the personal or political (Harris and Hickey-Moody). Indeed, feminist scholar Sara Ahmed's charge that "resignation is a feminist issue" when she resigned from her post at Goldsmiths, University of London, after a series of sexual harassment debacles, and her subsequent book *Living a Feminist Life* (2017) highlight the power and prevalence of popular/scholarly forms and strategies in today's feminist movement.

Contemporary feminism has many channels through which feminists can connect with each other and with feminist support literature, groups,

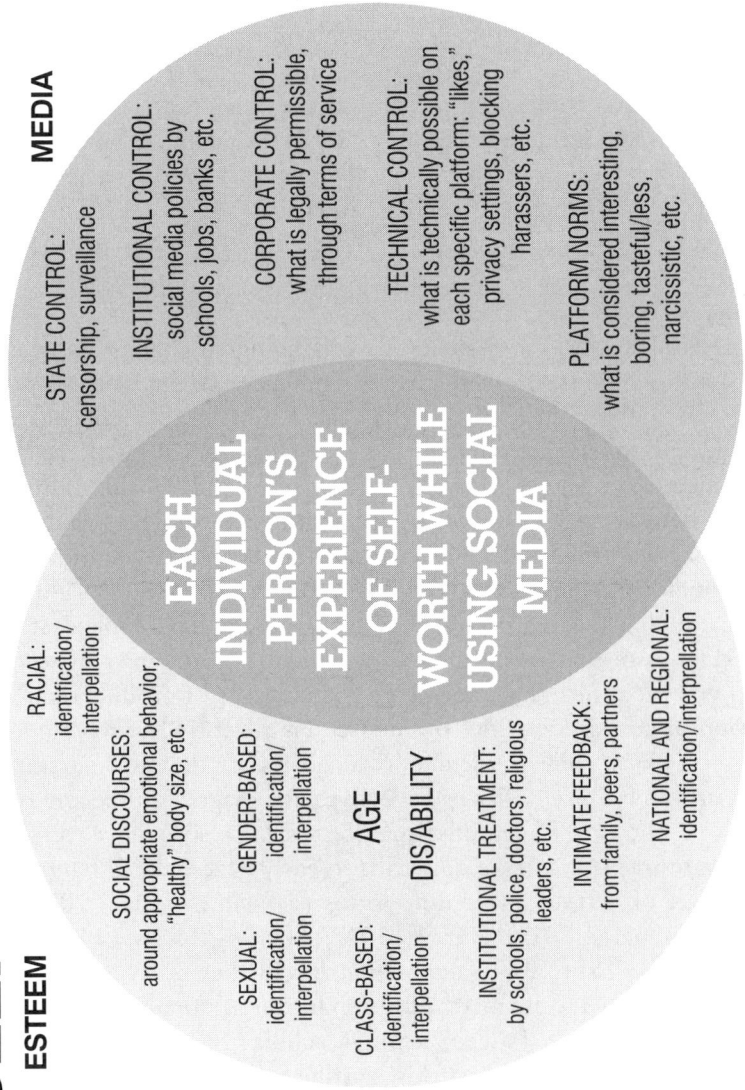

SOCIAL MEDIA

STATE CONTROL: censorship, surveillance

INSTITUTIONAL CONTROL: social media policies by schools, jobs, banks, etc.

CORPORATE CONTROL: what is legally permissible, through terms of service

TECHNICAL CONTROL: what is technically possible on each specific platform: "likes," privacy settings, blocking harassers, etc.

PLATFORM NORMS: what is considered interesting, boring, tasteful/less, narcissistic, etc.

EACH INDIVIDUAL PERSON'S EXPERIENCE OF SELF-WORTH WHILE USING SOCIAL MEDIA

SELF-ESTEEM

RACIAL: identification/ interpellation

SOCIAL DISCOURSES: around appropriate emotional behavior, "healthy" body size, etc.

GENDER-BASED: identification/ interpellation

SEXUAL: identification/ interpellation

AGE

CLASS-BASED: identification/ interpellation

DIS/ABILITY

INSTITUTIONAL TREATMENT: by schools, police, doctors, religious leaders, etc.

INTIMATE FEEDBACK: from family, peers, partners

NATIONAL AND REGIONAL: identification/interpellation

FIGURE 9.1 Self-worth and social media. Source: Theresa Senft. Used with permission.

and actions. Feminist scholars also focus on impact and networking, not just through academic channels but through popular media, social media, and online blogs, **vlogs,** and new outlets. There are many popular feminist websites that serve a range of these kinds of purposes. One example is VIDA, an initiative of the Australian Women's History Network that offers a collaborative blog about the research and practice of feminist history, with a specific focus on gender and women's history. Their goal is to create an open-access blog that makes contemporary understandings of global feminism (both historical and current)

> **Vlog (video blog):** A form of web broadcasting, dominated by feminists and other women online, that is usually personal or individual and sometimes uses text and other graphic enhancements.

accessible, approachable, and inspiring. Posts like "Feminist Digital Activism: The Revolution Is Being Streamed, Snapped and Tweeted" by indie feminist journalist Brigitte Lewis are typical of a new, 21st-century feminist consciousness and presence on the Internet (see *www.auswhn.org.au/blog/feminist-digital-activism*).

Feminist scholarship today is not and cannot be limited to scholarly communities and dissemination outlets. Contemporary global politics since September 11, 2001, have given rise to an increasing proliferation of online/off-line and public/scholarly ways of networking, protesting, and raising consciousness. Even those working from within "the academy" (universities and research institutions), such as the feminist researcher team of Emma Renold and Jessica Ringrose, work out into "real world" contexts for "real world" impact, such as in government presentations, art exhibitions, and street marches. Blurring lines between social activism, arts, and scholarly work, contemporary feminist research is an innovative blend of public scholarship and the critical perspectives needed to **curate** and interpret the constant flow of media representations of women's lives today. This chapter looks at some of those meeting points where politics, digital technology and media, popular culture, and **public intellectualism** overlap in addressing 21st-century feminist concerns.

Crunk, Punk, and Hip-Hop Feminisms

It's a great time for feminism in the public sphere. The proliferation of public journalistic and artistic feminist expressions and scholarly feminist outputs has never been more exciting. The expansion of **hip-hop feminism** (Love, 2012, 2017; Hodge, 2016; Saunders, 2016) and **crunk feminism**

(Cooper, 2016; Boylorn, 2013, 2011; Johnson & Boylorn, 2015) demonstrates in multiple popular cultural and scholarly forms the intersectionality of African American, gender, and sometimes queer oppressions. Jack Halberstam's work on Gaga and **punk feminisms** (2012) has also demonstrated for over a decade how generative are the intersections of gender and sexuality oppressions.

The development of digital technologies has helped bring such research to a public forum and widen its impact, offering new opportunities for immediate and broad-based responses to what in the past would have been invisible or minor transgressions against women, queers, people of color, and other minorities. Why write a scholarly article on African American feminisms when police brutality against young Black men is on the rise? Some scholars are finding not only community but additional global impact by disseminating their research online, and indeed writing for a range of forums, including both popular and scholarly books, online blogs/vlogs, magazines, newspapers, and Internet or television video interviews, all at the same time. In this way, scholarly feminism is performing a new role in the public sphere, thus expanding the feminist rallying cry of "the personal is political" in new and ever more widespread ways.

Today's feminist research is diverse, flexible, and agile in theoretical and methodological ways. One example, the Crunk Feminist Collective, is an online community begun in Atlanta, Georgia, whose tag line is "Where Crunk Meets Conscious and Feminism Meets Cool." With a hip-hop aesthetic, cultural and political orientation, and strong humorous side, this website and community explore issues of Black and African American womanhood and lived experience. Feminists of color like those who comprise the Collective and other groups bring to the forefront the range of diverse ways of having, and researching, feminist experience.

Pussy Riot, Femen, and New Digital Feminisms/ Feminist Activism

The Russian feminist "punk rock collective" Pussy Riot first burst onto the global stage with the arrest, trial, and ultimate imprisonment of three of its members in August 2012 (they were released on December 23, 2013). Their detractors critique their tendency to show lots of skin (what some call **activist porn**), videos and actions that some consider to be sexualizing of the activists, and the overwhelming whiteness of its interventions. They are an example of what some feminist scholars have written about as **riot grrrl feminism**.

Its newest video, *Straight Outta Vagina,* has become an instant pop classic that addresses classic feminist themes in a perfectly 21st-century digital manner through the use of a hip-hop music and aesthetic, trademark humor, ski masks, political critique, and their take-no-prisoners hard-hitting focus on the female form, in particular on genitals. Some of the bases for critiques of previous incarnations of the group as too White and too "femme" are in evidence in this video: there are muscles and cellulite, and a few people of color, but mostly the vibe is still uber-White old-school Pussy Riot.

While the video and song lyrics are a slap down of certain American leaders, group member and creator Nadya Tolokonnikova says it was also meant to celebrate the female anatomy, a simple gesture that is somehow still a political act.

The Russian context is not alone in demonstrating the ways in which "numerous studies have documented sex-based discrimination and misogyny in various Russian, Soviet, and post-Soviet Russian settings, from the family to the workplace and from politics to popular culture" (Sperling 2015, p. 67), yet at least in many Western nations, there has been a pervasive sense of complacency that "we are doing alright," that overall gains have been made, and that feminist violations lie mostly in other places around the globe, not right here at home.

For the last 30 years, the attention of feminist activism has focused more on female genital mutilation, child marriage, Muslim gendered practices of hijab wearing, and unequal educational opportunities for girls than on domestic violence, unequal pay for equal work, and other Western forms of gender inequity. Over the past 5 years, however, the eyes of the West have turned to Russia and other nations as their feminist movements have in some cases outshone Western ones, including Nigerian and other African feminist journalism, feminist activist art in China and Hong Kong, and of course Pussy Riot, Femen, and other strong online feminist presences.

Many Russian feminists continue to resist the Russian state responses to Pussy Riot and other feminist activist organizations. While many do not identify with Pussy Riot's brand of feminism, or even in some cases consider them a feminist organization, most supported a quick end to the band members' confinement in prison, another way in which popular media (and in particular, online cultures) have created wider movements than in the past, uniting generalist "human rights" believers behind movements they might not in the past have rallied behind. For example, an **eco-warrior** movement may post videos that attract likes and online participation from individuals who in the past would not have known about them or not have shown up in face-to-face contexts to join the movement. These patterns are easy to see across the board, but today no one movement is stronger or more fierce than feminisms.

Like other feminist activists and activist organizations, Pussy Riot became a flashpoint for a new wave of passionate debate about gender roles and gender inequality. And like other activist movements, their public actions quickly ignited violent responses from government and sometimes media outlets and their representatives. For example,

> At a picket in support of Pussy Riot in March 2012, Aleksander Bosykh, the assistant to Vice Premier Dmitri Rogozin and a leader of the right-wing nationalist Congress of Russian Communities, punched a Pussy Riot supporter, videographer Taisiia Krugovykh, in the head, while police at the scene stood by without acting to restrain him. As he later bragged (perhaps also trying to justify his violence), "A feminist lesbian attacked me, and got it in the face." (Sperling, 2015, p. 283)

Since Pussy Riot's first rush of fame due to a church protest and subsequent trial, they continue to fight gender inequality in a range of ways, including their own frequent self-portrayal as "unnatural" Russian women for being so outspoken and feminist. During Pussy Riot member Masha's trial, one interrogator asked her, "Do you dream of marrying and having a child?" She replied, "I don't. You will find that many women do not, and I'm one of them. Jail is not the worst place for a person who thinks."

It is instructive for activists and feminist researchers alike to watch the women's interviews from inside the courtroom cages where they were held during trial proceedings, surrounded by media. They appear so young (most in their early to mid-20s) and they are all so calm. It is not only inspiring, but also demonstrates their assiduous training in activist techniques. They come across as able professionals, doing a job to which they are utterly committed.

The documentary *Pussy Riot: A Punk Prayer* shows how incredibly seasoned they are as activists, impressive at such young ages, and demonstrates the **pedagogy of activism**—that there is training involved, capacity building, real transferable skills. Their work in the courtroom, which went on to inspire and inform countless others since then, shows the interconnection between feminist performance, politics, media, and scholarship. This brand of feminism, of which theatricality is inevitably a part, perfectly deploys a **theater of politics**. These feminist activists challenge every statement by the judge in the charging process in the courtroom, every word. Their very persistence is inspiring in its carefulness and its detail, especially in an era in which the persistence of women is a feminist meme.

The Pussy Riot exemplar really highlights the relationship between church and state, activism grounded in philosophy, the interconnection of all branches of the lives of feminist scholarship and other work that gets played out in public and critical contexts. For Pussy Riot and their supporters, their sexy, creative, and very public actions embodied a response to, and evocation of, the past, of the gulags, the show trials of communist Russia, invoking the vast fabric of cultural, historical, everyday Russianness, as all flashpoints, all zeitgeists, do. For that moment, Pussy Riot exemplified a new kind of 21st-century feminism. And what's amazing is that you can see it in the faces of those young women. The closing statements of all three Pussy Riot defendants are brilliant. Read them here: *http://nplusonemag. com/pussy-riot-closing-statements.*

"Revenge Porn" in/as Postfeminist Spaces

Certainly there have been widespread gender-related concerns about the Internet over the past decade, many of which are passed off as anxiety with new technology. But one area of ongoing gender-based harm is what is popularly known as "revenge porn," the practice of distributing pornographic images of someone without their consent (or sometimes without even their knowledge). Revenge porn is a form of sexual violence or abuse that is usually perpetrated within relationships or between current or ex-sexual partners. Gender and Internet scholars like Theresa Senft, Megan Boler, Ilona Hongisto, Jessica Ringrose, and Emma Renold have explored issues related to sexually explicit revenge or shaming behaviors online.

These investigations often move across multiple modalities and platforms, like the practices and artifacts they study. For example, Senft effectively uses social media platforms to gather, share, and discuss research into gendered and feminist practices in online spaces. Her group **Camgirl Collective**, her "Hey Girl Global" Facebook group, and the Facebook "PheMaterialisms" group, which explores the intersection of feminism and **new materialism** all work intersectionally

> **Feminist new materialism** is an interdisciplinary area of study situated at the nexus of feminism, posthumanism, science studies, and ecology, which generally asserts that agency is not a uniquely human attribute but is rather something inherent in all matter.

to expand knowledge about performances of gender, sexuality, and power in online and also hybrid online/off-line worlds. One aspect of these areas of study includes the ways in which girls and women are using practices like revenge porn too. Concerns with how, why, and when such practices are sometimes driven by girls and women themselves, and how porn studies can contribute to greater understanding of women's power and sexual agency but may simultaneously be perpetuating the sexualization and objectification of girls and women on social media and in misogynistic spaces more generally constitute a major focus of feminist media studies todays.

Feminist Vloggers

The world of vlogging (video blogging) has exploded over the past 5 years, which at first saw a narrowing of vlogging content due to the commercialization of the form, then more recently expanding out again to make room for more diverse purposes and vloggers. Certainly the majority of online vlogging stars are young, White, and heteronormative. But it does seem that currently vlogging is in a period of expansion, diversifying from gender-stereotyped possibilities for women vloggers (makeup, fashion, sex and dating tips) to include more activist and social-justice-oriented vloggers. The possibilities for feminist broadcasting through vlogging are rich and still underexplored.

Two examples are Laci Green (probably the world's most famous vlogger with nearly 1.5 million followers) and Kat Blaque (with just over 116,000 followers). Kat Blaque is a transgender African American vlogger, artist, and activist. Blaque's YouTube channel True Tea is primarily focused on answering questions from viewers on topics associated with Black culture, racism, and, to a lesser extent, gender identity. Laci Green has moved from being a pop teen vlogging hobbyist to a serious sex educator, both online and off. She identifies as pansexual, and her work is strongly oriented against **slut-shaming** and toward sex-positive messages. She has spoken on behalf of Planned Parenthood regularly.

Of course it's possible to argue that both of these vloggers are still in the category of gender-appropriate sex/dating genres, yet that would ignore their huge following and focus on sexual and gender diversity, myth busting about what a "woman" is, pleasure, and also feminism. The kinds of followings both Kat and Laci have online, and the number of views they record for vlogs about nonbinarism, women's sexual freedom, and racial and sexual diversity were not even imaginable a generation ago. As feminist research expands in scope and approach, we note that feminist vloggers have a unique role in addressing both political and apolitical topics of interest to women and girls, and are making a huge impact on the general public, and as public scholarship, vlogging is an unparalleled platform. Thanks Laci, Kat, and all you other feminist vloggers out there; we salute you!

Another effective online tool for feminist community building and commentary used by feminist researchers and activists is online magazines and websites. *Teen Vogue* (*www.teenvogue.com*) is one extremely influential online magazine that has really galvanized a generation of young women and girls, combining both beauty/makeup/dating concerns with hard-hitting political consciousness raising. Beyond just commenting on current affairs, their feminist features have helped call their young readers to action. Gone are the days when feminist work was not fashion-, sex-, or makeup-friendly. **Postfeminism** has contributed to breaking down those barriers with its crucial research on slut-shaming (Lumsden & Morgan, 2012; Ringrose & Barajas, 2011; Ringrose & Renold, 2012), sex-positiveness, and sexting (Jackson, Vares, & Gill, 2012; Dobson, 2011, 2014; Ringrose, Gill, Livingstone, & Harvey, 2012; Ringrose, Harvey, Gill, & Livingstone, 2013). Online magazines are more available, less expensive, and more universal than hard-copy "girls' magazines" used to be, and they are certainly more political.

Some online magazines are more overtly political in focus, including those like *Everyday Feminism,* which draws readers' attention to the interconnectedness of all oppressions (intersectionality) including class, race, religion, gender, sexuality, and ability. Like *Teen Vogue,* it is multimodal (room for visual and audio posts) and interactive. Both of these magazines (and the vast majority of online feminist magazines, such as *Bitch Media*) are American, and reflect primarily the perspectives and concerns of Americans and Western culture. Critics have identified this as a problem, reflecting a persistent lack of geo- and racial/cultural diversity in feminist communities. This is partly an economic issue, based on unequal access to the Internet and the hardware required for such endeavors.

Sexting, Selfies, and Other Digital (Post) Feminist Practices

The central concepts of postfeminism find new expression in the online practices of girls and young women, according to emerging scholarship (Krijnen & Van Bauwel, 2015; Ringrose et al., 2013; Krijnen & Bauwel, 2015; Harris, 2016a, 2016b; Bailey & Steeves, 2015) that seeks to understand new forms of digital self-representation and the ways in which still-patriarchal sociality frames them. **Trolling**, sexting, online rape threats, revenge porn, and **cyberbullying** are just some of the complications that emerge in parallel with self-representation of (young) women online and the misogynist pushback it garners. A whole new wave of feminist scholars is documenting and critically contextualizing this newest incarnation of feminist and antifeminist self-expression (Bailey & Steeves, 2015). Perhaps the most recognizable of all self-representational forms in the digital world are what have become known as **selfies** (Senft & Baym, 2015).

Amy Shields Dobson, perhaps one of the best-known scholars in **digital feminisms**, has written extensively about young women, feminisms, and self-representation online. Her work on "postfeminist networked publics" and what she calls "postfeminist self-making" is unique. She critically deconstructs discourses of "authentic" selves versus the performances of sexual selves online. She uses the term **heterosexy** (2015) for online social media representations that are acceptable versus those that are not. She is an expert on sexting and cybersafety, and draws critically and extensively on YouTube and other media forms of self-representation. She has been greatly influenced by gender scholar Rosalind Gill, and represents a new wave of digital (post)feminist scholars, including the prolific Jessica Ringrose, Emma Renold, Meg Barker, and other largely American, Canadian, and British scholars.

Led by Roz Gill, conferences, publications, and more public outputs on "digital cultures" and feminism continue to grow. One of Dobson's significant contributions is in her approach to the analysis of these media practices and products in ways that "take girls and young women seriously as media and cultural producers" (2015, p. 15), which she notes is often not the case. From moral panics to infantilization of women online, most mainstream media and scholars dismiss girls' and women's online content as amateurish and boring. Dobson's work and that of her colleagues is attempting to do the opposite: foreground girls' feminist and creative **prosumer practices** and outputs as serious and culturally significant work.

Some of the more sexual digital materials made by, for, and about girls and women (including sexting) have produced what some scholars have theorized as **moral panics** (McRobbie & Thornton, 1995; Barron & Lacombe, 2005). Moral panics are typified by social hysteria or social efforts to control women and their bodies such as the anti-abortion movement, the so-called slut-shaming discourse, and gender-unequal responses to "sexting," in which girls are shamed and boys' behaviors are left unanalyzed (Karaian, 2014). For more on moral panics, see the Suggested Resources section at the end of this chapter.

> **Moral panic** is a term used to describe public outcries about what is generally considered to be "proper" behavior, often relies on exaggerated anecdotes, and is often tied to propaganda and surveillance. Moral panics are concerned with social transgressions (like sexting) and what should be done to punish or bring transgressors into line.

Slut-Shaming, SlutWalks, and Digital Feminisms

Feminist sociologist Jessica Ringrose has defined slut-shaming this way:

> Slut is the signifier for the bad and excessive sexuality . . . [where] rela-
> tionships with boys can confer status and popularity onto girls, but . . .
> it is a high-risk game where those viewed as "slutty" are excluded by
> other girls . . . a notion that has recently been popularised to explore the
> dynamic of sexual regulation where a girl's reputation can be invoked
> and scrutinised to discipline her through codes of sexual conduct
> (Albury et al., 2011). Psychosocially slut-shaming appears to express a
> dynamic where jealousy gets sublimated into a socially acceptable form
> of social critique of girls' sexual expression (Ringrose & Renold, 2012).
> (Ringrose, 2013, p. 93)

For girls and young women, slut-shaming can have far-reaching consequences, both for individuals personally and for their communities. What
does it tell boys and men to blame females for attracting unwanted sexual
advances or attention, just by dressing or acting as they feel most comfortable? The impulse to control women's and adolescent girls' bodies is
as old as organized society itself, but postfeminist and related research
has finally systematically set about making it transparent. As Tanenbaum
(2000, 2015) and others have shown, the regulatory systems at work in
slut-shaming are just as pervasive among women's and girls' groups and
dynamics as they are with boys and men. This means that women and girls
participate in these harmful practices of "policing" each other, as much as
men and boys do.

Digital media is also playing an important role for **minoritarian
women,** making getting their stories out there more affordable and offering new (and not always mainstream) ways to get their stories out there
(Harris, 2012d, 2016b). When a group of Toronto-based women protested
in 2011 against a police comment that they should not "dress like sluts" if
they don't want to be sexually assaulted, the Toronto march, which became
known as SlutWalk, went viral, like the Women's March in Washington in
2017, and dozens of other SlutWalks were held in solidarity (Keller, 2016).
The opportunities afforded by digital and online media for organizing but
also for taking control of the means of (previously patriarchal) production,
are having powerful and expanding consequences.

Hacking Patriarchy

As Gill (2009, 2012) has pointed out, moving beyond a sexualization of
women's culture allows clearer critical perspectives on the ways in which

women from diverse practices and perspectives are still being relegated to supporting roles in the lives of men. For example, in hybrid activist cultures, do women participants negotiate both face-to-face and web-based practices of networking and movement building, or do they mostly perform invisible "supporting" roles? Tsing (2005) and others have written about conflicts that emerged between the ideals and manifest realities of the emphasis on *process*, and what time-consuming, horizontal, consensus-building practices meant for Occupy in terms of their function (1) as an ideal, (2) as a specific mode of organizational structure, and (3) as a facilitation tool of the consensus-building process.

Women's roles in activist movements (even feminist activist communities like the Women's March) often remain **invisible labor** within networked (online and off-line) communities. According to Occupy participants, gender itself was rarely if ever explicitly discussed within "formal" General Assembly discussions with their primary focus on capitalism.

To evaluate the compatibilities as well as frictions between theoretical frameworks that may be effectively brought together to examine the overlap of social movements with philosophies of media and technologies, it can be useful to contrast various theorists from the wide range of approaches to this work. For example, contrasting Jeffrey Juris's (2012) concept of the "logic of aggregation" with Lance Bennett's (Bennett & Segerberg, 2012) notion of the "logic of connective action" can result in feminist theoretics such as the "logic of connective labor" articulated by Boler et al. (2014).

Hybrid social movements and digital activism continue to show that new methods and theoretical frameworks are needed for understanding and interpreting these evolving practices and sites (Harris & Nyuon, 2012; Harris, 2012c).

Ecofeminism and 21st-Century Critical Feminisms

Ecofeminism is a social movement that connects the oppression of women and nature, and sometimes extends to a critique of the interconnected oppressions of gender, race, class, and nature.

Widespread protests against the Dakota Access Pipeline (DAPL) and the emergence of the powerful #NoDAPL Twitter hashtag is a fitting end to this chapter on public scholarship and critical perspectives, because it is a site of intersection for the oppression of women, nature, and indigenous peoples, and what some have come to term **ecofeminisms**. Fisher (2016) has written that the issue relates to a subgroup of radical feminism called ecofeminism, which links the exploitation of women and of nature, and the concept of biopiracy, or the commercial use of natural resources. These concepts are integral to the analysis of this event because of its exploitation of nature for monetary and material gains. (2016, n.p.)

This movement is important too for the ways in which the activists (who call themselves "water protectors" rather than protestors) have garnered crucial and lifesaving support for their in-person actions at the front lines and for their cause more generally.

The online *Brooklyn Magazine* published "In Protest: A Reading List for the Resistance" (Fustich, 2017), which draws attention to the continuing lack leadership by people of color in the Women's Marches and movement, especially the absence of indigenous women and what some have called indigenous concerns. The need to move from a march to a movement requires, according to many, education. Education in intersectionality. Education and solidarity that has been missing from feminist activism and scholarship for over 100 years.

The #NoDAPL protests have been started, organized, and led by Standing Rock Sioux tribal members (with representatives of over 100 tribes present), with a strong and distinctive cohort of Sioux women. *Bitch Media*—the feminism and pop culture online magazine—has covered the protest but also drawn important links to the ways in which Native activists have long led environmental protests, even if not always recognized for it. Many journalists, activists, and scholars have noted that Native women were the core of the Standing Rock resistance. Not that this should come as any surprise, because women have a long history of playing pivotal roles in activist movements, including ACT UP (AIDS activism), the Occupy movement (anti-capitalist activism), and Black Lives Matter (the ongoing antiracist movement), to name just a few. However, women have not always been acknowledged for their contributions, much less their leadership.

Many say that these indigenous women activists draw on matriarchal tribal structures to stand as the "core spiritual leaders strategizing how to block the 'black snake' pipeline and planning actions to stand up to a police force that has gone to great lengths to defend an oil corporation" (Levin, 2016, n.p.). In this case, the Water Protectors were able to stop—at least temporarily—the $3.7 billion project in the waning days of the Obama administration. The Army Corps of Engineers voted to not grant the permit for the pipeline to drill under the Missouri river, which effectively halted the work until more environmentally and culturally appropriate solutions could be found.

CONCLUSION

So where might the example of #NoDAPL be leading 21st-century feminism, in ways that previous middle-class White Western-dominated feminist movements and actions have not been able to do? To imagine what this future might look like, and how these diverse concerns are linked inexorably together, it's helpful to think about feminism now—perhaps as never before—as a popular cultural and intersectional movement. Feminism has not always been linked to pop culture, or seen as widely of interest to all women, or even a concern of our male allies, but it is now (Martin, Nickels, & Sharp-Grier, 2017; Trier-Bieniek, 2015).

Since our emergence into the second decade of the 21st century, throughout a series of hybrid activist movements that are able in some ways to counteract our raced, classed, and geo-political inequities, feminism has increasingly become a popular cultural concern and practice. Protests like #NoDAPL, #BlackLivesMatter, and the Women's Marches, through their digital flexibilities and capabilities, have become instant worldwide movements. Increasingly fought on both online and off-line platforms, these **hybrid movements** promise increased power for disenfranchised, marginalized, small, and remote communities and individuals. As this book has shown, the possibilities for feminism, feminist activism, and feminist research are growing every day, and their impact potential is growing just as fast.

DISCUSSION QUESTIONS

1. In what ways are indigenous/Native feminisms distinct from nonindigenous feminisms?
2. How has digital media (and social media in particular) changed the way feminist research is done?
3. Why might vlogging be a form of online self-representation that is more popular with women and girls than with men and boys?

ACTIVITIES

1. **Public feminist scholarship** is now enacted both in online and off-line contexts. Select one feminist activist movement or protest action and research as many forms of its public presence as possible: is it present on YouTube news/media clips but not in blogs/vlogs/social media? Make a précis of the forms of public scholarship that you found documenting this protest, and then comment on the different functions each form offers.

2. What is a **critical perspective** on feminist media? Pick one public figure (e.g., vlogger Laci Green, Elizabeth Warren, Pussy Riot) and research the range of perspectives available regarding that figure. For example, some see Pussy Riot as feminist heroes, but others have commented that they are upholding White, sexualized formations of women and that is the only reason they have such a large following. Research your own feminist figure, and the critical perspectives that surround her.

3. **Historical context:** It is just as important to understand the historical and cultural context of feminist scholarship and activism as it is to understand the people who do this work. Find an article or news piece about a feminist figure from more than 50 years ago. It can be a poster, news item, or speech clip. Repeat the exercise above, but note the public response to this historical feminist figure from her own time. To do so you may find it helpful to print out the article, poster, or other item and annotate the printout. Figures such as anarchist Emma Goldman, aviatrix Bessie Coleman, or Chinese feminist and revolutionary Qiu Jin would be rich examples of feminists who did much of the same work as our contemporary feminists such as Pakistani Malala Yousafzai, Oprah Winfrey, or Beyoncé, but operated in a different time.

SUGGESTED RESOURCES

Books

Davis, D.-A., & Craven, C. (2016). *Feminist ethnography: Thinking through methodologies, challenges, and responsibilities.* Lanham, MD: Rowman & Littlefield.

Gessen, M. (2014). *Words will break cement: The passion of Pussy Riot.* New York: Penguin.

A full treatment of the global movement spurred by the actions of a small feminist activist group in Russia.

Harris, A. (2016). *Creativity, religion and youth cultures.* New York: Routledge.

This creative, collaboratively written longitudinal project by the author and two groups of minoritarian young women details the interweaving of age, gender, race, and religion.

Marcus, S. (2010). *Girls to the front: The true story of the riot grrrl revolution.* New York: HarperCollins.

An excellent narrative of the power of the riot grrrl aesthetic and politic and how it has informed the contemporary resurgence of feminist activism.

Whiteley, S. (2013). *Sexing the groove: Popular music and gender.* London: Routledge.

Exploring the links between popular music culture and gender, with particular focus on the ways in which girls and women navigate these industries.

📖 Articles and Chapters

Barron, C., & Lacombe, D. (2005). Moral panic and the nasty girl. *Canadian Review of Sociology/Revue Canadienne de Sociologie, 42*(1), 51–69.

From the Canadian context, an essay on constructions of gendered vilification and sexual panic.

Bernstein, A. (2013). An inadvertent sacrifice: Body politics and sovereign power in the Pussy Riot affair. *Critical Inquiry, 40*(1), 220–241.

An analysis of the Russian Pussy Riot activist group and their pivotal social role in a reborn feminist movement.

Channell, E. (2014). Is sextremism the new feminism? Perspectives from Pussy Riot and Femen. *Nationalities Papers, 42*(4), 611–614.

Chidgey, R. (2014). Developing communities of resistance?: Maker pedagogies, do-it-yourself feminism, and DIY citizenship. In M. Ratto & M. Boler (Eds.), *DIY citizenship: Critical making and social media* (pp. 101–114). Cambridge, MA: MIT Press.

Details the links between DIY culture, gender, race, and critical scholarship.

Dobson, A. S. (2015). Girls' "pain memes" on YouTube: The production of pain and femininity in a digital network. In S. Baker, B. Robards, & B. Buttigieg (Eds.), *Youth cultures and subcultures: Australian perspectives*. Farnham, UK: Ashgate.

The relationship between pleasure, pain, and gender from this digital media and girlhood scholar.

Harris, A., & Roose, J. (2014). DIY citizenship amongst young Muslims: Experiences of the "ordinary." *Journal of Youth Studies, 17*(6), 794–813.

The extraordinary nature of scholarship on religion and gender in contemporary times.

Harris, A. (2006). Citizenship and the self-made girl. In M. Arnott & M. Mac an Ghaill (Eds.), *RoutledgeFalmer reader in gender and education* (pp. 268–282). London: Routledge.

A leader in girlhood studies addresses feminist forms of citizenship.

Harris, A. (2017, Spring). An adoptee autoethnographic femifesta. *International Review of Qualitative Research, 10*(1), 24–28.

A call to arms for queer, adopted and other minoritarian feminists.

Harris, A. (2009). "You could do with a little more Gucci": Ethnographic documentary talks back. *Creative Approaches to Research, 2*(1), 18–34.

A collaborative ethnographic study on race, gender and sexuality in Australia.

Love, B. (2016). Complex personhood of hip hop and the sensibilities of the culture that fosters knowledge of self and self-determination. *Equity and Excellence in Education, 49*(4), 414–427.

A leading critical race education scholar extends the tradition of scholarship on political public forms such as hip-hop, and their gendered and racialized nature.

McRobbie, A., & Thornton, S. L. (1995). Rethinking "moral panic" for multi-mediated social worlds. *British Journal of Sociology, 46*(4), 559–574.

The gendered bias of the idea of "moral panic" in online worlds is explored.

Prozorov, S. (2014). Pussy Riot and the politics of profanation: Parody, performativity, veridiction. *Political Studies, 62*(4), 766–783.

What role has this feminist activist group played in global politics?

Ringrose, J., Harvey, L., Gill, R., & Livingstone, S. (2013). Teen girls, sexual double standards and "sexting": Gendered value in digital image exchange. *Feminist Theory, 14*(3), 305–323.

This article from leading feminist scholars explores the politics of gender in social media and adolescence.

Seal, L. (2013). Pussy Riot and feminist cultural criminology: A new "femininity in dissent"? *Contemporary Justice Review, 16*(2), 293–303.

Details some characteristics of the new activist feminist movement.

☐ Digital Resources

Leslie Feinberg (*www.lesliefeinberg.net*), "This Is What Solidarity Looks Like" (slide show). In addition to her pivotal transgender text *Stone Butch Blues,* this powerful teaching and organizing tool from transgender activist Leslie Feinberg shows how a mass liberation movement can start from a single community to achieve a global reach.

Journal of Resistance Studies, Vol. 2, no. 2
http://resistance-journal.org/product/volume-2-number-2-2016

Feministki community (Russian feminist web community—an online "safe space")
www.ravnopravka.ru

Pussy Riot: A Punk Prayer
www.youtube.com/watch?v=tH4hjg83Mt8

Pussy Riot: The Movement
www.snagfilms.com/films/title/pussy_riot_the_movement

"Make America Great Again" (Pussy Riot)
www.youtube.com/watch?v=s-bKFo30o2o

"I Can't Breathe" (Pussy Riot)
www.youtube.com/watch?v=dXctA2BqF9A

Feminist Scholars
by Discipline or Area of Study

Note: Dates refer to works in the reference list for which the listed scholar is the sole or lead author.

- *Activism*
  - Cari L. Gulbrandsen (2012)—how women mediate power within feminist activism
  - Clare Hemmings (2012)—affective solidarity, reflexivity, and politics

- *Art*
  - Michelle Meagher (2011)—feminist art, theory, storytelling
  - Margaret E. Toye (2010)—poststructuralist feminist ethics and literary creation ("poethics")
  - Keila E. Tyner (2009)—textiles and clothing ("dressing the female body")

- *Cultural Studies*
  - Crystal Abadin
  - Kath Albury
  - Amy Dobson
  - Theresa Senft

- *Education*
  - Gail Cannella—higher education patriarchy, capitalism, violence, power
  - Cynthia Dillard
  - Michelle Fine
  - Patti Lather (2012)—"becoming feminist"

243

- *Feminist Social Research*
  - Myfanwy Franks (2002)—standpoint theory, feminist social research
  - MacGregor (2009)—feminist social research on climate change

- *Gender and Queer Studies*
  - Sara Ahmed
  - Jack Halberstam
  - Hesford (2005)—the specter of feminism-as-lesbian
  - Landstrom (2007)—queering feminist technology studies
  - Lombardo (2010)—gender equality politics, feminist taboos
  - Cris Mayo
  - Jasbir Puar
  - Vernet (2011)—men and feminisms

- *Geography*
  - Bhog (2012)—education, feminist readings of geography textbooks
  - Bondi (2009)—reflexivity and habits of gender/geography in HE

- *Globalization/Transnationalism /Race and Whiteness*
  - Deepak (2011)
  - Mitra (2011)—Indian feminists
  - Jasbir Puar (2007)
  - White (2006)—African American feminists

- *Health*
  - Hankivsky (2010)—intersectionality and women's health research

- *Higher Education and Adult Learning*
  - Carpenter (2012)—Marxist–feminist theory in adult learning

- *Intersectionality*
  - Alexander-Floyd (2012)—intersectionality in the social sciences/post-Black feminist era
  - Carbin (2013)—intersectionality
  - Hankivsky (2010)—intersectionality and women's health research

- *Methods*
  - Brisolara (2014)—feminist evaluation
  - Carroll (2013)—emotional labor/feminist research methodologies
  - Hesse-Biber (2012)—triangulation/mixed-methods research
  - Keary (2013)—feminist genealogical methodologies

- Mertens (2009)—transformative research
- Smart (2009)—qualitative methods
- Spierings (2012)—quantitative techniques in feminist research

- *New Materialisms*
  - Karen Barad
  - Jane Bennett
  - Hinton (2015)—feminist materialisms
  - Jessica Ringrose
  - Kathrin Thiele
  - Iris van der Tuin

- *Organizational feminism*
  - Buzzanell—human relations/organizational feminism, marketplace
  - Gouin (2011)—participatory action research/social justice organizations
  - Mackay (2010)—feminist institutionalism/political science.

- *Philosophy*
  - Karen Barad
  - Megan Boler
  - Elizabeth Grosz
  - Donna Haraway
  - Sandra Hardin—philosophy of science

- *Postcolonial Feminisms*
  - Gloria Anzaldúa
  - Sylvanna M. Falco—Latina feminisms/sociology
  - AnaLouise Keating
  - Rio (2011)—feminist economics and race/Whiteness

- *Power*
  - Cannella—higher education patriarchy, capitalism, violence, power
  - Deepak (2011)—globalization, power, social work, transnationalism
  - Gulbrandsen (2012)—how women mediate power within feminist activism
  - Holland (2010)
  - Karnieli-Miller et al (2009)—power and qualitative research
  - Majic (2014)—sex work

- *Psychology*
  - Sheriff (2009)—discourse analysis, psychology, postmaternity
  - Yoder (2012)—feminist multicultural competence and psychological well-being

- *Religion/Theology*
    - Fiorenza (2013)—critical feminist studies in religion
    - Gebara (2008)—feminist theology/Latin America
    - Hopkins (2009)—gender, emotion, feminist geographies of religion
    - Scholz (2010)—feminist sociology, biblical research, hermeneutics

- *Rhetoric*
    - Royster (2012)—feminist rhetorical practices

- *Social Work and Family Studies*
    - Archer (2009)—social work, ethnography
    - Basile (2013)—intimate partner violence

- *Sociology*
    - Kum-Kum Bhavnani
    - Dana Collins
    - Bev Skeggs
    - Ward (2009)—heteronormativity and sociology

- *Technology*
    - Schuster (2013)—social media, political science

- *War/Crime/Violence/Military*
    - Basile (2013)—intimate partner violence
    - Cannellla—higher education patriarchy, capitalism, violence, power
    - DeKeseredy (2011)—aggression, violence, abuse
    - Henry (2014)—wartime rape, international criminal law
    - Stachowitsch (2012)—foreign policy, international relations, gender and the military
    - Wattanaporn (2014)—feminist criminology
    - Weber (2012)—feminist military families

- *Youth Studies*
    - Holland (2010)—youth, power, participatory qualitative research

References

Abbott, H. P. (2008). *The Cambridge introduction to narrative* (2nd ed.). Cambridge, UK: Cambridge University Press.

Adams, C. J., & Gruen, L. (2014). *Ecofeminism: Feminist intersections with other animals and the Earth*. London: Bloomsbury.

Adams, T. (2008). A review of narrative ethics. *Qualitative Inquiry, 14*(2), 175–194.

Adams, T., Holman Jones, S., & Ellis, C. (2015). *Autoethnography: Understanding qualitative research*. New York: Oxford University Press.

Addams, J. (1899, May). The function of the social settlement. *Annals of the American Academy of Political and Social Science, 13*, 33–44.

Adler, E. S., & Clark, R. (2011). *An invitation to social research: How it's done* (4th ed.). Belmont, CA: Wadsworth.

Ahmad, H. (2010). *Postnational feminisms: Postcolonial identities and cosmopolitanism*. New York: Peter Lang.

Ahmed, S. (2010). *The promise of happiness*. Durham, NC: Duke University Press.

Ahmed, S. (2017). *Living a feminist life*. Durham, NC: Duke University Press.

Alaimo, S., & Hekman, S. (Eds.). (2008). *Material feminisms*. Bloomington: Indiana University Press.

Alcoff, L. (2006). *Visible identities: Race, gender, and the self*. New York: Oxford University Press.

Alexander-Floyd, N. G. (2012). Disappearing acts: Reclaiming intersectionality in the social sciences in a post-Black feminist era. *Feminist Formations, 24*(1), 1–25.

Allen, M. (2011). Violence and voice: Using a feminist constructivist grounded theory to explore women's resistance to abuse. *Qualitative Research, 11*(1), 23–45.

Andalzúa, G. (2002). Preface: (Un)natural bridges, (un)safe spaces. In G. Andalzúa, & A. Keating (Eds.), *This place we call home: Radical visions for transformation* (pp. 1–5). New York: Routledge.

Anderson, K., & Jack, D. (1991). Learning to listen: Interview techniques and analysis. In S. Gluck & D. Patai (Eds.), *Women's words: The feminist practice of oral history* (pp. 11–26). New York: Routledge.

Angelique, H. L., & Culley, M. R. (2000). Searching for feminism: An analysis of community psychology literature relevant to women's concerns. *American Journal of Community Psychology, 28,* 793–813.

Anyiwo, U. M. (2016). The female vampire in popular culture: Or what to read or watch next. In A. Hobson & U. M. Anyiwo (Eds.), *Gender in the vampire narrative* (pp. 173–192). Rotterdam, The Netherlands: Sense Publishers.

Anzaldúa, G., & Keating, A. (Eds.). (2002). *This bridge we call home: Radical visions for transformation.* New York: Routledge.

Archer, J. (2009). Intersecting feminist theory and ethnography in the context of social work research. *Qualitative Social Work, 8*(2), 143–160.

Armitage, S. (2011). The stages of women's oral history. In D. A. Ritchie (Ed.), *The Oxford handbook of oral history* (pp. 169–185). New York: Oxford University Press.

Arthurs, J. (2008). *Sex and the City* and consumer culture: Remediating postfeminist drama. In C. Brundson & L. Spigel (Eds.), *Feminist television criticism: A reader* (pp. 29–40). New York: Open University Press.

Arvin, M., Tuck, E., & Morrill, A. (2013). Decolonizing feminism: Challenging connections between settler colonialism and heteropatriarchy. *Feminist Formations, 25*(1), 8–34.

Australian Women's History Network/VIDA. Retrieved from *www.auswhn.org.au/blog/history-domestic-violence.*

Babbie, E. (2013). *The practice of social research* (13th ed.). Belmont, CA: Wadsworth, Cengage Learning.

Bailey, C. A. (1996). *A guide to field research.* Thousand Oaks, CA: Pine Forge Press.

Bailey, C. A. (2007). *A guide to qualitative field research.* Thousand Oaks, CA: Pine Forge Press.

Bailey, J., & Steeves, V. (Eds.). (2015). *Egirls, ecitizens.* Ottawa, ON, Canada: University of Ottawa Press.

Baker, J. (2008, February). The ideology of choice. Overstating progress and hiding injustice in the lives of young women: Findings from a study in North Queensland, Australia. *Women's Studies International Forum, 31*(1), 53–64.

Banet-Weiser, S. (2007). What's your flava?: Race and postfeminism in media culture. In Y. Tasker & D. Negra (Eds.), *Interrogating postfeminism* (pp. 201–226). Durham, NC: Duke University Press.

Banyard, K. (2010). *The equality illusion: The truth about women and men today.* London: Faber and Faber.

Barad, K. (2007). *Meeting the universe halfway: Quantam physics and the entanglement of matter and meaning.* Durham, NC: Duke University Press.

Barron, C., & Lacombe, D. (2005). Moral panic and the nasty girl. *Canadian Review of Sociology/Revue Canadiene de Sociologie, 42*(1), 51–69.

Barron, M., & Kimmel, M. (2000). Sexual violence in three pornographic media: Toward a sociological explanation. *Journal of Sex Research, 37*(2), 161–168.

Basile, K. C., Hall, J. E., & Walters, M. L. (2013). Expanding resource theory and feminist-informed theory to explain intimate partner violence perpetration by court-ordered men. *Violence Against Women, 19*(7), 848–880.

Battles, K., & Hilton-Morrow, W. (2002). Gay characters in conventional spaces: *Will and Grace* and the situation comedy genre. *Critical Studies in Media Communication, 19,* 87–105.

Beardsley, R., & Miller, M. (2002). Revisioning the process: A case study in feminist program evaluation. In D. Seigart & S. Brisolara (Eds.), *Feminist evaluation: Explorations and experiences. New Directions for Evaluation, 96,* 57–70. San Francisco: Jossey-Bass.

Behar, R. (1995). Introduction: Out of exile. In R. Behar & D. A. Gordon (Eds.), *Women writing culture* (pp. 1–29). Berkeley: University of California Press.

Bell, L. (2014). Ethics and feminist research. In S. N. Hesse-Biber (Ed.), *Feminist research practice: A primer* (2nd ed., pp. 73–106). Thousand Oaks, CA: SAGE.

Bennett, J. (2009). *Vibrant matter: A political ecology of things.* Durham, NC: Duke University Press.

Bennett, J. (2016). *Feminist fight club: An office survival manual (for a sexist workplace).* New York: Penguin.

Bennett, W. L., & Segerberg, A. (2012). The logic of connective action: Digital media and the personalization of contentious politics. *Information, Communication and Society, 15*(5), 739–768.

Berger Gluck, S. (1977). What's so special about women?: Women's oral history. *Frontiers: A Journal of Women Studies, 2*(2), 3–17.

Bhavnani, K. (2001). *Feminism and 'race.'* New York: Oxford University Press.

Bhavnani, K., & Coulson, M. (1997). Transforming socialist feminism: The challenge of racism. In H. S. Mirza (Ed.), *Black British feminism* (pp. 59–62). New York: Routledge.

Bhog, D., Bharadwaj, P., & Mullick, D. (2012). Plotting the contours of the modern nation: A Feminist reading of geography textbooks. *Contemporary Education Dialogue, 9*(1), 39–61.

Biemer, P., & Lyberg, L. E. (2003). *Introduction to survey quality.* Hoboken, NJ: Wiley.

Bird, L. C. (2004). A queer diversity: Teaching difference as interrupting intersections. *Canadian Online Journal of Queer Studies in Education, 1*(1).

Boler, M. (1997). The risks of empathy: Interrogating multiculturalism's gaze. *Cultural Studies, 11*(2), 253–273.

Boler, M. (1999). *Feeling power: Emotions and education.* New York: Routledge.

Boler, M., Macdonald, A., Nitsou, C., & Harris, A. (2014). Connective labor and social media: Women's roles in the "leaderless" Occupy movement. *Convergence, 20*(4), 438–460.

Boler, M., & Nitsou, C. (2014). Women activists of Occupy Wall Street: Consciousness-raising and connective action in hybrid social movements. *Cyberactivism on the participatory Web.* New York: Routledge.

Bondi, L. (2002). *Subjectivities, knowledges, and feminist geographies: The subjects and ethics of social research.* Lanham, MD: Rowman & Littlefield.

Borland, K. (1991). "That's Not What I Said": Interpretive conflict in oral narrative research. In S. Berger Gluck & D. Patai (Eds.), *Women's words: The feminist practice of oral history* (pp. 63–75). New York: Routledge.

Bowen, K. (2011, November). *Evaluation of a rural methamphetamine treatment program: Intensive outpatient therapy using the matrix model retrospective gender analysis in an Appalachian context.* Presented at the annual meeting of the American Evaluation Association, Anaheim, CA.

Boyd, M. R. (2014). Community-based research: Understanding the principles, practices, challenges, and rationale. In P. Leavy (Ed.), *The Oxford handbook of qualitative research* (pp. 498–517). New York: Oxford University Press.

Boyd, P. R. (2015). Paradoxes of feminism. In A. Trier-Bieniek (Ed.), *Feminist theory and pop culture* (pp. 103–114). Rotterdam, The Netherlands: Sense Publishers.

Boyle, K. (2008). Feminism without men: Feminist media studies in a post-feminist age. In C. Brundson & L. Spigel (Eds.), *Feminist television criticism: A reader* (pp. 174–190). New York: Open University Press.

Boylorn, R. M. (2011). Gray or for colored girls who are tired of chasing rainbows: Race and reflexivity. *Cultural Studies → Critical Methodologies, 11*(2), 178–186.

Boylorn, R. M. (2013). Blackgirl blogs, auto/ethnography, and crunk feminism. *Liminalities: A Journal of Performance Studies, 9*(2), 73–82.

Boylorn, R. M. (2014). Working while black: 10 microaggressions experienced in the workplace. Crunk Feminist Collective. Retrieved from *www.crunkfeministcollective.com/2014/11/11/working-while-black-10-racial-microaggressions-experienced-in-the-workplace.*

Braidotti, R. (1996). Cyberfeminism with a difference. In M. Peters, M. Olssen, & Lankshear, C. (Eds.), *Futures of critical theory: Dreams of difference* (pp. 239–260). Lanham, MD: Rowman & Littlefield.

Braidotti, R. (2011). *Nomadic subjects: Embodiment and sexual difference in contemporary feminist theory* (2nd ed.). New York: Columbia University Press.

Brannen, J., & O'Connell, R. (2015). Data analysis I: Overview of data analysis strategies. In S. Hesse-Biber & R. B. Johnson (Eds.), *The Oxford handbook of multimethod and mixed methods research inquiry* (pp. 257–274). New York: Oxford University Press.

Brennan, S. (1999). Recent work in feminist ethics. *Ethics, 109,* 858–893.

Brinkerhoff, R. O. (2005). The success case method: A strategic evaluation approach to increasing the value and effect of training. *Advances in Developing Human Resources, 7*(1), 86–101.

Brisolara, S. (2014). Feminist theory: Its domains and applications. In S. Brisolara, D. Siegart, & S. SenGupta (Eds.), *Feminist evaluation and research: Theory and practice* (pp. 3–41). New York: Guilford Press.

Brisolara, S., & Seigart, D. (2012). Feminist evaluation research. In S. N. Hesse-Biber (Ed.), *Handbook of feminist research: Theory and praxis* (2nd ed., pp. 135–153). Thousand Oaks, CA: SAGE.

Britzman, D. (2011). *Freud and education.* New York: Routledge.

Bruce, T. (2013). Reflections on communication and sport: On women and femininities. *Communication and Sport, 1*(1–2), 125–137.

Buch, E. D., & Staller, K. M. (2014). What is feminist ethnography? In S. Hesse-Biber (Ed.), *Feminist research practice: A primer* (pp. 107–144). Thousand Oaks, CA: SAGE.

Buist, C., & Sutherland, J. (2015). Warning!: Social construction zone. In A.

Trier-Bieniek (Ed.), *Feminist theory and pop culture* (pp. 77–88). Rotterdam, The Netherlands: Sense Publishers.

Butler, J. (1988). Performative acts and gender constitution: An essay in phenomenology and feminist theory. *Theatre Journal, 40*(4), 519–531.

Butler, J. (1990a). *Gender trouble: feminism and the subversion of identity.* New York: Routledge.

Butler, J. (1990b). Performative acts and gender constitution: An essay in phenomenology and feminist theory. In S. E. Case (Ed.), *Performing feminisms: Feminist critical theory and theatre* (pp. 270–282). Baltimore: Johns Hopkins University Press.

Butler, J. (1993). *Bodies that matter: On the discursive limits of sex.* New York: Routledge.

Butler, J., & Athanasiou, A. (2013). *Dispossession: The performative in the political.* New York: Wiley.

Campbell, R. (2002). *Emotionally involved: The impact of researching rape.* New York: Routledge.

Campbell, R., Shaw, J., & Fehler-Cabral, G. (2015). Shelving justice: The discovery of thousands of untested rape kits in Detroit. *City and Community, 14,* 151–166.

Carbin, M., & Edenheim, S. (2013). The intersectional turn in feminist theory: A dream of a common language? *European Journal of Women's Studies, 20*(23), 233–248.

Carey, M. (1994). Forms of interviewing. *Qualitative Health Research, 5*(4), 413–416.

Carpenter, L. (1998). From girls to women: Scripts for sexuality and romance in *Seventeen* magazine, 1974–1994. *Journal of Sex Research, 35*(2), 158–169.

Carpenter, S. (2012). Centering Marxist-feminist theory in adult learning. *Adult Education Quarterly, 62*(1), 19–35.

Carroll, K. (2013). Infertile?: The emotional labour of sensitive and feminist research methodologies. *Qualitative Research, 13*(5), 546–561.

Caulley, D. N. (2008). Making qualitative research reports less boring: The techniques of writing creative nonfiction. *Qualitative Inquiry 4*(3), 424–449.

Chafetz, J. S. (2004). Bridging feminist theory and research methodology. *Journal of Family Issues, 25*(7), 953–967.

Charmaz, K. (2007). What's good writing in feminist research?: What can feminist researchers learn about good writing? In S. N. Hesse-Biber (Ed.), *Handbook of feminist research: Theory and praxis* (pp. 443–458). Thousand Oaks, CA: SAGE.

Charmaz, K. (2008). Grounded theory as an emergent method. In S. N. Hesse-Biber & P. Leavy (Eds.), *Handbook of emergent methods* (pp. 155–170). New York: Guilford Press.

Charmaz, K. (2012). Writing feminist research. In S. N. Hesse-Biber (Ed.), *Handbook of feminist research: Theory and praxis* (pp. 475–494). Thousand Oaks, CA: SAGE.

Chen, Y. (2012). *Women in Chinese martial arts films in the new millennium: Narrative analyses and gender politics.* Lanham, MD: Lexington Books.

Chilisa, B. (2012). *Indigenous research methodologies.* Thousand Oaks, CA: SAGE.

Chilton, G., & Leavy, P. (2014). Arts-based research practice: Merging social research and the creative arts. In P. Leavy (Ed.), *The Oxford handbook of qualitative research* (pp. 403–422). New York: Oxford University Press.

Chilton, M., Rabinowich, J., Council, C., & Breaux, J. (2009). Witnesses to hunger: Participation through Photovoice to ensure the right to food. *Health and Human Rights, 11*(1), 73–85.

Chin, A. (2013). The neoliberal institutional review board, or why just fixing the rules won't help feminist (activist) ethnographers. In C. Craven & D. Davis (Eds.), *Feminist activist ethnography: Counterpoints to neoliberalism in North America* (pp. 201–216). Langham, MD: Lexington Books.

Chmielewski, J. F., & Yost, M. R. (2013). Psychosocial influences on bisexual women's body image. *Psychology of Women Quarterly, 37*(2), 224–241.

Choi, Y., Steiner, L., & Kim, S. (2005, August). *Claiming feminist space in Korean cyber territory.* Presented at the Association for Education in Journalism and Mass Communication Conference, San Antonio, TX.

Cipriani, C. (2015, February 10). Sorry, ladies: Study on women in film and television confirms the worst. Indiewire. Retrieved from *www.indiewire.com/2015/02/sorryladies-study-on-women-in-film-and-television-confirms-the-worst-65220.*

Cixous, H. (2003). *Rootprints: Memory and life writing.* London: Routledge.

Clavio, G., & Eagleman, A. N. (2011). Gender and sexually suggestive images in sports blogs. *Journal of Sports Management, 7,* 295–304.

Coffey, A. (1999). *The ethnographic self: Fieldwork and the representation of identity.* London: SAGE.

Colby, A., & Kohlberg, L. (1987). *The measurement of moral judgment: Vol. 1. Theoretical foundations and research validation.* Cambridge, UK: Cambridge University Press.

Cole, A. L., & Knowles, J. G. (2001). Qualities of inquiry: Process, form, and "goodness." In L. Nielsen, A. L. Cole, & J. G. Knowles (Eds.), *The art of writing inquiry* (pp. 211–229). Halifax, NS, Canada: Backalong Books.

Collective, C. R. (1977). 'A Black Feminist Statement' (pp. 210–218).

Collins, D. (Ed.). (2011). *New directions in feminism and human rights.* London: Routledge.

Collins, P. H. (2008). *Black feminist epistemology.* Routledge: New York.

Collins, P. H. (2009). *Black feminist thought: Knowledge, consciousness and the politics of empowerment* (2nd ed.). New York: Routledge.

Collins, P. H., & Bilge, S. (2016). *Intersectionality.* Hoboken, NJ: Wiley.

Commeyras, M., & Alvermann, D. (1996). Reading about women in world history textbooks from one feminist perspective. *Gender and Education, 8*(1), 31–48.

Connell, R. W. (1987/2007). *Southern theory: The global dynamics of knowledge in social science.* Crows Nest, Australia: Allen & Unwin.

Connell, R. W. (2014). *Gender and power: Society, the person and sexual politics.* Cambridge, UK: Polity Press.

Cooper, B. (2016). Feminism for badasses. *Signs: Journal of Women in Culture and Society, 41*(3), 704–705.

Crave, C., & Davis, D. (2016). *Feminist ethnography: Thinking through methodologies, challenges, and possibilities.* Langham, MD: Rowman & Littlefield.

Crenshaw, K. (1989). Demarginalizing the intersection of race and sex: A Black feminist critique of antidiscrimination doctrine, feminist theory and antiracist politics. *University of Chicago Legal Forum, 140,* 139–167.

Creswell, J. W. (2014). *Research design: Qualitative, quantities, and mixed methods approaches* 4th ed.). Thousand Oaks, CA: SAGE.

Crotty, M. (1998). *The foundations of social research: Meaning and perspective in the research process.* Thousand Oaks, CA: SAGE.

Cuklanz, L. M., & Moorti, S. (2006). Television's "new" feminism: Prime-time representations of women and victimization. *Critical Studies in Mass Communication, 23,* 302–321.

Currie, D. (1999). *Girl talk: Adolescent magazines and their readers.* Buffalo, NY: University of Toronto Press.

Davies, R., & Dart, J. (2005). The most significant change technique: A guide to its use. Retrieved from *https://www.researchgate.net/publication/275409002_ The_%27Most_Significant_Change%27_MSC_Technique_A_Guide_to_ Its_Use.*

de Freitas, E. (2003). Contested positions: How fiction informs empathetic research. *International Journal of Education and the Arts* 4(7). Retrieved from *www.ijea.org/v4n7.*

De Lauretis, T. (1984). *Alice doesn't: Feminism, semiotics, cinema.* Bloomington: Indiana University Press.

De Lauretis, T. (1991). (Ed.). Queer theory: Lesbian and gay sexualities [Special issue]. *Differences: A Journal of Feminist Cultural Studies.*

DeCarvalho, L. J., & Cox, N. B. (2015). Queerness (un)shackled. In A. Trier-Bieniek (Ed.), *Feminist theory and pop culture* (pp. 65–76). Rotterdam, The Netherlands: Sense Publishers.

Deepak, A. C. (2011). Sustainability and population growth in the context of globalization: A postcolonial feminist social work perspective. *Journal of Research on Women and Gender, 3,* 1–22.

DeKeseredy, W. S. (2011). Feminist contributions to understanding woman abuse: Myths, controversies, and realities. *Aggression and Violent Behavior, 16*(4), 297–302.

D'Enbeau, S., & Buzzanell, P. M. (2013). Constructing a feminist organization's identity in a competitive marketplace: The intersection of ideology, image, and culture. *Human Relations, 66*(11), 1447–1470.

DeShong, H. A. F. (2013). Feminist reflexive interviewing: Researching violence against women in St. Vincent and the Grenadines. *Caribbean Review of Gender Studies, 7,* 1–24.

Devault, M. L., & Gross, G. (2007). Feminist interviewing: Experience, talk and knowledge. In S. N. Hesse-Biber (Ed.), *Handbook of feminist research: Theory and praxis* (pp. 173–197). Thousand Oaks, CA: SAGE.

Dicker, R. (2016). *A history of US feminisms* (rev. ed.). Berkeley, CA: Seal Press.

Dickson-Swift, V. (2008). *Undertaking sensitive research in the health and social sciences.* Cambridge, UK: Cambridge University Press.

Dickson-Swift, V., James, E., & Kippen, S. (2009). Researching sensitive topics: Qualitative research as emotion work. *Qualitative Research, 9*(1), 61–79.

Dillard, C. B. (2000). The substance of things hoped for, the evidence of things not seen: Examining an endarkened feminist epistemology in educational research and leadership. *International Journal of Qualitative Studies in Education, 13*(6), 661–681.

Dillard, C. B. (2006). *On spiritual strivings: Transforming an African American woman's academic life.* Albany: SUNY Press.

Dillard, C. B. (2008). When the ground is black, the ground is fertile: exploring darkened feminist epistemology and healing methodologies of the spirit. In N. Denzin, Y. Lincoln, & L. Tuhiwai Smith (Eds.), *Handbook of critical indigenous methodologies* (pp. 277–292). Thousand Oaks, CA: SAGE.

Dillard, C. B. (2012). *Learning to (re)member the things we've learned to forget: Endarkened feminisms, spirituality, and the sacred nature of (re)search and teaching.* New York: Peter Lang.

Dillard, C. B. (2016). Turning the ships around: A case study of (re)membering as transnational endarkened feminist inquiry and praxis for black teachers! *Educational Studies, 52*(5), 406–423.

Dillard, C. B., & Okpalaoka, C. (2011). The sacred and spiritual nature of endarkened transnational feminist praxis in qualitative research. In N. Denzin & Y. Lincoln (Eds.), *The SAGE handbook of qualitative research* (4th ed., pp. 147–162). Los Angeles: SAGE.

Dobson, A. S. (2011, November). Hetero-sexy representation by young women on MySpace: The politics of performing an "objectified" self. *Outskirts: Feminisms along the Edge, 25.*

Dobson, A. S. (2014). Performative shamelessness on young women's social network sites: Shielding the self and resisting gender melancholia. *Feminism and Psychology, 24*(1), 97–114.

Dobson, A. S. (2016). *Postfeminist digital cultures: Femininity, social media, and self-representation.* New York: Palgrave Macmillan.

Dobson, A. S., & Ringrose, J. (2016). Sext education: Pedagogies of sex, gender and shame in the schoolyards of Tagged and Exposed. *Sex Education, 16*(1), 8–21.

Doucet, A. (2008). "From Her Side of the Gossamer Wall(s)": reflexivity and relational knowing. *Qualitative Sociology, 31,* 73–87.

Dow, B. (1990). Hegemony, feminist criticism, and *The Mary Tyler Moore Show. Critical Studies in Mass Communication, 7,* 261–274.

Duggan, L., & Muñoz, J. E. (2009). Hope and hopelessness: A dialogue. *Women and Performance: A Journal of Feminist Theory, 19*(2), 275–283.

Duong, L. P. (2012). *Treacherous subjects: Gender, culture and trans-Vietnamese feminism.* Philadelphia: Temple University Press.

Dutro, E. (2008). "That's why I was crying in this book": Trauma as testimony to children's responses to literature. *Changing English, 15,* 423–434.

Ebert, T. L. (1996). *Ludic feminism and after: Postmodernism, desire, and labor in late capitalism.* Ann Arbor: University of Michigan Press.

Edwards, R., & Mauthner, M. (2002). Ethics and feminist research: Theory and practice. In M. Mauthner, M. Birch, J. Jessop, & T. Miller (Eds.), *Ethics in qualitative research* (pp. 14–31). London: SAGE.

Eichler, M. (1988). *Nonsexist research methods. A practical guide.* New York: McGraw-Hill.

Eisenhart, M. (2001). Changing conceptions of culture and ethnographic methodology: Recent thematic shifts and their implications for research on teaching. In V. Richardson (Ed.), *Handbook of research on teaching* (4th ed., pp. 209–225). Washington, DC: American Educational Research Association.

Ellis, C. (2004). *The ethnographic I: The methodological novel about autoethnography.* New York: AltaMira Press.

Ellis, C. (2007). Telling secrets, revealing lives: Relational ethics in research with intimate others. *Qualitative Inquiry, 13*(1), 3–29.

Enloe, C. (2014). *Bananas, beaches and bases: Making feminist sense of international politics*. Berkeley: University of California Press.

Esposito, J. (2009). What does race have to do with *Ugly Betty?*: An analysis of privilege and postracial representations on a television sitcom. *Television and New Media, 10,* 521–535.

Etherington, K. (2007). Ethical research in reflexivity relationships. *Qualitative Inquiry, 13*(5), 599–616.

Etter-Lewis, G. (1991). Black women's life stories: Reclaiming self in narrative texts. In S. Gluck & D. Patai (Eds.), *Women's words: The feminist practice of oral history* (pp. 43–58). New York: Routledge.

Eurostat Statistics Explained. (2016, March). The unadjusted gender pay gap. Retrieved from *http://ec.europa.eu/eurostat/statistics-explained/index.php/ File:The_unadjusted_gender_pay_gap,_2014_(¹)_(difference_between_ average_gross_hourly_earnings_of_male_and_female_employees_ as_%25_of_male_gross_earnings_new.png#filelinks.*

Evans, L., & Davies, K. (2000). No sissy boys here: A content analysis of the representation of masculinity in elementary school reading textbooks. *Sex Roles: A Journal of Research, 42,* 255–270.

Evans, R. (1994). The negation of powerlessness: Maori feminism, a perspective. *Hecate, 20*(2), 53.

Evans-Winters, V. E. (2011). *Teaching black girls: Resiliency in urban classrooms* (rev. ed.). New York: Peter Lang.

Evans-Winters, V. E. (2015). Black feminism in qualitative education research: A mosaic for interpreting race, class, and gender in education. In V. E. Evans-Winters & B. L. Love (Eds.), *Black feminism in education: Black women speak back, up, and out* (pp. 129–142). New York: Peter Lang.

Fahs, B. (2016). Methodological mishaps and slippery subjects: Stories of first sex, oral sex, and sexual trauma in qualitative sex research. *Qualitative Psychology, 3*(2), 209–225.

Falcon, S. M. (2008). Mestiza double consciousness: The voices of Afro-Peruvian women on gendered racism. *Gender and Society, 22*(5), 660–680.

Fallon, M. (2016). *Writing quantitative research*. Rotterdam, The Netherlands: Sense Publishers.

Faulkner, S. L., & Squillante, S. (2016). *Writing the personal: Getting your stories onto the page*. Leiden, The Netherlands: Brill-Sense.

Faundez, A., & Abarca, H. (2011). *Principales Hellazgos de la Sistematizacion de Evaluanciones con Enfoque de Igualdad de Genero y Dereches Humanos en America Latina* (Document for discussion at the Forum on Evaluations with Gender Equality and Human Rights Approach in Latin America, RELAC, Latin American and Caribbean Evaluation network).

Figiel, S. (1996/2014). *Where we once belonged*. Auckland, NZ: Pasifika Press.

Fine, M. (1992). *Disruptive voices: The possibilities of feminist research*. Ann Arbor: University of Michigan Press.

Fine, M. (1994). Working the hyphens: Reinventing self and other in qualitative research. In N. K. Denzin & Y. S. Lincoln (Eds.), *The handbook of qualitative research* (pp. 70–82). Thousand Oaks, CA: SAGE.

Fine, M. (2004). Witnessing whiteness/gathering intelligence. In M. Fine, L. Weiss, L. Powell Pruitt, & A. Burns (Eds.), *Off white: Readings on power, privilege, and resistance* (2nd ed., 245–256). New York: Routledge.

Fine, M., Torre, M. E., Boudin, K., Bowen, I., Clark, J., & Hylton, D. (2003). Participatory action research: From within and beyond prison bars. In P. Camic, J. E. Rhodes, & L. Yardley (Eds.), *Qualitative research in psychology: Expanding perspectives in methodology and design* (pp. 173–198). Washington, DC: American Psychological Association.

Fiorenza, E. S. (2013). Critical feminist studies in religion. *Critical Research on Religion, 1*(1), 43–50.

Fisher, C. B. (2000). Relational ethics in psychological research: One feminist's journey. In M. M. Brabeck (Ed.), *Practicing feminist ethics in psychology* (pp. 125–142). Washington, DC: American Psychological Association.

Fisher, J. (2016). *"Ecofeminism and the Dakota Access Pipeline" in FemGeniuses: Where feminism meets genius!* Retrieved from *https://femgeniuses. com/2016/11/03/ecofeminism-and-the-dakota-access-pipeline.*

Fowler, F. J. (1984). *Survey research methods.* Beverly Hills, CA: SAGE.

Fowler, F. J., Jr. (2009). *Survey research methods* (4th ed.). Thousand Oaks, CA: SAGE.

Fowler, F. J., Jr. (2014). *Survey research methods* (5th ed.). Thousand Oaks, CA: SAGE.

Franks, M. (2002). Feminisms and cross-ideological feminist social research: Standpoint, situatedness and positionality—developing cross-ideological feminist research. *Journal of International Women's Studies, 3*(2), 40–53.

Fraser, N., & Nicholson, L. J. (1990). Social criticism without philosophy: An encounter between feminism and postmodernism. In L. J. Nicholson (Ed.), *Feminism/postmodernism* (pp. 19–38). New York: Routledge.

Freeman, D. (1999). *The fateful hoaxing of Margaret Mead: A historical analysis of her Samoan research* (p. 208). Boulder, CO: Westview Press.

Fresno-Calleja, P. (2014). Talking back, fast, and beyond: Selina Tusitala Marsh's poetry and the performance of Pasifika Identities. *Contemporary Women's Writing, 8*(3), 354–372.

Frost, N., & Elichaoff, F. (2014). Feminist postmodernism, poststructuralism, and critical theory. In S. Hesse-Biber (Ed.), *Feminist research practice: A primer* (2nd ed., pp 42–72). Thousand Oaks, CA: SAGE.

Fustich, K. (2017, February 1). "In protest: A reading list for the resistance." Retrieved from *www.bkmag.com/2017/02/01/protest-reading-list-resistance.*

Gamble, S. (Ed.). (2001). *The Routledge companion to feminism and postfeminism.* London: Routledge.

Gamson, J. (1999). Taking the talk show challenge: Television, emotion, and public spheres. *Constellations, 6*(2), 190–205.

Gannon, S., & Davies, B. (2012). Postmodern, post-structural, and critical theories. In S. N. Hesse-Biber (Ed.), *The handbook of feminist research: Theory and praxis* (2nd ed., pp. 65–91). Thousand Oaks. CA: SAGE.

Gardner, R. P. (2015). If you listen, you will hear: Race, place, gender, and the trauma of witnessing through listening in research contexts. In V. E. Evans-Winters & B. L. Love (Eds.), *Black feminism in education: Black women speak back, up, and out* (pp. 121–128). New York: Peter Lang.

Gay, R. (2014). *Bad feminism.* New York: Corsair/HarperCollins.

Gebara, I. (2008). Feminist theology in Latin America: A theology without recognition. *Feminist Theology, 16*(3), 324–331.

Geertz, C. (1973). *The interpretations of cultures.* New York: Basic Books.

Genz, S. (2006). Third Way/ve: The politics of postfeminism. *Feminist Theory,* 7(3), 333–353.

Giddings, P. (1984). *When and where I enter: The impact of black women on race and sex in America.* New York: Morrow.

Gilbert, M. R., & Masucci, M. (2006). The implication of including women's daily lives in a feminist GIScience. *Transactions in GIS, 10,* 751–761.

Gill, R. (2009). Beyond the "sexualization of culture" thesis: An intersectional analysis of "sixpacks," "midriffs," and "hot lesbians" in advertising. *Sexualities, 12*(2), 137–160.

Gill, R. (2012). Media, empowerment and the "sexualization of culture" debates. *Sex Roles, 66*(11–12), 736–745.

Gill, R. (2016). Post-postfeminism?: New feminist visibilities in postfeminist times. *Feminist Media Studies, 16*(4), 610–630.

Gill, R., & Scharff, C. (2011). Introduction. In R. Gill & C. Scharff (Eds.), *New femininities: Postfeminism, neoliberalism and subjectivity.* Basingstoke, UK: Palgrave.

Gilligan, C. (1982). *In a different voice: Psychological theory and women's development.* Cambridge, MA. Harvard University Press.

Gilligan, C. (1995). Moral orientation and moral development. In V. Held (Ed.), *Justice and care: Essential readings in feminist ethics* (pp. 31–46). Boulder, CO: Westview Press.

Glaser, B. G., & Strauss, A. (1967). *The discovery of grounded theory: Strategies for qualitative research.* New York: Aldine.

Golde, P. (1970). *Women in the field: Anthropological experiences.* Chicago: Aldine.

Gonick, M. (2004). The "Mean Girl" crisis: Problematizing representations of girls' friendships, *Feminism and Psychology, 14*(3), 395–400.

Gonick, M., Renold, E., Ringrose, J., & Weems, L. (2009). Rethinking agency and resistance: What comes after girl power? *Girlhood Studies, 2*(2), 1–9.

Gossett, J. L., & Byrne, S. (2002). "Click here": A content analysis of Internet rape sites. *Gender and Society, 16*(5), 689–709.

Gouin, R. R., Cocq, K., & McGavin, S. (2011). Feminist participatory research in a social justice organization. *Action Research, 9*(3), 261–281.

Greene, J. (1995, November). *Evaluators as advocates.* Presented at the annual meeting of the American Evaluation Association, Vancouver, BC, Canada.

Griffin, C., Szmigin, S. C., Bengry-Howell, A., Hackley, C., & Mistral, W. (2013). Inhabiting youthful femininity as an impossible space: Hypersexual femininity and the culture of intoxication among young women in the UK. *Feminism and Psychology, 23*(2), 167.

Griffin, R. A. (2015). Olivia Pope as problematic and paradoxical. In A. Trier-Bieniek (Ed.), *Feminist theory and pop culture* (pp. 35–48). Rotterdam, The Netherlands: Sense Publishers.

Griffiths, J. L. (2009). *Traumatic possessions: The body and memory in African American women's writing and performance.* Charlottesville: University of Virginia Press.

Grosz, E. (2011). *Becoming undone: Darwinian reflections on life, politics and art.* Durham, NC: Duke University Press.

Gulbrandsen, C. L., & Walsh, C. A. (2012). It starts with me: Women mediate power within feminist activism. *Affilia, 27*(3), 275–288.

Gullion, J. S. (2016). *Writing ethnography*. Rotterdam, The Netherlands: Sense Publishers.

Gutkind, L. (1997). *The art of creative nonfiction: Writing and selling the literature of reality*. New York: Wiley.

Halberstam, J. (1993). Imagined violence/queer violence: Representation, rage and resistance. *Social Text, 37*, 187–201.

Halberstam, J. (1998). *Female masculinity*. Durham, NC: Duke University Press.

Halberstam, J. (2005). *In a queer time and place: Transgender bodies, subcultural lives*. New York: NYU Press.

Halberstam, J. (2011). *The queer art of failure*. Durham, NC: Duke University Press.

Halberstam, J. (2012). *Gaga feminism: Sex, gender, and the end of normal* (Vol. 7). Boston: Beacon Press.

Hall, E. J., & Shepherd Stolley, K. (1997). A historical analysis of the presentation of abortion and adoption in marriage and family textbooks: 1950–1987. *Family Relations, 46*, 73–82.

Halpin, T. (1989). Scientific objectivity and the concept of "the other." *Women's Studies International Forum, 12*(3), 285–294.

Halsanger, S. (Ed.). (2005). *Theorizing feminisms: A reader*. London: Oxford University Press.

Halse, C., & Honey, A. (2005). Unravelling ethics: Illuminating the moral dilemmas of research ethics. *Signs: Journal of Women in Culture and Society, 30*, 2141–2162.

Handyside, S., & Ringrose, J. (2017). Snapchat memory and youth digital sexual cultures: Mediated temporality, duration and affect. *Journal of Gender Studies*.

Hankivsky, O., Reid, C., Cormier, R., Varcoe, C., Clark, N., Benoit, C., & Brotman, S. (2010). Exploring the promises of intersectionality for advancing women's health research. *International Journal for Equity in Health, 9*(1), 5.

Haraway, D. (1991). *Simians, cyborgs, and women: The reinvention of nature*. New York: Routledge.

Haraway, D. (2014). Situated knowledges: The science question in feminism and the privilege of partial perspective. In A. Jaggar (Ed.), *Just methods: An interdisciplinary feminist reader* (2nd ed., pp. 346–351). Boulder, CO: Paradigm.

Harding, R., & Peel, E. (2007). Heterosexism at work: Diversity training, discrimination law and the limits of liberal individualism. In V. Clarke & E. Peel (Eds.), *Out in psychology: Lesbian, gay, bisexual, trans and queer perspectives* (pp. 247–271). London: Wiley.

Harding, S. (1987). *Feminism and methodology*. Bloomington: Indiana University Press.

Harding, S. (1998). *Is science multicultural?: Postcolonialisms, feminism, and epistemologies*. Bloomington: Indiana University Press.

Harding, S. (2004). "Introduction: Standpoint theory as a site of political, philosophic, and scientific debate. In *The feminist standpoint theory reader: Intellectual and political controversies* (pp. 1–15). New York: Routledge.

Harding, S. (2012). Feminist standpoints. In S. N. Hesse-Biber (Ed.), *The handbook of feminist research: Theory and praxis* (2nd ed., pp. 46–64). Thousand Oaks, CA: SAGE.

Harmon, D., & Boeringer, S. B. (2004). A content analysis of Internet-accessible written a pornographic depictions. In S. Hesse-Biber & P. Leavy (Eds.), *Approaches to qualitative research: A reader on theory and practice* (pp. 402–407). New York: Oxford University Press.

Harper, B. A. (2014). *Scars: A Black lesbian experience in rural White New England.* Leiden, The Netherlands: Brill-Sense.

Harris, A. (Ed.). (2004). *All about the girl: Culture, power and identity.*. New York: Routledge.

Harris, A. (2012a). (All the) Single Ladies: diasporic women are doing it for themselves. *Australian Feminist Studies, 27*(72), 157–170.

Harris, A. (2012b). Blame it on Tyra: Race, refugeity and sexual representation. *Sex Education: Sexuality, Society and Learning, 12*(1), 79–94.

Harris, A. (2012c). *Ethnocinema: Intercultural arts education.* The Netherlands: Springer.

Harris, A. (2012d). Truth or dare: Sex, race, and mockumentary film. *Feminist Media Studies, 13*(3), 540–556.

Harris, A. (2016a). *Creativity, religion and youth cultures.* New York: Routledge.

Harris, A. (2016b). Love has a body that feels like heat: (Extra)ordinary affects and genderqueer love. In *Departures in Critical Qualitative Research, 5*(4), 24–41.

Harris, A. (2016c). *Video as method.* London: Oxford University Press.

Harris, A. (2017). An adoptee autoethnographic femifesta. *International Review of Qualitative Research, 10*(1), 24–28.

Harris, A., & Holman Jones, S. (2016). *Writing for performance.* Rotterdam, The Netherlands: Sense Publishers.

Harris, A., & Holman Jones, S. (2017). Feeling fear, feeling queer: The peril and potential of queer terror. *Cultural Studies, Critical Methodologies.*

Harris, A., & Nyuon, N. (2012). People get tired: African Australian cross-cultural dialogue and ethnocinema. In P. Vannini (Ed.), *Popularizing research: Engaging new media, new audiences, new genres* (pp. 19–24). New York: Peter Lang,

Harrison, F. V. (1995). Writing against the grain: Cultural politics of difference in the work of Alice Walker. In R. Behar & D. A. Gordon (Eds.), *Women writing culture* (pp. 233–245). Berkeley: University of California Press.

Hartsock, N. (1983). The feminist standpoint: Developing the ground for a specifically feminist historical materialism. In S. Harding & M. B. Hintikka (Eds.), *Discovering reality, second edition: Feminist perspectives on epistemology, metaphysics, methodology, and philosophy of science* (pp. 283–310). Dordrecht, The Netherlands: Kluwer Academic Publishers.

Hekman, S. (2008). Constructing the ballast: An ontology for feminism. In S. Alaimo & S. Hekman (Eds.), *Material feminisms* (pp. 95–119). Bloomington, IN: Indiana University Press.

Held, V. (2006). *The ethics of care: Personal, political, and global.* Oxford, UK: Oxford University Press.

Helgren, J., & Vasconcellos, C. A. (Eds.). (2010). *Girlhood: A global history.* New Brunswick NJ: Rutgers University Press.

Hemmings, C. (2012). Affective solidarity: Feminist reflexivity and political transformation. *Feminist Theory, 13*(2), 147–161.

Henry, N. (2014). The fixation on wartime rape: Feminist critique and international criminal law. *Social and Legal Studies, 23*(1), 93–111.

Hertz, R. (1997). *Reflexivity and voice.* London: SAGE.

Hesford, V. (2005). Feminism and its ghosts: The spectre of the feminist-as-lesbian. *Feminist Theory, 6*(3), 227–250.

Hesse-Biber, S. N. (1996). *Am I thin enough yet?: The cult of thinness and the commercialization of identity.* New York: Oxford University Press.

Hesse-Biber, S. N. (2006). *The cult of thinness* (2nd ed.) New York: Oxford University Press.

Hesse-Biber, S. N. (2012). *The handbook of feminist research theory and praxis* (2nd ed.). London: SAGE.

Hesse-Biber, S. N. (Ed.). (2013a). *Feminist research practice: A primer* (2nd ed.). Thousand Oaks, CA: SAGE.

Hesse-Biber, S. N. (2013b). A re-invitation to feminist research. In S. N. Hesse-Biber (Ed.), *Feminist research practice: A primer* (2nd ed., pp. 1–13). Thousand Oaks, CA: SAGE.

Hesse-Biber, S. N., & Leavy, P. (2005). *The practice of qualitative research.* Thousand Oaks, CA: SAGE.

Hesse-Biber, S., & Leavy, P. (2011). *The practice of qualitative research* (2nd ed.). Thousand Oaks, CA: SAGE.

Hesse-Biber, S. N., & Piatelli, D. (2007). From theory to method and back again: The synergistic practice of theory and method. In N. Hesse-Biber (Ed.), *Handbook of feminist research: Theory and praxis* (pp. 143–153). Thousand Oaks, CA: SAGE.

Hickey-Moody, A. (2007). *Intellectual disability, Sensation and thinking through affect.* In A. Hickey-Moody & P. Malins (Eds.), *Deleuzian encounters.* New York: Palgrave Macmillan.

Hickey-Moody, A. (2016). A femifesta for posthuman art education: Visions and becomings. In C. A. Taylor & C. Hughes (Eds.), *Posthuman research practices in education* (pp. 258–266). Basingstoke, UK: Palgrave Macmillan UK.

Hinton, P., Treusch, P., van der Tuin, I., Dolphijn, R., & Sauzet, S. (2015). Teaching with gender: European women's studies in international and interdisciplinary classrooms. *ATGENDER, 12.* Retrieved from *atgender.eu/vol-12-teaching-with-feminist-materialisms.*

Hochschild, A. (2003.) *The managed heart: Commercialization of human feeling* (2nd ed.). Berkeley: University of California Press.

Hodge, D. (2016). *Home with hip hop feminism: Performances in communication and culture, by Aisha S. Durham.* New York: Peter Lang.

Holland, S., Renold, E., Ross, N. J., & Hillman, A. (2010). Power, agency and participatory agendas: A critical exploration of young people's engagement in participative qualitative research. *Childhood, 17*(3), 360–375.

Holm, G. (2008). Visual research methods: Where are we and where are we going? In S. N. Hesse-Biber & P. Leavy (Eds.), *Handbook of emergent methods* (pp. 325–342). New York: Guilford Press.

Holman Jones, S. (2005). Autoethnography: Making the personal political. In N.

K. Denzin & Y. S. Lincoln (Eds.), *Handbook of qualitative research* (3rd ed., pp. 763–791), Thousand Oaks, CA: SAGE.

Holmes, M. (2010). The emotionalization of reflexivity. *Sociology, 44*(1), 139–154.

Holmes, S. (2016). Blindness to the obvious?: Treatment experiences and feminist approaches to eating disorders. *Feminism and Psychology, 26*(4), 464–486.

hooks, b. (1982). *Ain't I a woman: Black women and feminism.* Boston: South End Press.

hooks, b. (1994). *Teaching to transgress: Education as the practice of freedom.* New York: Routledge.

hooks, b. (2000a). *Feminist theory: From margin to center.* London: Pluto Press.

hooks, b. (2000b). *Feminism is for everybody: Passionate politics.* London: Pluto Press.

Hopkins, P. E. (2009). Women, men, positionalities and emotion: Doing feminist geographies of religion. *ACME: An International Journal for Critical Geographies, 8*(1), 1–17.

Householder Kalogeropoulos, A. (2015). Girls, grrrls, girls. In A. Trier-Bieniek (Ed.), *Feminist theory and pop culture* (pp. 19–34). Rotterdam, The Netherlands: Sense Publishers.

Hsu, W. F. (2014). Digital ethnography toward augmented empiricism: A new methodological framework. *Journal of Digital Humanities, 3*(1). Retrieved from *http://journalofdigitalhumanities.org/3-1/digital-ethnography-toward-augmented-empiricism-by-wendy-hsu.*

Hunsinger, J., & Senft, T. M. (2013). *The social media handbook.* New York: Routledge.

Iosefo, F. (2016). Third spaces: Sites of resistance in higher education? *Higher Education Research and Development, 35*(1), 189–192.

Irigaray, L. (1985). *This sex which is not one* (Catherine Porter, Trans.). Ithaca, NY: Cornell University Press.

Israel, B., Eng, E., Schultz A., & Parker, E. (2005). *Methods in community-based participatory research for health.* San Francisco: Jossey-Bass.

Jackson, S., Vares, T., & Gill, R. (2012). The whole playboy mansion image: Girls' fashioning and fashioned selves within a postfeminist culture. *Feminism and Psychology, 23*(2), 143–162.

Jaggar, A. M. (Ed.). (2014). *Just methods: An interdisciplinary feminist reader* (2nd ed.). New York: Pluto Press.

Jayaratne, T. E., Thomas, N. G., & Trautmann, M. T. (2003). An intervention program to keep girls in the science pipeline: Outcome differences by ethnic status. *Journal of Research in Science Teaching, 40,* 393–414.

Jenkins, K., & Pihama, L. (2001). Matauranga Wahine: Teaching Maori women's knowledge alongside feminism. *Feminism and Psychology, 11*(3), 293–303.

Johnson, A., & Boylorn, R. M. (2015). Digital media and the politics of intersectional queer hyper/in/visibility in Between Women. *Digital Media, 11*(1).

Johnson, J. M. (2002). In-depth interviewing. In J. F. Gubrium & J. A. Holstein (Eds.), *Handbook of interview research: Context and method* (pp. 103–120). Thousand Oaks, CA: SAGE.

Johnson, L. (2000). *Placebound: Australian feminist geographies.* Oxford, UK: Oxford University Press.

Junqueira, E. S. (2009, Spring). Feminist ethnography in education and the challenges of conducting fieldwork: Critically examining reciprocity and relationships between academic and public interests. *Perspectives on Urban Education, 6*(1), 73–79.

Juris, J. (2012). Reflections on #occupy everywhere. *American Ethnologist, 39*(2), 259–279.

Kaiser, K., & Skoglund, E. (2006). *Prominence of men and women in newspaper sports coverage as an indicator of gender equality pre- and post-Title IX.* Paper presented at the annual meeting of the Association for Education in Journalism and Mass Communication Convention, San Francisco, CA.

Karaian, L. (2014). Policing "sexting": Responsibilization, respectability and sexual subjectivity in child protection/crime prevention responses to teenagers' digital sexual expression. *Theoretical Criminology, 18*(3), 282–299.

Karnieli-Miller, O., Strier, R., & Pessach, L. (2009). Power relations in qualitative research. *Qualitative Health Research, 19*(2), 279–289.

Karon, S. (1992). The politics of naming: Lesbian erasure in a feminist context. In S. Reinharz & E. Stone (Eds.), *Looking at invisible women: An exercise in feminist pedagogy*. Washington, DC: University Press of America.

Keary, A. (2013). Feminist genealogical methodologies. *Feminist Theology, 21*(2), 126–144.

Keating, A., & Anzaldúa, G. (Eds.). (2002). *This bridge we call home: Radical visions for transformation*. New York: Routledge.

Keller, J. (2016). Making activism accessible: Exploring girls' blogs as sites of contemporary feminist activism. In C. Mitchell & C. Rentschler (Eds.), *Girlhood and the politics of place* (pp. 261–278). London: Berghahn Books.

Kelly, A. (1978). Feminism and research. *Women's Studies International Quarterly, 1*, 225–232.

Kilbourne, J. (1999). *Deadly persuasion: Why women and girls must fight the addictive power of advertising*. New York: Free Press.

Kilbourne, J. (2000). *Can't buy me love: How advertising changes the way we think and feel*. New York: Simon & Schuster.

Kitzinger, J. (1994). The methodology of focus groups: The importance of interaction between research participants. *Sociology of Health and Illness, 16*, 103–121.

Ko, D., & Zheng, W. (2006). Introduction: Translating feminisms in China. *Gender and History, 18*(3), 463–471.

Kohlberg, L. (1981). *Essays on moral development: Vol. 1. The philosophy of moral development: Moral stages and the idea of justice*. New York: Harper & Row.

Krijnen, T., & Van Bauwel, S. (2015). *Gender and media: Representing, producing, consuming*. Abingdon, VA: Routledge.

Krimsky, S. (2000). Transdisciplinarity for problems at the interstices of disciplines. In M. A. Somerville & D. J. Rapport (Eds.), *Transdisciplinarity: Recreating integrated knowledge* (pp. 109–114). Oxford, UK: EOLSS.

Kristeva, J. (1981). Women's time. *Journal of Women in Culture and Society, 7*, 13–35.

Kwan, M. P. (2002). Feminist visualization: Re-envisioning GIS as a method in feminist geographic research. *Annals of the Association of American Geographers, 92*, 645–661.

Ladson-Billings, G. (2000). Racialized discourses and ethnic epistemologies. In N. Denzin & Y. Lincoln (Eds.), *Handbook of qualitative research* (2nd ed., pp. 257–277). Thousand Oaks, CA: SAGE.

Landström, C. (2007). Queering feminist technology studies. *Feminist Theory, 8*(1), 7–26.

Langhout, R. D., Fernandez, J. S., Wyldebore, D., & Savala, J. (2016). Photovoice and house meetings as tools within participatory action research. In L. A. Jason & D. S. Glenwick (Eds.), *Handbook of methodological approaches to community-based research: Qualitative, quantitative, and mixed methods* (pp. 81–91). New York: Oxford University Press.

Lather, P. (1991). *Getting smart, feminist research and pedagogy with/in the postmodern.* New York: Routledge.

Lather, P. (2000, April). *The possibilities of paradigm proliferation.* Paper presented at the annual meeting of the American Educational Research Association, New Orleans, LA.

Lather, P. (2007). *Getting Lost: Feminist efforts toward a double(d) science.* Albany: State University of New York Press.

Lather, P. (2008a). Getting lost: critiquing across difference as methodological practice. In K. Gallagher (Ed.), *The methodological dilemma: Creative, critical and collaborative approaches to qualitative research* (pp. 219–231). Abingdon, VA: Routledge.

Lather, P. (2008b). (Post) feminist methodology. *International Review of Qualitative Research, 1*(1), 55–64.

Lather, P., & Smithies, C. S. (1997). *Troubling the angels: Women living with HIV/AIDS.* New York: Westview Press.

Latour, B. (2004). Why has critique run out of steam?: From matters of fact to matters of concern. *Critical inquiry, 30*(2), 225–248.

Leavy, P. (2000). Feminist content analysis and representative characters. *The Qualitative Report, 5*(1), 1–16.

Leavy, P. (2006). Ally McBeal as a site of postmodern bodily boundaries and struggles over cultural interpretation: The hysteric as a site of feminist resistance. In E. Watson (Ed.), *Searching the soul of Ally McBeal: Critical essays* (pp. 19–35). Jefferson, NC: McFarland & Co.

Leavy, P. (2007). The practice of feminist oral history and focus group interviews. In S. Hesse-Biber & P. L. Leavy (Eds.), *Feminist research practice: A primer* (pp. 149–186). Thousand Oaks, CA: SAGE.

Leavy, P. (2009). *Method meets art: Arts-based research practice.* New York: Guilford Press.

Leavy, P. (2011a). *Essentials of transdisciplinary research: Using problem-centered methodologies.* Walnut Creek, CA: Left Coast Press.

Leavy, P. (2011b). *Oral history: Understanding qualitative research.* New York: Oxford University Press.

Leavy, P. (2013). *Fiction as research practice: Short stories, novellas, and novels.* Walnut Creek, CA: Left Coast Press/Routledge.

Leavy, P. (2015). *Method meets art: Arts-based research practice* (2nd ed.). New York: Guilford Press.

Leavy, P. (2016). A commentary on academic publishing: Insider tips. *The*

Qualitative Report, 21(6). Retrieved from *http://nsuworks.nova.edu/tqr/vol21/iss6/6*.

Leavy, P. (2017) *Research design: Quantitative, qualitative, mixed methods, arts-based, and community-based participatory research approaches*. New York: Guilford Press.

Leavy, P., & Hastings, L. (2010, May 3). Body image and sexual identity: An interview study with lesbian, bisexual and heterosexual college age women. *Electronic Journal of Human Sexuality, 13*. Retrieved from *www.ejhs.org/volume13/bodyimage.htm*.

Leavy, P., & Sardi Ross, L. (2006). The matrix of eating disorder vulnerability: Oral history and the link between personal and social problems. *Oral History Review, 33*(1), 65–81.

Leavy, P., & Scotti, V. (2017). *Low-fat love stories*. Rotterdam, The Netherlands: Sense Publishers.

Lee-Koo, K., & D'Costa, B. (2008). *Gender and global politics in the Asia Pacific*. New York: Palgrave Macmillan.

Letiecq, B., & Schmalzbauer, L. (2012). Community-based participatory research with Mexican migrants in a new rural destination. *Action Research, 10*(3), 244–259.

Levin, S. (2016). At Standing Rock, women lead fight in face of mace, arrests, and strip searches. Retrieved from *www.theguardian.com/us-news/2016/nov/04/dakota-access-pipeline-protest-standing-rock-women-police-abuse*.

Levin, D. E., & Kilbourne, J. (2009). *So sexy so soon: The new sexualized childhood and what parents can do to protect their kids*. New York: Random House.

Lewin, E. (2006). *Feminist anthropology: A reader*. Oxford, UK: Blackwell.

Loftin, W. A., Barnett, S. K., Bunn, P. S., & Sullivan, P. (2005). Recruitment and retention of rural African Americans in diabetes research: lesson learned. *Diabetes Educator, 31*(2), 251–259.

Lombardo, E., Meier, P., & Verloo, M. (2010). Discursive dynamics in gender equality politics: What about "feminist taboos"? *European Journal of Women's Studies, 17*(2), 105–123.

Lorde, A. (1984). *Sister outsider: Essays and speeches*. Trumansburg, NY: Crossing Press.

Love, B. L. (2012). *Hip hop's li'l sistas speak: negotiating hip hop identities and politics in the new South*. New York: Peter Lang.

Love, B. L. (2017). Difficult knowledge: When a black feminist educator was too afraid to #SayHerName. *English Education, 49*(2), 197–208.

Lumpkin, A. (2009). Female representation in feather articles published by *Sports Illustrated* in the 1990s. *Women in Sport and Physical Activity Journal, 18*(2), 38–51.

Lumsden, K., & Morgan, H. M. (2012, October 26). *"Fraping," "Sexting," "Trolling" and "Rinsing": Social networking, feminist thought and the construction of young women as victims or villains*. Paper presented at Proceedings of Forthcoming Feminisms: Gender Activism, Politics, and Theory, Leeds, UK.

Luttrell, W. (2000). "Good enough" methods for ethnographic research. *Harvard Educational Review, 70*(4), 499–523.

Lykke, N. (2010). *Feminist studies: A guide to intersectional theory, methodology and writing.* New York: Routledge.

MacGregor, S. (2009). A stranger silence still: The need for feminist social research on climate change. *Sociological Review, 57*(2), 124–140.

Mackay, F., Kenny, M., & Chappell, L. (2010). New institutionalism through a gender lens: Towards a feminist institutionalism? *International Political Science Review, 31*(5), 573–588.

Magar, V. (2012). Rescue and rehabilitation: A critical analysis of sex workers' antitrafficking response India. *Signs, 37,* 619–644.

Magill, D. (2015). Racial hybridity and the reconstruction of white masculinity in *Underworld.* In U. M. Anyiwo (Ed.), *Race in the vampire narrative* (pp. 81–90). Rotterdam, The Netherlands: Sense Publishers.

Majic, S. (2014). Beyond "victim-criminals" sex workers, nonprofit organizations, and gender ideologies. *Gender and Society, 28*(3), 463–485.

Malhotra, S., & Rowe, A. C. (Eds.). (2013). *Silence, feminism, power: Reflections at the edges of sound.* Basingstoke, UK: Palgrave/Springer.

Mark, J. (1988). *A stranger in her native land: Alice Fletcher and the American Indians.* Lincoln: University of Nebraska Press.

Martin, E. (1999). The egg and the sperm: How science has constructed a romance based on stereotypical male-female roles. In S. Hesse-Biber, C. Gilmartin, & R. Lyndenberg (Eds.), *Feminist approaches to theory and methodology: An interdisciplinary reader* (pp. 15–25). New York: Oxford University Press.

Martin, J. L., Nickels, A. E., & Sharp-Grier, M. (2017). *Feminist pedagogy, practice, and activism: Improving lives for girls and women.* New York: Routledge.

Martineau, H. (1998). *How to observe morals and manners.* New Brunswick, NJ: Transaction Books. (Original work published 1838)

Masini, E. B. (1991). The household, gender, and age project. In E. Masini & S. Stratigos (Eds.), *Women, households and change* (pp. 3–17). Tokyo: United Nations University Press.

Masini, E. B. (2000). Transdisciplinarity, futures studies, and empirical research. In M. A. Somerville & D. J. Rapport (Eds.), *Transdisciplinarity: ReCreating integrated knowledge,* (pp. 117–124). Oxford, UK: EOLSS.

Mathison, S. (2014). Research and evaluation: Intersections and divergence. In S. Brisolara, D. Siegart, & S. SenGupta (Eds.), *Feminist evaluation and research: Theory and practice* (pp. 42–58). New York: Guilford Press.

McDowell, L. (2013). *Gender, identity and place: Understanding feminist geographies.* Cambridge, UK: Polity Press.

McHugh, M. C. (2014). Feminist qualitative research: Toward transformation of science and society. In P. Leavy (Ed.), *Oxford handbook of qualitative research* (pp. 137–164). New York: Oxford University Press.

McIntosh, H., & Cuklanz, L. M. (2014). Feminist media research. In S. N. Hesse-Biber (Ed.), *Feminist research practice: A primer* (2nd ed., pp. 264–295). Thousand Oaks, CA: SAGE.

McKinlay, E., Gan, M., Buntting, C., & Jones, A. (2015). New Zealand: Towards inclusive STEM education for all students. In B. Freeman, S. Marginson, & R. Tytler (Eds.), *The age of STEM: Educational policy and practice across the world in science, technology, engineering and mathematics* (pp. 201–214). New York: Routledge.

McLafferty, S. (2002). Women and GIS: Geospatial technologies and feminist geographies. *Cartographica, 40*(4), 37–45.

McNicholas, P. (2004, July 6). *Maori feminism: A contribution to accounting research and practice.* Paper presented at the Fourth Asia Pacific Interdisciplinary Research in Accounting Conference, Singapore.

McRobbie, A. (2000). *Jackie* magazine: Romantic individualism and the teenage girl. In A. McRobbie (Ed.), *Feminism and youth culture* (pp. 67–117). New York: Routledge.

McRobbie, A. (2004). Notes on postfeminism and popular culture: Bridget Jones and the new gender regime. In A. Harris (Ed.), *All about the girl: Culture, power and identity* (pp. 3–14). New York: Routledge.

McRobbie, A. (2008). *The aftermath of feminism: Gender, culture and social change.* London: SAGE.

McRobbie, A., & Thornton, S. L. (1995). Rethinking "moral panic" for multi-mediated social worlds. *British Journal of Sociology, 46*(4), 559–574.

Meade, C. D., Menard, J. M., Luque, J. S., Martinez-Tyson, D., & Gwede, C. K. (2009). Creating community–academic partnerships for cancer disparities research and health promotion. *Health Promotion Practice. 12*(3), 456–462.

Meagher, M. (2011). Telling stories about feminist art. *Feminist Theory, 12*(3), 297–316.

Mertens, D. M. (2005). *Research and evaluation in education and psychology: Integrating diversity with quantitative, qualitative, and mixed methods* (2nd ed.). Thousand Oaks, CA: SAGE.

Mertens, D. M. (2008). *Transformative research and evaluation.* New York: Guilford Press.

Mertens, D. (2010). *Research and evaluation in education and psychology: Integrating diversity with quantitative, qualitative, and mixed methods* (3rd ed.). Thousand Oaks, CA: SAGE.

Mertens, D. M. (2014). A transformative feminist stance: Inclusion of multiple dimensions of diversity with gender. In S. Brisolara, D. Siegart, & S. SenGupta (Eds.), *Feminist evaluation and research: Theory and practice* (pp. 95–112). New York: Guilford Press.

Mertens, D. M., & Stewart, N. (2014). The feminist practice of program evaluation. In S. N. Hesse-Biber (Ed.), *Feminist research practice: A primer* (2nd ed., pp. 330–362). Thousand Oaks, CA: SAGE.

Miller, T., & Boulton, M. (2007). Changing constructions of informed consent: Qualitative research and complex social worlds. *Social Science and Medicine, 65,* 2199–2211.

Mills, G. E. (2007). *Action research: A guide for the teacher researcher.* Upper Saddle River, NJ: Pearson.

Miner, K., & Jayaratne, T. (2014). Feminist survey research. In S. Hesse-Biber (Ed.), *Feminist research practice: A primer* (pp. 296–329). Thousand Oaks, CA: SAGE.

Miner, K., Jayaratne, T., Pesonen, A., & Zurbrugg, L. (2011). Using survey research as a quantitative method for feminist social change. In S. Hesse-Biber (Ed.),

Handbook of feminist research: Theory and praxis (2nd ed., pp. 237–263). Thousand Oaks, CA: SAGE.

Miner-Rubino, K., Jayaratne, T. E., & Konik, J. (2007). Using survey research as a quantitative method for feminist social change. In S. Nagy Hesse-Biber (Ed.), *Handbook of feminist research. theory and praxis* (pp. 199–222). Thousand Oaks, CA: SAGE.

Minh-ha, T. T. (1987). Difference: A special Third World women issue. *Feminist Review, 25*(1), 5–22.

Minh-ha, T. T. (2009). *Woman, native, other: Writing postcoloniality and feminism.* Bloomington: Indiana University Press.

Minister, K. (1991). A feminist frame for the oral history interview. In S. Gluck & D. Patai (Eds.), *Women's words: The feminist practice of oral history* (pp. 27–42). New York: Routledge.

Minkler, M. (2004). Ethical challenges for the "outside" researcher in community-based participatory action research. *Health Education and Behavior, 31*(6), 684–697.

Mitra, A. (2011). To be or not to be a Feminist in India. *Affilia, 26*(2), 182–200.

Mohanram, R. (1996). The construction of place: Maori feminism and nationalism in Aotearoa/New Zealand. *NWSA Journal, 8*(1), 50–69.

Moloney, S. (2011). Focus groups as transformative spiritual encounters. *International Journal of Qualitative Methods, 10*(1), 58–72.

Montoya, M. J., & Kent, E. E. (2014). Dialogical action: Moving from community-based to community-driven participatory research. *Qualitative Health Research, 21*(7), 1000–1011.

Moraga, C., & Anzaldúa, G. (Eds.). (1983). *This bridge called my back: Writings by radical women of color.* New York: Kitchen Table Press.

Morgan, D. (1996). Focus groups. *Annual Review of Sociology, 22,* 129–152.

Morgan, D., & Krueger, R. (1993). When to use focus groups and why. In D. Morgan (Ed.), *Successful focus groups: Advancing the state of the art* (pp. 3–19). Newbury Park, CA: SAGE.

Morse, J. M. (2010). Sampling in grounded theory. In A. Bryant & K. Charmaz (Eds.), *The SAGE handbook of grounded theory* (pp. 229–244). London: SAGE.

Moss, P., & Al-Hindi, K. F. (Eds.). (2008). *Feminisms in geography: Rethinking space, place, and knowledges.* Lanham, MD: Rowman & Littlefield.

Motzafi-Haller, P. (1997). Writing birthright: On native anthropologists and the politics of representation. In D. Reed-Danahay (Ed.), *Auto/ethnography: Rewriting the self and the social* (pp. 195–222). Oxford, UK: Berg.

Mulvey, L. (1975). Visual pleasure and narrative cinema. *Screen, 16*(3), 6–18.

Naples, N., & Gurr, B. (2014). Feminist empiricism and standpoint theory: Approaches to understanding the social world. In S. Hesse-Biber (Ed.), *Feminist research practice: A primer* (2nd ed., pp. 14–41). Thousand Oaks, CA: SAGE.

Nelson, L., & Seager, J. (Eds.). (2008). *A companion to feminist geography.* Malden, MA: Wiley.

Neroni, H. (2005). *The violent woman: Femininity, narrative, and violence in contemporary American cinema.* Albany: State University of New York Press.

Newbury, J., & Hoskins, M. (2010). Relational inquiry: Generating new knowledge with adolescent girls who use crystal meth. *Qualitative Inquiry, 16*(8), 642.

Ngozi Adichie, C. (2015). *We should all be feminists*. New York: Anchor Books.

Nichols, T. (2014). Measuring gender inequality in Angola: A feminist-ecological model for evaluation. In S. Brisolara, D. Siegart, & S. SenGupta (Eds.), *Feminist evaluation and research: Theory and practice* (pp. 176–196). New York: Guilford Press.

Nicol, R. (2016). "You were such a good girl when you were human": Gender and subversion in *The Vampire Diaries*. In A. Hobson & M. U. Anyiwo (Eds.), *Gender in the vampire narrative* (pp. 145–160). Leiden, The Netherlands: Brill-Sense.

Nip, J. (2004). The Queer Sisters and its electronic bulletin board: A study of the Internet for social movement mobilization. *Information, Communication, and Society, 7*(1), 23–49.

Noddings, N. (1984). *Caring: A feminine approach to ethics and moral education*. Berkeley: University of California Press.

Noddings, N. (2003). *Caring: A feminine approach to ethics and moral education* (2nd ed.). Berkeley, CA: University of California Press.

Nussbaum, M. (1999, February). The professor of parody: The hip defeatism of Judith Butler. *New Republic, 22,* 37–45.

Oakley, A. (1981). Interviewing women: A contradiction in terms. In H. Roberts (Ed.), *Doing feminist research* (pp. 30–61). London: Routledge and Kegan Paul.

Ogles, J. (2016, June 13). There were straight victims in Orlando too. *The Advocate*. Retrieved from *www.advocate.com/crime/2016/6/13/there-were-straight-victims-orlando-too*.

Oliveira, D. L. (2011). The use of focus groups to investigate sensitive topics: An example taken from research on adolescent girls' perceptions about sexual risks. *Ciência & Saúde Coletiva, 16*(7), 3093–3102.

Parker, R. S. (1990). Nurses' stories: The search for a relational ethic of care. *Advances in Nursing Science, 13*(1), 31–40.

Patton, M. Q. (2008). *Utilization focused evaluation*. Thousand Oaks, CA: SAGE.

Patton, M. Q. (2015). *Qualitative research and evaluation methods* (4th ed.). Thousand Oaks, CA: SAGE.

Pederson, P. M. (2002). Examining equity in newspaper photographs. *International Review for the Sociology of Sport, 34,* 303–318.

Peirce, L. M. (2011). The American mother: A feminist analysis of the Kleenex "Get-Mommed" campaign. *Journal of Media and Communication Studies, 3,* 118–122.

Pfohl, S. (1992). *Death at the parasite café*. New York: St. Martin's Press.

Pfohl, S. (2007). The reality of social constructions. In J. A. Holstein & J. F. Gubrium (Eds.), *Handbook of constructionist research* (pp. 645–688). New York: Guilford Press.

Phillips, D. C., & Burbules, N. C. (2000). *Postpositivism and educational research*. Lanham, MD: Rowman & Littlefied.

Piepmeier, A. (2007). Postfeminism vs. the Third Wave. *Electronic Book Review*.

Retrieved from *www.electronicbookreview.com/thread/writingpostfeminism/reconfiguredrip2*.

Pillow, W. S., & Mayo, C. (2007). Toward understandings of feminist ethnography. In S. Hesse-Biber (Ed.), *Handbook of feminist research: Theory and praxis* (pp. 155–172). Thousand Oaks, CA: SAGE.

Pink, S. (2007). *Doing visual ethnography* (2nd ed.). Thousand Oaks, CA: SAGE.

Pink, S. (2009). *Doing sensory ethnography*. Thousand Oaks, CA: SAGE.

Pink, S., Horst, H. A., Postill, J., Hjorth, L., Lewis, T., & Tacchi, J. (2015). *Digital ethnography: Principles and practice*. Thousand Oaks: SAGE.

Pinnick, C. L., Koertge, N., & Almeder, R. F. (2003). *Scrutinizing feminist epistemology: An examination of gender in science*. New Brunswick, NJ: Rutgers University Press.

Podems, D. (2010). Feminist evaluation and gender approaches: There's a difference? *Journal of MultiDisciplinary Evaluation, 6*(14), 1–17.

Podems, D. (2014). Feminist evaluation for nonfeminists. In S. Brisolara, D. Siegart, & S. SenGupta (Eds.), *Feminist evaluation and research: Theory and practice* (pp. 113–142). New York: Guilford Press.

Pohl, C., & Hadorn, G. H. (2007). *Principles for designing transdisciplinary research* (A. B. Zimmermann, Trans.). Munich, Germany: Oekom Gesell F. Oekolog.

Pozner, J. L. (2010). *Reality bites back: The troubling truth about guilty pleasure TV*. Berkeley, CA: Seal Press.

Preissle, J. (2007). Feminist research ethics. In S. N. Hesse-Biber (Ed.), *Handbook of feminist research: Theory and praxis* (pp. 515–532). Thousand Oaks, CA: SAGE.

Projansky, S. (2007). Mass magazine cover girls: Some reflections on postfeminist girls and postfeminism's daughters. In Y. Tasker & D. Negra (Eds.), *Interrogating postfeminism* (pp. 40–72). Durham, NC: Duke University Press.

Projansky, S. (2011). Girl's sexualities in The Sisterhood of the Travelling Pants universe: Feminist challenges and missed opportunities. In H. Radner & R. Stringer (Eds.), *Feminism at the movies: Understanding gender in contemporary popular culture* (pp. 134–148). New York: Routledge.

Puar, J. K. (2007). *Terrorist assemblages: Homonationalism in queer times*. Durham, NC: Duke University Press.

Radner, H. (2011). Speaking the name of the father in the neo-romantic comedy: 13 Going on 30 (2004). In H. Radner & R. Stringer (Eds.), *Feminism at the movies: Understanding gender in contemporary popular culture* (pp. 134–148). New York: Routledge.

Rajan, G., & Desai, J. (Eds.). (2013). *Transnational feminism and global advocacy in South Asia*. Abingdon, VA: Routledge.

Ramji, H. (2008). Exploring commonality and difference in in-depth interviewing: A case-study of researching British Asian women. *British Journal of Sociology, 59*(1), 99–116.

Reason, P., & Bradbury, H. (Eds.). (2008). *The SAGE handbook of action reseach: Participative inquiry and practice*. Thousand Oaks CA: SAGE.

Reinharz, S. (1992). *Feminist methods in social research*. New York: Oxford University Press.

Reinharz, S., & Kulick, R. (2007). Reading between the lines: Feminist content analysis into the second millennium. In. S. N. Hesse-Biber (Ed.), *Handbook of feminist research: Theory and praxis* (pp. 257–276). Thousand Oaks, CA: SAGE.

Renold, E., & Ringrose, J. (2011). Schizoid subjectivities?: Re-theorizing teen girls' sexual cultures in an era of "sexualization." *Journal of Sociology, 47*(4), 389–409.

Retallack, H., Ringrose, J., & Lawrence, E. (2016). "Fuck your body image": Teen girls' Twitter and Instagram feminism in and around school. In *Learning Bodies* (pp. 85–103). Singapore: Springer.

Richardson, L. (1981). Gender stereotyping in the English language adapted from *The Dynamics of Sex and Gender: A Sociological Perspective* (3rd ed.). Boston: Houghton Mifflin.

Richardson, L. (1997). *Fields of play: Constructing an academic life*. New Brunswick, NJ: Rutgers University Press.

Ringrose, J. (2007). Successful girls?: Complicating post-feminist, neoliberal discourses of educational achievement and gender equality. *Gender and Education, 19*(4), 471–489.

Ringrose, J. (2011). Are you sexy, flirty, or a slut?: Exploring "sexualization" and how teen girls perform/negotiate digital sexual identity on social networking sites. In R. Gill & C. Scharff (Eds.), *New femininities: Postfeminism, neoliberalism, and subjectivity* (pp. 99–116). Basingstoke, UK: Palgrave Macmillan.

Ringrose, J. (2013). *Postfeminist education?: Girls and the sexual politics of schooling*. New York: Routledge.

Ringrose, J., & Barajas, K. E. (2011). Gendered risks and opportunities?: Exploring teen girls' digitized sexual identities in postfeminist media contexts. *International Journal of Media and Cultural Politics, 7*(2), 121–138.

Ringrose, J., Gill, R., Livingstone, S., & Harvey, L. (2012). *A qualitative study of children, young people and "sexting": A report prepared for the NSPCC*. London: National Society for the Prevention of Cruelty to Children.

Ringrose, J., Harvey, L., Gill, R., & Livingstone, S. (2013). Teen girls, sexual double standards and "sexting": Gendered value in digital image exchange. *Feminist Theory, 14*(3), 305–323.

Ringrose, J., & Renold, E. (2012). Slut-shaming, girl power and "sexualisation": Thinking through the politics of the international SlutWalks with teen girls. *Gender and Education, 24*(3), 333–343.

Ringrose, J., & Renold, E. (2016). Teen feminist killjoys?: Mapping girls' affective encounters with femininity, sexuality, and feminism at school. In C. Mitchell & C. Rentscheler (Eds.), *Girlhood and the politics of place* (pp. 104–121). New York: Berghahn Books.

Rio, C. (2012). Whiteness in feminist economics: The situation of race in bargaining models of the household. *Critical Sociology, 38*(5), 669–685.

Roberts, J. M., & Sanders, T. (2005). Before, during and after: Realism, reflexivity and ethnography. *Sociological Review, 53*, 294–313.

Rodriguez, C. R., Tsikata, D., & Ampofo, A. A. (Eds.). (2015). *Transatlantic feminisms: Women and gender studies in Africa and the diaspora*. New York: Lexington Books.

Roller, M. R., & Lavrakas, P. J. (2015). *Applied qualitative research design: A total quality framework approach*. New York: Guilford Press.

Roof, J. (2007). Authority and representation in feminist research. In S. N. Hesse-Biber (Ed.), *The handbook of feminist research: Theory and praxis* (pp. 425–442). Thousand Oaks, CA: SAGE.

Roof, J. (2012). Authority and representation in feminist research. In S. N. Hesse-Biber (Ed.), *The handbook of feminist research: Theory and praxis* (2nd ed., pp. 520–543). Thousand Oaks, CA: SAGE.

Rose, D. (2000). Analysis of moving images. In M. W. Bauer & G. Gaskell (Eds.), *Qualitative researching with text, image and sound* (pp. 246–262). London: SAGE.

Rosenberg, M. (1990). Reflexivity and emotions. *Social Psychology Quarterly, 53*(1), 3–12.

Ross, G. V. (2003, May). *Cuestiones de ética, politica y poder en mi investigación autobiografica con las mujeres viviendo con VIH en la ciudad de La Paz.* Paper presented at the Regional Meeting "Sexuality, Health and Human Rights in Latin America," Lima, Peru.

Rosser, S. V. (2014). *Breaking into the lab: Engineering progress for women in science.* New York: NYU Press.

Rowe, A. C. (2000). Locating feminism's subject: The paradox of white femininity and the struggle to forge feminist alliances. *Communication Theory, 10*(1), 64–80.

Rowe, A. C. (2005). Be longing: Toward a feminist politics of relation. *NWSA Journal, 17*(2), 15–46.

Rowe, A. C. (2008). *Power lines: On the subject of feminist alliances.* Durham, NC: Duke University Press.

Rowe, A. C. (2009). Subject to power—Feminism without victims. *Women's Studies in Communication, 32*(1), 12–35.

Rowe, A. C., & Lindsey, S. (2003). Reckoning loyalties: White femininity as "crisis." *Feminist Media Studies, 3*(2), 173–191.

Royster, J. J., & Kirsch, G. E. (2012). *Feminist rhetorical practices: New horizons for rhetoric, composition, and literacy studies.* Carbondale, IL: SIU Press.

Ruel, E., Wagner, W. E., III, & Gillespie, B. J. (2016). *The practice of survey research: Theory and applications.* Thousand Oaks, CA: SAGE.

Saidel, R. G. (2004). *The Jewish women of Ravensbrück Concentration Camp.* Madison, WI: University of Wisconsin Press.

Saini, A. (2009). Annals of the Black superheroine. *Bitch: Feminist response to popular culture, 45,* 35–41.

Saldaña, J. (2003). Dramatizing data: A primer. *Qualitative Inquiry, 9*(2), 218–236.

Saldaña, J. (2009). *The coding manual for qualitative researchers.* Thousand Oaks, CA: SAGE.

Saldaña, J. (2014). Coding and analysis strategies. In P. Leavy (Ed.), *The Oxford handbook of qualitative research* (pp. 581–605). New York: Oxford University Press.

Salinas Mulder, S., & Amariles, F. (2014). Latin American feminist perspectives on gender power issues in evaluation. In S. Brisolara, D. Siegart, & S. SenGupta (Eds.), *Feminist evaluation and research: Theory and practice* (pp. 224–254). New York: Guilford Press.

Salinas Mulder, S., Rance, S., Serrate Suarez, M., & Castro Condori, M. (2000).

Unethical ethics?: Reflections on intercultural research practices. *Reproductive Health Matters, 8*(15), 104–122.

Sandberg, S. (2013). *Women, work and the will to lead.* London: W. H. Allen.

Sampson, H., Bloor, M., & Fincham, B. (2008). A price worth paying?: Considering the "Cost" of reflexive research methods and the influence of feminist ways of "Doing." *Sociology, 42*(5), 919–933.

Saunders, T. (2016). Towards a transnational hip-hop feminist liberatory praxis: A view from the Americas. *Social Identities, 22*(2), 178–194.

Schlenker, J., Caron, S., & Halteman, W. (1998). A feminist analysis of *Seventeen* magazine: Content analysis from 1945 to 1995. *Sex Roles, 38*(1–2), 135–149.

Scholz, S. (2010). A third kind of feminist reading: Toward a feminist sociology of biblical hermeneutics. *Currents in Research, 9*(1), 9–32.

Schuster, J. (2013). Invisible feminists?: Social media and young women's political participation. *Political Science, 65*(1), 8–24.

Scott, J. (2011). *The fantasy of feminist history.* Durham, NC: Duke University Press.

Scott-Dixon, K. (Ed.). (2006). *Trans/forming feminisms: Trans/feminist voices speak out.* Toronto, ON, Canada: Sumach Press.

Scriven, M. (1997). Truth and objectivity in evaluation. In E. Chelimsky & W. Shadish (Eds.), *Evaluation for the 21st century: A handbook* (pp. 477–500). Thousand Oaks, CA: SAGE.

Sedgwick, E. K. (1990). *Epistemology of the closet.* Berkeley: University of California Press.

Sedgwick, E. K. (1997). Paranoid reading and reparative reading, or, you're so paranoid, you probably think this introduction is about you. In E. K. Sedgwick (Ed.), *Novel gazing: Queer readings in fiction* (pp. 123–151). Durham, NC: Duke University Press.

Seigart, D. M. (1999). *Participatory evaluation and community learning: Sharing knowledge about school-based health care.* Unpublished master's thesis. Cornell University, Ithaca, NY.

Seigart, D. (2005). Feminist evaluation. In S. Mathison (Ed.), *Encyclopedia of evaluation* (pp. 154–157). Thousand Oaks, CA: SAGE.

Seigart, D. (2014). Feminist research approaches to studying school-based health care: A three-country comparison. In S. Brisolara, D. Siegart, & S. SenGupta (Eds.), *Feminist evaluation and research: Theory and practice* (pp. 263–283). New York: Guilford Press.

Senft, T. M. (2000). Baud girls and cargo cults. In A. Herman & T. Swiss (Eds.), *The World Wide Web and contemporary cultural theory* (pp. 183–206). London: Routledge.

Senft, T. M. (2008). *Camgirls: Celebrity and community in the age of social networks.* New York: Peter Lang.

Senft, T. M., & Baym, N. K. (2015). Selfies introduction—What does the selfie say?: Investigating a global phenomenon. *International Journal of Communication, 9*, 19.

Serano, J. (2016a). *Outspoken: A decade of transgender activism and trans feminism.* Oakland, CA: Switch Hitter Press.

Serano, J. (2016b). *Whipping girl: A transsexual woman on sexism and the scapegoating of femininity* (2nd ed.). Berkeley, CA: Seal Press.

Sheriff, M., & Weatherall, A. (2009). A feminist discourse analysis of popular-press accounts of postmaternity. *Feminism and Psychology, 19*(1), 89–108.

Signorielli, N., & Bacue, A. (1999). Recognition and respect: A content analysis of prime-time television characters across three decades. *Sex Roles, 40*(7), 527–544.

Silver, C. (2010, April). *CAQDAS tools for visual analysis.* Paper presented at the Mixed Methods Seminar "Using Software Tools In Visual Analyses," Surrey, UK.

Skeggs, B. (2005). The making of class and gender through visualizing moral subject formation. *Sociology, 39*(5), 965–982.

Slater, R. (2000). Using life histories to explore change: Women's urban struggles in Cape Town, South Africa. *Gender and Development, 8*(2), 38–46.

Smart, C. (2009). Shifting horizons: Reflections on qualitative methods. *Feminist Theory, 10*(3), 295–308.

Smith, D. (1987). *The everyday world as problematic: A feminist sociology.* Boston: Northeastern University Press.

Spalter-Roth, R., & Hartmann, H. (1996). Small happinesses: The feminist struggle to integrate social research and social activism. In H. Gottfried (Ed.), *Feminism and social change: Bridging theory and practice* (pp. 206–224). Urbana: University of Illinois Press.

Sparkes, A. C. (1994). Self, silence, and invisibility as a beginning teacher: A life history of lesbian experience. *British Journal of Sociology of Education, 15*(1), 93–119.

Sperling, V. (2015). *Sex, politics, and Putin: Political legitimacy in Russia.* Oxford, UK: Oxford University Press.

Spierings, N. (2012). The inclusion of quantitative techniques and diversity in the mainstream of feminist research. *European Journal of Women's Studies, 19*(3), 331–347.

Spivak, G. C. (1988). Can the subaltern speak? In G. Nelson & L. Grossberg (Eds.), *Marxism and the interpretation of culture* (pp. 271–313). Urbana: University of Illinois Press.

Spivak, G. C., & Grosz, E. (1990). Criticism, feminism, and the institution. *The Post-Colonial Critic: Interviews, Strategies, Dialogues,* 1–16.

Sprague, J. (2016). *Feminist methodologies for critical researchers: Bridging differences* (2nd ed.). London: Rowman & Littlefield.

Stacey, J. (1991). Can there be a feminist ethnography? In S. Gluck & D. Patai (Eds.), *Women's words: The feminist practice of oral history* (pp. 111–120). New York: Routledge.

Stachowitsch, S. (2012). Military gender integration and foreign policy in the United States: A feminist international relations perspective. *Security Dialogue, 43*(4), 305–321.

Stanley, L., & Wise, S. (2002). *Breaking out again: Feminist ontology and epistemology.* London: Routledge.

Steinberg, S., & Cannella, G. S. (Eds.). (2012). *Critical qualitative research reader.* New York: Peter Lang.

Steinberg, S. J., & Steinberg, S. L. (2011). Geospatial analysis technology and social science research. In S. N. Hesse-Biber (Ed.), *The handbook of emergent technologies in social research* (pp. 563–591). New York: Oxford University Press.

Stephens, D. P., & Phillips, L. D. (2003). Freaks, gold diggers, divas and dykes: The socio-historical development of African American female adolescent scripts. *Sexuality and Culture, 7*, 3–47.

Stephens, J. (2010). Our remembered selves: Oral history and feminist memory. *Oral History, 38*(1), 81–90.

Stoeker, R. (2008). Challenging institutional barriers to community-based research. *Action Research, 6*(1), 49–67.

St. Pierre, E. A. (2000). Poststructural feminism in education: An overview. *International Journal of Qualitative Studies in Education, 13*(5), 477–515.

St. Pierre, E. A., & Pillow, W. (Eds.). (2000). *Working the ruins: Feminist poststructural theory and methods in education.* New York: Routledge.

Strauss, A. (1987). *Qualitative analysis for social scientists.* Cambridge, UK: Cambridge University Press.

Stryker, S. (2009). *Transgender history.* Berkeley, CA: Seal Press.

Stryker, S., & Whittle, S. (Eds.). (2013). *The transgender studies reader.* New York: Routledge.

Stuart, C., & Whitmore, E. (2006). Using reflexivity in a research methods course: Bridging the gap between research and practice. In S. White, J. Fook, & F. Gardner (Eds.), *Critical reflection in health and social care* (pp. 156–171). Berkshire, UK: Open University Press.

Sturgeon, N. (1997/2016). *Ecofeminist natures: Race, gender, feminist theory and political action.* New York: Routledge.

Sumerau, J. E. (2017). *Cigarettes and wine.* Leiden, The Netherlands: Brill-Sense.

Tanenbaum, L. (2000). *Slut: Growing up female with a bad reputation.* New York: HarperCollins.

Tanenbaum, L. (2015). *I am not a slut: Slut-shaming in the age of the internet.* New York: HarperCollins.

Tasker, Y., & Negra, D. (2007). Introduction: Feminist politics and postfeminist culture. In Y. Tasker & D. Negra (Ed.), *Interrogating postfeminism: Gender and the politics of popular culture* (pp. 1–26). Durham, NC: Duke University Press.

Taylor, C. A., & Hughes, C. (2016). *Posthuman research practices in education.* London, UK: Palgrave MacMillan.

Teaiwa, T. K. (2014a). The ancestors we get to choose: White influences I won't deny. In A. Simpson & A. Smith (Eds.), *Theorizing native studies* (pp. 43–55). Durham, NC: Duke University Press.

Teaiwa, T. K. (2014b). Same sex, different armies: Sexual minority invisibility among Fijians in the Fiji military forces and British army. In N. Besnier & K. Alexeyeff (Eds.), *Gender on the edge: Transgender, gay and other Pacific Islanders* (pp. 266–292). Honolulu: University of Hawai'i Press.

Teaiwa, T. K., & Slatter, C. N. (2013). Samting Nating: Pacific WAVES at the margins of feminist security studies. *International Studies Perspectives, 14*(4), 447–450.

Tenni, C., Smith, A., & Boucher, C. (2003). The researcher as autobiographer: Analyzing data written about oneself. *Qualitative Report, 8*(1), 1–12.

Thiele, K. (2014). Ethos of diffraction: New paradigms for a (post) humanist ethics. *Parallax, 20*(3), 202–216.

Thurston, L. P. (1989). *Girls, computers, and amber waves of grain: Computer equity programming for rural teachers.* Presented at the National Women's Studies Association Conference, Manhattan, KS.

Thurston, L. P., Cauble, B., & Dinkel, J. (1998, March 25–28). *Beyond bells and whistles: Using multimedia for preservice and inservice education.* Paper presented at the Conference Proceedings of the American Council on Rural Special Education, Charleston, SC.

Thurston, L. P., & Dasta, K. (1990). An analysis of in-home parent tutoring procedures: Effects on children's academic behavior at home and in school and on parents' tutoring behaviors. *Remedial and Special Education, 11*(4), 41–52.

Toft, D. (2011, October 3). New sports press survey: Newspapers focus narrowly on sports results. *Play the Game.* Retrieved February 3, 2017, from *www.playthegame.org/news/news-articles/2011/new-sports-press-survey-newspapers-focus-narrowly-on-sports-results.*

Tolman, D. L. (2009). *Dilemmas of desire: Teenage girls talk about sexuality.* Cambridge, MA: Harvard University Press.

Tong, R. (2013). *Feminist thought: A more comprehensive introduction* (4th ed.). Boulder, CO: Westview Press.

Tong, R., & Williams, N. (2009). Feminist ethics. In E. N. Zalta (Ed.), *The Stanford encyclopedia of philosophy.* Retrieved from *http://plato.stanford.edu/entries/feminism-ethics.*

Tourangeau, R., & Yan, T. (2007). Sensitive questions in surveys. *Psychological Bulletin, 133*(5), 859–883.

Toye, M. E. (2010). Towards a poethics of love poststructuralist feminist ethics and literary creation. *Feminist Theory, 11*(1), 39–55.

Trent, A., & Cho, J. (2014). Evaluating qualitative research. In P. Leavy (Ed.), *The Oxford handbook of qualitative research* (pp. 677–696). New York: Oxford University Press.

Trier-Bieniek, A. (Ed.). (2015). *Feminist theory and pop culture.* Rotterdam, The Netherlands: Sense.

Tsing, A. (2005). *Friction: An ethnography of global connection.* Princeton, NJ: Princeton University Press.

Tuchman, G. (1978). Introduction: The symbolic annihilation of women by the mass media. In G. Tuchman, A. Kaplan Daniels, & J. Benet (Eds.), *Hearth and home: Images of women in the mass media* (pp. 3–38). New York: Oxford University Press.

Tuck, E. (2009). Suspending damage: A letter to communities. *Harvard Educational Review, 79*(3), 409–428.

Tuck, E., & McKenzie, M. (2015). *Place in research: Theory, methodologies and methods.* New York: Routledge.

Tuck, E., & Yang, K. W. (2012). Decolonization is not a metaphor. *Decolonization: Indigeneity, Education and Society, 1*(1), 1–40.

Tuiwai Smith, L. (1999). *Decolonizing methodologies: Research and indigenous peoples.* Dunedin, NZ: University of Otago Press.

Tuiwai Smith, L. (2002). *Decolonizing methodologies: Research and indigenous peoples*. London, UK: Zed Books.

Tuiwai Smith, L. (2012). *Decolonizing methodologies: Research and indigenous peoples* (2nd ed.). London: Zed Books.

Tupuola, A.-M. (1998). Fa'aSamoa in the 1990s: Young Samoan women speak. *Feminist Thought in Aotearoa/New Zealand, 51–57.*

Tupuola, A.-M. (2004). Talking sexuality through an insider's lens: The Samoan experience. In A. Harris (Ed.), *All about the girl: Culture, power and identity* (pp. 115–127). New York: Routledge.

Turnbull, A. (2000). Collaboration and censorship in the oral history interview. *International Journal of Research Methodology, 3*(1), 15–34.

Turner, J., & Stets, J. (2005). *The sociology of emotions*. Cambridge, UK: Cambridge University Press.

Tyner, K. E., & Ogle, J. P. (2009). Feminist theory of the dressed female body: A comparative analysis and applications for textiles and clothing scholarship. *Clothing and Textiles Research Journal, 27*(2), 98–121.

Van der Tuin, I. (2015). *Generational feminism: New materialist introduction to a generative approach*. Lanham, MD: Lexington Books.

Van der Tuin, I., & Dophijn, R. (2012). *New materialism: Interviews and cartographies*. Utrecht, The Netherlands: Open Humanities Press.

Vernet, J. P., Vala, J., & Butera, F. (2011). Can men promote feminist movements?: Outgroup influence sources reduce attitude change toward feminist movements. *Group Processes and Intergroup Relations, 14*(5), 723–733.

Villenas, S. (1996). The colonizer/colonized chicana ethnographer: Identity, marginalization, and co-optation in the field. *Harvard Educational Review, 66*(4), 711–731.

Visweseran, K. (1994). *Fictions of feminist ethnography*. Minneapolis: University of Minnesota Press.

Vogt, W. P., Vogt, E. R., Gardner, D. C., & Haeffele, L. M. (2014). *Selecting the right analyses for your data: Quantitative, qualitative, and mixed methods*. New York: Guilford Press.

Wachholz, S., & Mullaly, B. (2000). The politics of a textbook: A content analysis of the coverage and treatment of feminist, radical, and anti-racist social work scholarship in American introductory social work textbooks published between 1988 and 1997. *Journal of Progressive Human Services, 11*(2), 51–76.

Walker, M. U. (2007). *Moral understandings: A feminist study in ethics* (2nd ed.). Oxford, UK: Oxford University Press.

Walkerdine, V. (1984). Developmental psychology and the child-centred pedagogy: The insertion of Piaget into early education. In J. Henriques, W. Hollway, C. Urwin, C. Venn, & V. Walkerdine (Eds.), *Changing the subject: Psychology, social regulation and subjectivity* (pp. 153–201). London: Methuen.

Walkerdine, V. (1997). *Daddy's girl: Young girls and popular culture*. Cambridge: Harvard University Press.

Walkerdine, V. (2001). Safety and danger: Childhood, sexuality, and space at the end of the millenium. In K. Kultqvist & G. Dahlberg (Eds.), *Governing the child in the new millenium* (pp. 15–34). New York: Routledge.

Walkerdine, V. (2012). *Counting girls out: Girls and mathematics* (2nd ed.). London: Falmer Press.

Walters, S. D. (1995). *Materials girls: Making sense of feminist cultural theory.* Berkeley: University of California Press.

Wang, C. C. (2005). Photovoice: Social change through photography. Retrieved from *www.photovoice.com/method/index.html.*

Wang, C. C., & Burris, M. A. (1994). Empowerment through photo novella: Portraits of participation. *Health Education and Behavior, 21,* 171–186.

Wang, C. C., Burris, M. A., & Ping, X. Y. (1996). Chinese village women as visual anthropologists: A participatory approach to reaching policymakers. *Social Science and Medicine, 42,* 1391–1400.

Ward, J., & Schneider, B. (2009). The reaches of heteronormativity: An introduction. *Gender and Society, 23*(4), 433–439.

Ward, K. (2002). Reflections of a job done: Well? In D. Seigart & S. Brisolara (Eds.), Feminist evaluation: Explorations and experiences. *New Directions for Evaluation, 96,* 41–56.

Waring, M. (1988). *If women counted: A new feminist economics.* San Francisco: Harper & Row.

Waring, M. (2014). Counting for something!: Recognizing women's contribution to the global economy through alternative accounting systems. In A. M. Jaggar (Ed.), *Just methods: An interdisciplinary feminist reader* (pp. 97–104). New York: Routledge.

Warren, S. (2004). The utopian potential of GIS. *Cartographica: The International Journal for Geographic Information and Geovisualization, 39*(1), 5–16.

Watson, A. (2016). Directions for public sociology: Novel writing as a creative approach. *Cultural Sociology, 10*(4), 431–447.

Wattanaporn, K. A., & Holtfreter, K. (2014). The impact of feminist pathways research on gender-responsive policy and practice. *Feminist Criminology, 9*(3), 1–17.

Wax, R. H. (1952, Fall). Field methods and techniques: Reciprocity as a field technique. *Human Organization, 11*(3), 34–37.

Weber, C. D. (2012). Putting the family into the military mission: A feminist exploration of a national guard family program. *Cultural Studies? Critical Methodologies, 12*(5), 424–437.

Weber, J. D., & Carini, R. M. (2013). Where are the female athletes in *Sports Illustrated*?: A content analysis of covers (2000–2011). *International Review for the Sociology of Sport, 48*(2), 196–203.

Weiss, R. (1994). *Learning from strangers: The art and method of qualitative interview studies.* New York: Free Press

West, C., & Zimmerman, D. H. (1987). Doing gender. *Gender and society, 1*(2), 125–151.

Weuve, C., Pitney, W. A., Martin, M., & Mazerolle, S. M. (2014). Athletic trainers in the collegiate setting. *Journal of Athletic Training, 49*(5), 696–705.

White, A. M. (2006). Racial and gender attitudes as predictors of feminist activism among self-identified African American feminists. *Journal of Black Psychology, 32*(4), 455–478.

Whitmore, E. (2014). Researcher/evaluator roles and social justice. In S. Brisolara,

D. Seigart, & S. SenGupta (Eds.), *Feminist evaluation and research: Theory and practice* (pp. 59–94). New York: Guilford Press.

Williams, M. L., & Tyree, T. C. M. (2015). The "Un-quiet queen." In A. Trier-Bieniek (Ed.), *Feminist theory and pop culture* (pp. 49–64). Rotterdam, The Netherlands: Sense Publishers.

Wilson, C. (2013). *That's my stuff: Pasifika literature and Pasifika identity.* Retrieved from *http://researcharchive.vuw.ac.nz/handle/10063/3726.*

Wolcott, H. (1994). *Transforming qualitative data: Description, analysis, and interpretation.* Thousand Oaks, CA: SAGE.

Women's Media Center. (2015). Divided 2015: The media gender gap. Retrieved from *www.womensmediacenter.com/reports/2015-wmc-divided-media-gender-gap.*

Wright, M. (2008). Craven emotional warriors. *Antipode, 40,* 376–382.

Wu, H. (2011). *Once iron girls: Essays on gender by post-Mao Chinese literary women.* Langham, UK: Lexington Books.

Wyatt, J. (2006). Psychic distance, consent, and other ethical issues: Reflections on the writing of "A Gentle Going?" *Qualitative Inquiry, 12*(4), 813–818.

Yin, R. (2006). Mixed methods research: Are the methods genuinely integrated or merely parallel? *Research in the Schools, 13*(1), 41–47.

Yoder, J. D., Snell, A. F., & Tobias, A. (2012). Balancing multicultural competence with social justice: Feminist beliefs and optimal psychological functioning. *Counseling Psychologist, 40*(8), 1101–1132.

Zylinksa, J. (2005). *The ethics of cultural studies.* New York: Continuum.

Author Index

Note. *n* or *t* following a page number indicates a note or a table.

Subject Index

Note. *f*, *n*, *b*, or *t* following a page number indicates a figure, a note, a box, or a table.

About the Authors

Patricia Leavy, PhD, is an independent sociologist and former Chair of Sociology and Criminology and Founding Director of Gender Studies at Stonehill College in Easton, Massachusetts. She is the author, coauthor, or editor of over 25 books, and the creator and editor of seven book series. Known for her commitment to public scholarship, she is frequently contacted by the U.S. national news media and has regular blogs for *The Creativity Post* and *We Are the Real Deal.* She is also cofounder and coeditor-in-chief of the journal *Art/Research International.* Dr. Leavy has received numerous awards for her work in the field of research methods, including the New England Sociologist of the Year Award from the New England Sociological Association, the Special Achievement Award from the American Creativity Association, the Egon Guba Memorial Keynote Lecture Award from the American Educational Research Association Qualitative Special Interest Group, the Special Career Award from the International Congress of Qualitative Inquiry, the Significant Contribution to Educational Measurement and Research Methodology Award from the American Educational Research Association, and the Distinguished Contributions Outside the Profession Award from the National Art Education Association. In 2016, Mogul, a global women's empowerment platform, named her an "Influencer." In 2018, she was honored by the National Women's Hall of Fame and SUNY New Paltz established the annual Patricia Leavy Award for Art and Social Justice. Dr. Leavy delivers invited lectures and keynote addresses at universities and conferences. Her website is *www.patricialeavy.com.*

Anne Harris, PhD, is Associate Professor and Vice Chancellor's Senior Research Fellow at RMIT University in Melbourne, Australia, and Australian Research

301

Council Future Fellow (2017–2021) studying intercultural creativity. She is Honorary Research Fellow at the University of Nottingham (United Kingdom) and Adjunct Professor at Monash University (Australia). She conducts research in the areas of gender, creativity, diversity, performance, and emerging digital ethnographies. She has worked as a playwright, teaching artist, and journalist in the United States and Australia. Dr. Harris has authored or coauthored over 60 articles and 13 books on gender and sexuality, creativity, the arts, and nondominant culture formations. She is the creator and series editor of the Palgrave book series *Creativity, Education and the Arts*, and recently completed an Australian Research Council Discovery Early Career Researcher Award on the commodification of creativity. Her intercultural, collaborative arts-based research can be seen at *www.creativeresearchhub.com.*